Neoplasms of the
Foot and Leg

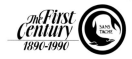

Neoplasms of the Foot and Leg

Edited by

Donald R. Cole, M.D.

Consultant to the President
Associate Director
Division of Institutional Research
New York College of Podiatric Medicine
New York, New York

Thomas M. DeLauro, D.P.M.

Executive Vice-President for Academic & Clinical Affairs
Professor, Divisions of Medical and Surgical Sciences
New York College of Podiatric Medicine
New York, New York

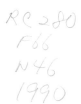 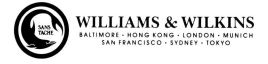

WILLIAMS & WILKINS
BALTIMORE · HONG KONG · LONDON · MUNICH
SAN FRANCISCO · SYDNEY · TOKYO

Editor: Carol-Lynn Brown
Associate Editor: Victoria M. Vaughn
Copy Editor: Peter W. Binns
Designer: Wilma Rosenberger
Illustration Planner: Ray Lowman
Production Coordinator: Barbara Felton

Copyright © 1990
Williams & Wilkins
428 East Preston Street
Baltimore, Maryland 21202, USA

Accurate indications, adverse reactions, and dosage schedules for drugs are provided in this book, but it is possible that they may change. The reader is urged to review the package information data of the manufacturers of the medications mentioned.

Printed in the United States of America

Library of Congress Cataloging in Publication Data

Neoplasms of the foot and leg / edited by Donald R. Cole, Thomas M.
DeLauro.
    p. cm.
   Includes bibliographical references.
   ISBN 0-683-02055-2
   1. Foot—Tumors. 2. Leg—Tumors. I. Cole, Donald R.
II. DeLauro, Thomas M.
   [DNLM: 1. Bone Neoplasms. 2. Foot Diseases. 3. Leg. 4. Soft
Tissue Neoplasms. WE 880 N438]
   RC280.F66N46   1990
   616.99'298—dc20
   DNLM/DLC
   for Library of Congress   90-12034
                                         CIP

90 91 92 93 94
1 2 3 4 5 6 7 8 9 10

To my co-pilot for the trip through life, Carol, and
my children—Debra, Alyson, and Jonathan

D.R.C.

For my wife, Isabelle
my children—Nicole and Lauren—and
Mom and Dad

T.M.D.

Foreword

Tumors of the lower extremities are a unique entity; they are uncommon. Few texts on tumors of the foot and the lower extremity have been published. This book will fill a void in podiatric literature so that podiatrists, podiatric residents, and students will have a readily available text to help them in understanding tumors of the lower extremity.

Malignant tumors affecting the foot and the lower extremity, are rare, but there has been a steady increase over the last several decades, particularly in the occurrence of skin cancers. Tumors of the foot present significant problems. Their diagnosis may be quite difficult because of particular locations on weight-bearing surfaces and their clinical appearance. Sometimes a skin tumor may appear to be hyperkeratosis. Malignancies of the foot, even though rare, create dramatic problems for the clinician because of the complications related to their treatment.

Unlike other foot problems, tumorous lesions of the foot present many different signs and symptoms. For example, one of the first clinical signs of a Morton-type neuroma is cramping. Another good example is warty-appearing lesions of the skin that in reality are malignant lesions and are only diagnosed on biopsy evaluation. Treatment of tumors of the foot might differ from treatment of that tumor in other areas of the body. Bone tumors, on the other hand, are extremely rare in the foot but continuous recognition and documentation in podiatric texts are extremely important.

Podiatric medicine is a young health profession. It is through texts such as this and the efforts of all the authors involved that podiatric oncology will be better understood. An appreciation of podiatric pathology as related to other areas of the body, such as its relationship to internal organs from metastatic spread, will enhance the readers' skills.

This text fills a void in the libraries of all podiatrists. Whereas research in podiatric oncology is ongoing, this text will serve the general podiatric practitioner and medical clinician. Hopefully, this book will help stimulate others working in lower extremity tumors and podiatric pathology in general.

Drs. Cole and DeLauro are to be congratulated for the completion and editing of such a large-scale undertaking; all who read this work and, ultimately, their patients will reap the benefits.

Steven J. Berlin, D.P.M., F.A.C.F.S.

Preface

While preparing to teach an oncology course, the senior author (D.R.C.) became aware of the paucity of up-to-date, complete texts on neoplasms of the foot and leg. This text aims to fill that void and provide the practitioner with a current, comprehensive review of available material. Emphasis is on proper diagnosis and adequate treatment without mutilation. Doctors must remember to treat the *patient*, not just the neoplasm. Only then will we avoid mutilation in this often recurring problem. Benefit/risk factors are critical.

Doctors dealing primarily with feet have a crucial role in disease prevention because many neoplasms are seen there in the earliest, and most "curable" phase. As Dr. George T. Pack stated in *Tumors of the Hands and Feet*, "Perhaps no other region or organs in the body are so readily favored for the early detection of tumors as are the hands and feet."

Contributors

Hal F. Abrahamson, D.P.M.
Podiatric Orthopedic Resident
New York College of Podiatric Medicine
New York, New York

Carl Abramson, Ph.D.
Professor
Department of Microbiology, Immunology
  and Pathology
Pennsylvania College of Podiatric
  Medicine
Philadelphia, Pennsylvania

Stephen A. Appelbaum, Ph.D.
Psychotherapy Training Program
Menniger Foundation
University of Missouri School of Medicine
Kansas City, Kansas

Carol Cambas, Ph.D.
Adjunct Assistant Professor of
  Anthropology
School of Continuing Education
New York University
New York, New York

Mary Ann Cardile, D.P.M.
Podiatric Surgical Resident
New York College of Podiatric Medicine
New York, New York

Donald R. Cole, M.D.
Consultant to the President
Associate Director
Division of Institutional Research
New York College of Podiatric Medicine
New York, New York

Thomas M. DeLauro, D.P.M.
Vice President and Professor
Division of Surgical Sciences
New York College of Podiatric Medicine
New York, New York

Frank A. Spinosa, D.P.M.
Associate Professor
Division of Medicine
New York College of Podiatric Medicine
New York, New York

Mark A. Kosinski, D.P.M.
Clinical Assistant Professor
Division of Medicine
New York College of Podiatric Medicine
New York, New York

W. Clark Lambert, M.D., Ph.D.
Director
Division of Dermatopathology
Department of Pathology
Professor and Vice Chairman
Division of Dermatology
New Jersey Medical School
Newark, New Jersey

Daniel J. McCarthy, D.P.M., Ph.D.
Chief, Podiatric Section
Veterans Administration Medical Center
Baltimore, Maryland

Robert A. Schwartz, M.D., M.P.H.
Professor and Chairman
Division of Dermatology
New Jersey Medical School
Newark, New Jersey

Christopher W. Sciales, M.D.
Clinical Instructor
Division of Dermatology
New Jersey Medical School
Newark, New Jersey

Roy E. Shore, Ph.D., Dr.P.H.
Professor
Institute of Environmental Medicine
New York University Medical Center
New York, New York

C. Harris, D.P.M.
Associate Professor
Division of Medicine
New York College of Podiatric Medicine
New York, New York

German C. Steiner, M.D.
Associate Director of Pathology and
  Laboratory Medicine
Hospital for Joint Diseases Orthopedic
  Institute
Associate Professor of Surgical Pathology
New York University School of Medicine
Professor of Pathology
New York College of Podiatric Medicine
New York, New York

Arthur Steinhart, D.P.M.
Professor and Chairman
Division of Medical Sciences
New York College of Podiatric Medicine
New York, New York

Donnamarie Stewart, D.P.M.
Associate Professor
Department of Medicine
New York College of Podiatric Medicine
New York, New York

Gerald A. Weber, D.P.M.
Associate Professor
Division of Medicine and Surgery
New York College of Podiatric Medicine
New York, New York

Contents

Foreword vii
Preface ix
Contributors xi

1/ Current Etiologic Theories of Neoplasia 1
Carl Abramson and Daniel J. McCarthy

2/ Epidemiology of Neoplasms of the Foot 24
Roy E. Shore

3/ Psychologic Aspects of Cancer 33
Stephen A. Appelbaum

4/ Differentiation between Benign and Malignant Neoplasia:
Primary and Secondary 40
Donald R. Cole

5/ Soft-tissue Neoplasia 45
Part A/ Vascular Neoplasia 45
Mark A. Kosinski
Part B/ Muscle 63
C. Harris
Part C/ Tenosynovial Neoplasia 79
Thomas M. DeLauro
Part D/ Neural Neoplasms of the Lower Extremity 97
Gerald A. Weber and Mary Ann Cardile
Part E/ Fibrous Tumors of the Foot and Leg 120
Donnamarie Stewart and Hal F. Abrahamson
Part F/ Lower Extremity Soft-tissue Tumors of Adipose Tissue 143
Arthur Steinhart
Part G/ Cutaneous Neoplasms of the Foot and Leg 149
Christopher W. Sciales, Robert A. Schwartz, and W. Clark Lambert

6/ Cysts and Cyst-like Lesions 163
Frank A. Spinosa

7/ Cartilaginous and Osseous Neoplasms 186
German C. Steiner

8/ Summary 208
Carol Cambas

Index 211

Current Etiologic Theories of Neoplasia

—Carl Abramson
—Daniel J. McCarthy

The exponential growth of the art and practice of podiatric medicine and surgery makes it inevitable that practitioners will be called upon to deal with malignancy. Skin cancers and malignancies of bone, muscle, and connective tissue occur with varying degrees of frequency, and acquired immune deficiency syndrome (AIDS), caused by infection with the human immunodeficiency virus (HIV-1), generates an increased incidence of opportunistic infections and neoplastic diseases such as Kaposi's sarcoma and lymphomas. Diminished control of immunologic regulatory mechanisms and immunosuppression caused by HIV infection, as well as a concomitant increase of latent diseases and neoplasms, should give researchers new opportunities to increase their scientific base of knowledge regarding host control and activation of these mechanisms.

Oncogenesis is the result of multifactorial events, the mechanisms of which are largely unknown to the scientific community. However, as advanced technologies are introduced, new answers to old questions are being found, and the mechanisms of oncogenesis are beginning to be clarified because of breakthroughs in researchers' understandings of molecular, immunologic, and genetic factors and how they interact with host, microbial, and environmental factors. Evidence exists that neoplastic transformation most likely requires the activation of a synergistic or sequential cascade of events requiring predisposing genetic factors and internal and external substances called growth factors, regulators, repressors, suppressors, initiators, promotors, proto-oncogenes, oncogenes, and carcinogens (1–3). This chapter reviews relative factors currently regarded as contributing to the multifactorial neoplastic transformational event.

ONCOGENES

Oncogenes code for products, the specific function(s) of which may lead to neoplastic transformation of human or animal cells in vivo or in vitro. The precursor of the oncogene is a proto-oncogene. These two terms are often used interchangeably; however, once a proto-oncogene is activated, it is called an oncogene. Proto-oncogenes are normal cellular genes (c-oncogenes) believed to play an important role in the regulation of differentiation and proliferation of normal cells (4). A number of factors and events, e.g., viral transduction, chromosomal translocations, or chemical carcinogens, can activate and change the program of the proto-oncogene, resulting in variable production of gene products which can ultimately alter the cell cycle (4). When the c-oncogene (*c-onc*) is transduced by a retrovirus and becomes part of its genetic library, it is called a viral oncogene (*v-onc*) and can induce viral oncogenesis (5). We will discuss this process, as well as the products and functions of different oncogenes as they affect the cell, and the involvement of oncogenes in the sequence of events contributing to normal and abnormal cell differentiation and proliferation. Activated oncogenes have been reported to occur in 15–20% of human tumors and approximately 40 oncogenes have been identified.

Historical Background

In 1911, Dr. Peyton Rous showed that a cell-free filtrate extracted from an avian sarcoma resulted in tumor formation when inoculated into tumor-free chickens. He postulated that the transmissible agent was a "filterable virus" that was oncogenic (6); it was eventually called the Rous sarcoma virus (RSV). In the 1970s, a single gene, named *src* for sarcoma, was identified as the structure responsible for the onco-

1

genic potential of RSV. Three other genes have also been found in the genome of the RSV-RNA-retrovirus: (a) gag gene, which codes for the capsid protein; (b) pol gene, which codes for "reverse transcriptase" (RNA-directed DNA polymerase); and (c) env gene, which codes for the outer envelope. Of the four genes, only the v-src (viral sarcoma) oncogene codes for a protein required for oncogenesis. Normal chicken embryo fibroblast cells are transformed by transfection with v-src product but not with env, pol, or gag products (7). The src gene may be removed or the gene product inactivated, but the RSV still functions and replicates, although it is not oncogenic. The v-src gene is thereby identified to be the oncogene. It was assumed that oncogenes originated in viruses, specifically retroviruses, and were transmitted to mammals by infection. A complementary gene was found in mammalian DNA (8) by a technique called "molecular hybridization" which uses an isolated, cloned, and tagged v-src gene as a probe. Because the probe was v-src, the complementary mammalian gene was termed c-src. The normal cellular gene was given the name "cellular oncogene" (c-onc), or proto-oncogene (9). It was postulated that the c-onc preceded the v-onc and that the viral gene incorporated the c-onc during infection of the susceptible host, where it functioned as a proto-oncogene.

Proto-oncogenes

Proto-oncogenes are localized compartmentally and produce products which affect cell proliferation in the normal cell cycle by (a) interacting with the cell membrane to create "first messenger" signal transduction through that membrane, (b) transducing the signal from the inner leaflet of the plasma membrane and transmitting it as a "second messenger" to the nucleus, and (c) initiating DNA transcription and replication resulting in cell division (10). External signals which regulate the cell cycle are provided by mitogens such as peptides, steroid hormones, lymphokines, or growth factors. One example, epidermal growth factor (EGF), binds to EGF receptors to activate signal transduction, transferring the message through the membrane into the cytoplasm and, eventually, to the nucleus.

Some proto-oncogenes code for protein kinases, which catalyze the transfer of phosphate groups to certain proteins at the threonine, serine, or tyrosine residues. These resi-

dues serve as receptors. Activated oncogene products, mimicking external mitogenic signals, can overstimulate or deregulate DNA synthesis, replication, and cell division, resulting in a loss of control of the cell cycle. Once the cell is transformed, autocrine secretion of growth factors can result in uncontrolled cell proliferation. Therefore, prior to neoplastic transformation and tumor progression, some genetic event must occur which alters the proto-oncogene, resulting in an activated oncogene which then codes for a variable or altered product that contributes to the cascade of events that changes a regulated cell cycle to one which becomes abnormally irregular (11).

Oncogene Products, Functions, and Growth Factors

Oncogene-encoded products differ in their biochemical properties and activities and seem to be necessary for controlled or uncontrolled regulation of cellular differentiation and/or proliferation. Activated, mutated oncogene products that disrupt cellular regulation may lead to the premalignant or malignant process of neoplastic transformation. The products of oncogenes can be distinguished from one another by what roles they play in signal transduction or can be grouped on a functional or mechanistic basis according to their subcellular location. The first group consists of DNA-binding proteins, which occur in the nucleus, and includes ski, c-myc, L-myc, N-myc, fos, myb, erb A, and cea 1. Since these are only found in the nucleus, it is believed that they bind to DNA or DNA-associated nuclear proteins and cause deregulation of the mitotic process by interacting with it. These oncogenes have been associated with, but not limited to, neuroblastoma, retinoblastoma, small-cell lung carcinoma, sarcomas, myelocytic leukemia, myeloblastic leukemia, and osteosarcoma (10, 12). The second group of products are the GTP (guanine triphosphate)-binding or ras proteins coded for by the ras family of oncogenes (13). The family includes (a) H-ras (derived from Harvey rat sarcoma, a v-onc), (b) K-ras (derived from Kirsten rat sarcoma, a v-onc), and (c) N-ras (derived from a nonviral source by tranfection of DNA from human neuroblastomas (Non-ras). The ras proteins, purified and cloned, with a molecular weight of 21 kilodaltons (p21) were found to have intrinsic GTPase activity. The normal protein binds GTP at the inner surface of the plasma membrane, has GTPase activity, and is believed to play a role in transduction of cell surface signals that regulate adenylate cyclase activity. Activated *ras* oncogene product (p21) results in a decrease in GTPase activity with increased binding of GTP that is believed to be responsible for its transforming capability. The cell responds as though the external signal is continuous. Based on the kinetics of equilibrium between GDP and GTP, GTPase may be in an inactive or active form and regulation responds accordingly (14). Human neoplasms associated with activated cellular *ras* genes are bladder, lung, colon, gall bladder, pancreatic, renal pelvic, ovarian and gastric carcinoma, melanoma, fibrosarcoma, rhabdomyosarcoma, and acute lymphocytic, chronic myelocytic and acute myelocytic leukemia (15).

A third group of oncogenes code for protein kinases, which phosphorylate proteins at threonine, serine, or tyrosine amino acid targets in cell membrane. Serine or threonine kinases are encoded for by the Maloney murine sarcoma virus *(v-mos)* and 3611 murine sarcoma virus *(raf)*. Tyrosine phosphorylation is carried out by the protein kinases of the Rous sarcoma virus oncogene *(v-src)*, its normal cellular proto-oncogene *(c-src)*, and the Abelson leukemia oncogene *(abl)*, which is associated with chronic myelogenous leukemia. Other oncogenes in this *src* gene family are *yes* (avian sarcoma) and *fes* (feline sarcoma) (16). The *v-src* and the *c-src* differ from each other by point mutations and genetic substitutions although there is extensive sequence homology. The *src* gene product is a phosphoprotein called pp 60^{SRC}, having a molecular weight of 60 kilodaltons. Vinculin, a cytoskeletal protein of mesenchymal cells, which is localized in focal adhesion plaques interposed between the ends of action bundles and cellular plasma membrane, connects bundles of cytoskeletal figments to the plasma membrane-anchoring proteins. It is a substrate for the *src* oncogene-transforming product of tyrosine kinase pp 60^{SRC}, which is found to contain up to 10–20-fold more phosphate following transformation than do non-transformed controls. Increased phosphorylation of vinculin results in anchorage-independent growth associated with malignant tumors. Lipid and protein binding are suggested as *src* oncogene-induced uncontrolled growth (17). Also, in this protein kinase

group are oncogenes which phosphorylate tyrosine targets. This class of oncogene protein product is reported to be homologous to, or to mimic, certain growth factors or to indirectly influence gene expression that codes for growth factors (18, 19). Platelet derived growth factor (PDGF), epidermal growth factor (EGF), and colony-stimulating factor-1 (CSF-1) are reported to be associated with oncogene products. For example, PDGF, which is also a mitogen, has a β-chain almost structurally identical to the protein product encoded for by the *v-sis* oncogene of simian sarcoma virus (20). It is regarded as a transforming retrovirus gene derived from the normal *c-sis* proto-oncogene which encodes PDGF (21). Activation of *c-sis* and subsequent production of PDGF will not transform normal cells unless other growth factors are present, e.g. transforming growth factors TGF-α and TGF-β and insulin-like growth factors (22).

Human tumor cells, e.g., osteosarcoma, fibrosarcoma, and gliomas, have PDGF receptors and *c-sis* oncogenes. When stimulated by a PDGF-like mitogen, they produce polypeptides related to PDGF, which is continuously kept in an activated state and results in unregulated cell division (23). EGF binds to a specific tyrosine kinase cell surface receptor, embedded in the plasma membrane, which is called the epidermal growth factor receptor (EGFR). The binding increases tyrosine-specific protein kinase activity, and phosphorylation is accomplished (24). This delivers a signal across the membrane, ultimately stimulating DNA synthesis and cell division. Therefore, EGF has been called a progression factor. The EGFR binds EGF and TGF-α and is composed of a transmembrane and a cytoplasmic area. The cytoplasmic part is a functional homolog of the truncated protein product coded for by the *v-erb* oncogene. EGFR-positive breast cancers are reported to occur as larger tumors with a poor prognosis. It is, therefore, suggested that the EGFR marker be used as a predictor of a more aggressive tumor, and that clinicians be advised to institute heroic intensive therapeutic measures (25).

Colony-stimulating factors regulate the production and function of mature hematopoietic cells that act through specific receptors on specific cells. Human granulocyte CSF (G-CSF), granulocyte-macrophage CSF (GM-CSF), multilineage CSF (Multi-CSF or interleukin 3), and macrophage CSF (M-CSF or CSF-1) are factors that have been genetically cloned and characterized and have had their biologic activity studied (26). It is suggested that some CSFs and their receptors may be involved in the pathogenesis of leukemia, whereas others function to enhance the hemopoietic host response in intracellular and extracellular infections (27). One part of this dichotomy is explained by the finding that some of the CSFs, e.g., CSF-1 receptor, are homologous to the retroviral oncogene *v-fms* product; insertion of this oncogene into a dependent cell line resulted in leukemogenesis. Autocrine production of CSFs from leukemic clones have also been reported (26, 28). During certain infectious processes, the CSFs stimulate the production and functional activity of granulocytes and mononuclear cells which contribute to the enhancement of host complement receptor expression, phagocytosis, and cytotoxicity. Cloned CSFs have been used therapeutically to correct blood cell deficiencies, augment host defense in infection, and stimulate hyperproduction of primal effector cells in the treatment of malignancies and AIDS (29).

Oncogene Activation

Chromosomal aberrations, abnormalities, or disrupting events may alter the molecular and genetic structures of the proto-oncogene and result in the activation of cellular oncogenes. Once activated, they are likely to produce a different or amplified product which could contribute to the neoplastic cascade of events (15).

There are three basic mechanisms which can induce genetic changes in proto-oncogenes or their products that can lead to activated oncogenes.

(a) Activation of proto-oncogenes by point mutations or structural alteration involving as few as only one amino acid can lead to transforming activity. The cellular *ras* oncogene has been reported to be the best example of oncogene activation by structural alteration(s), specifically nucleotide point mutation (13). Substitutions of a single amino acid, except proline, for the normal glycine in codon 12 confers transforming activity. Mutated *ras* genes (*H-ras* and *K-ras*) have been reported in a large variety of human malignancies, e.g., bladder, lung, colon, leukemia, and neuroblastomas. *K-ras* is reported in 50% of adenocarcinomas and in 30–40% of colonic tumors. In one experiment, the chemical carcinogen nitrosomethylurea (NMU) was used to induce mammary tumors in rats. Of those genes that were transformed, 87% showed a mutation in the 12th codon, suggesting that mutations can be induced in proto-oncogenes by certain chemical carcinogens (14, 30). Some mutations can be detected by transfection studies, especially at codon 12.

(b) Chromosomal rearrangement or translocations have been shown to activate cellular proto-oncogenes at a high frequency. This displacement is usually next to strong promoter/enhancer elements or after the proto-oncogenes have been removed from the influence of their regulatory genes. Their biochemical functions may also be altered if fusion takes place with different genetic nucleotides. An example of altered expression of an oncogene because of translocation is the B cell neoplastic disease of Burkitt's lymphoma. The normal location of the *c-myc* oncogene is at the distal end of the long arm of chromosome 8. Eighty-five percent of the reciprocal translocations of the oncogene that occur in Burkitt's lymphoma occur between chromosome 8 and chromosome 14. Occasionally, exchange may occur with either chromosome 2 or 22. If translocation takes place between 8 and 14, the *c-myc* locus on chromosome 8 is placed in close proximity to the immunoglobulin heavy chain (IgH) gene. This region, which undergoes increased transcriptional activity, adversely affects and alters normal regulation of the translocated *c-myc* locus. This diminishes its function and expression of gene product (31).

A second example of chromosomal translocation is the pluripotent stem-cell disease, chronic myelocytic leukemia. The characteristic abnormal small chromosome in the leukemic cells is the Philadelphia (Ph 1) chromosome. It is the result of a reciprocal translocation of the *c-abl* oncogene on chromosome 9 to chromosome 22. The translocated *c-abl* locus fuses with a small DNA segment on chromosome 22 called the breakpoint cluster region *(bcr)*, now known as *phl* (32). An *abl-phl* hybrid gene is formed, which codes for a chimeric abnormal protein with tyrosine kinase activity, unlike the normal *c-abl* or *phl* sequences which do not code for tyrosine kinase. It is important to note that transforming *v-abl* (viral, not cellular oncogene) does code for tyrosine kinase. Thus, the translocated *c-abl* gene encodes similarly to the transforming *v-abl* gene, except the *c-abl* expression is abnormal (33).

(c) Gene overexpression, caused by amplification or other mechanisms, can also activate the transformation of proto-oncogenes to tumorigenic oncogenes or activated oncogenes. This leads to a corresponding quantitative overexpression of the activated gene product. This process occurs during the formation of a number of human tumors and can result in up to a several hundredfold increase of the product. The amplified oncogene may be detected molecularly or observed cytogenetically in the form of extra chromosomal double-minutes (reduplication of genes) or as a chromosomally integrated homogenous-staining region (34). Mechanisms other than amplification that can cause increased expression of genes are chromosomal duplication or mutations in regulatory sequences (31). Amplification of *N-myc* oncogenes, resulting in 3–300 copies are reported to occur in 38% of all neuroblastoma tumors (34, 35). The tumor's aggressiveness and the resultant poor prognosis for the patient seems to be directly related to the degree of amplification of the *N-myc* oncogene. *L-myc* and *c-myc* amplification is also observed in small-cell lung carcinoma, retinoblastoma, colon carcinoma, and gastric adenocarcinoma (36).

A second example of amplification relates to the *c-neu* oncogene, which is associated with 30% of breast cancers (37). The activated *c-neu* oncogene expresses a product which chemically resembles EGFR. Because of this biochemical structural similarity, the *c-neu* product and EGFR bind to a shared site on the tumor, stimulating increased tumor growth. Under this stimulation, autocrine production of TGF-α has been shown to contribute to the enhancement of tumor growth. The expression of EGFR, amplified *c-neu* product, and TGF-α on breast cancer cells suggests advanced-stage disease and poor prognosis (38).

Antioncogenes or Suppressor Genes (Oncosuppressor Genes)

Activated proto-oncogenes can be converted by point mutation, gene amplification, or translocation into oncogenes that code for products reported to be involved in the pathogenesis of cancer. There are also other genes that down-regulate normal cell growth by selective suppression. These are "antioncogenes" or "tumor suppressor genes" because their inactivation or loss is shown to be associated with the malignant process (39). Others propose the term "oncosuppressor" gene and show both oncogenes and oncosuppressor genes to be highly conserved among eukaryotes (1, 40). This suggests they may play an important role in normal cell regulation, growth, and differentiation. Mutations which activate proto-oncogenes to oncogenes or inactivate or delete oncosuppressor genes may alter normal cell regulation and ultimately lead to the neoplastic process. Mutations in antioncogenes may be inherited as a heterozygous trait (one allele is inactivated) resulting in the progeny carrying a predisposition for tumor development. If a second mutation inactivates or deletes the second copy of the gene (allele), the patient is then homozygous for that locus. The loss of heterozygosity for selected loci is shown to be associated with certain cancers (2, 41). Oncosuppressor or antioncogenes are implicated in retinoblastoma and osteosarcoma, Wilms' tumor, hepatoblastoma, rhabdomyosarcoma, familial adenomatous polyposis, bilateral neurofibromatosis, and multiple endocrine neoplasia types 1, 2, and 2A, as well as breast, lung, and colon cancers (1–3).

Retinoblastoma, the childhood tumor of embryonic neural retina, occurs in heritable and nonheritable forms and is a classic example of antionocogene expression. In the heritable form, the Rb gene on chromosome 13 has a chromosomal deletion resulting from a germline mutation. The child is born with one defective and one normal copy of the gene. If a second mutation occurs at the normal Rb locus, the patient becomes homozygous for the mutant allele and the result is retinoblastoma (42). The mechanism of the normal Rb gene protein product binds to DNA and represses DNA synthesis, thereby acting as an antioncogene. This was determined from studies of transforming proteins of SV40 and adenovirus, both of which are DNA viruses. These transforming proteins bind to specific host cell nuclear proteins, which results in the inactivation of the bound host cellular proteins. The target of these DNA oncogenic viruses has been identified as an inhibitor or neutralizer of the antioncogene-Rb protein product (43, 44). This selective inhibition or inactivation of an oncosuppressor gene product by an oncogenic gene product may explain another step in the cascade of events leading to neoplastic transformation (45, 46).

Cell Cycle

"Cell cycle" is defined as the period of time a cell takes to pass through two successive cell divisions beginning and ending with mitosis. Parameters of this process are materially altered in malignancy. Four phases, G_1, S, G_2, and M, are identified. G_1 is that variable period of time between the conclusion of mitosis and the initiation of DNA replication (G = gap). The S phase marks that period of 8–10 hours when the genome is replicated (DNA synthesis). G_2 is a 2- or 3-hour period marking the time between replication of DNA and initiation of mitosis. M, or mitosis, is a 1- or 2-hour period initiated by condensation of DNA and completion of new cell membranes at the close of replication (47).

A special fifth metabolic compartmental phase, identified as G_0, is represented by the pool of nonreplicating cells that remain quiescent until called upon to enter the replicative cycle. These cells are essentially blocked from replication; this feature, along with modulations of the cell cycle, has important implications for tumorigenesis and neoplasia. G_0-state cells have DNA content identical to that of G_1-state cells, but appear to have been blocked in cell division to a limited number of specific control points. Investigators of cancer therapies and oncogenic processes may do well to study the biochemical characteristics of these areas. Many tumors take a constant time to double, which differs in different types of human tumors. Tumors that are responsive to anticancer drugs grow more rapidly than do less responsive slow-growing (slow-doubling time) tumors.

G_1 cells and reversibly quiescent G_0 cells contain diploid DNA, so it is difficult to differentiate them. Moreover, it is not always clear whether or not G_0-state cells differ from G_1-state cells or if they are parts of the same continuum. Cells in the G_1 state may represent that period of the cell cycle during which control of replication is established. Tumor cells demonstrate inactivation of regulatory elements and imbalances of biosynthetic activity. They tend to accumulate abnormal amounts of cell products at inappropriate times within the cell cycle. Tumor cells do not react normally to the usual parameters that control cell differentiation or replication. They may become quiescent or nonproliferative due to poor nutrition or differentiation, or they may just die, as noted histologically by the presence of necrosis or of pyknotic cells.

The mechanism for transforming the quiescent G_0 cells into replicative G_1 cells is unknown. However, it is known that the regulation of cell division takes place between the G_0 and G_1 states and that it may be at this point in the cell cycle that cell proliferation may be initiated.

Tumorigenesis may be characterized by an increased span of cell life, a decreased cell cycle time, or a decrease in G_0 cells with an accompanying increase in the number of replicating cells. Tumor growth is often erratic and occasionally even involves regression. Tumors may initially have clonal origins but become progressively diverse over time (48).

VIRAL ONCOGENESIS

The origins and concepts of oncogenesis can be traced back to Hippocrates and his coworkers, who believed a healthy body was the result of a balance between the body humors. An imbalance was thought to result in inflammatory and malignant tumors. It was not until 1911 when Rous' experiments demonstrated the induction of tumors by cell-free extracts that viral oncology became a valid new science. A recent review, a "portrait of Rous Sarcoma Virus," emphasizes the importance of this first model for providing the evidence needed to recognize and identify a viral transforming gene (49). Other animal viruses that have been studied and shown to cause tumors in vitro and/or in vivo are listed in Table 1.1.

Human tumor viruses are classified according to their nucleic acid type, i.e., RNA or DNA. The RNA viruses belong to the Retroviridae family and the DNA viruses to the Papovaviridae, Herpesviridae and Hepandnaviridae families. Another DNA virus, the adenovirus, is shown to cause malignant transformation of laboratory animal models and/or tissue culture systems, but is not yet shown to be involved in human tumor transformation (50).

RNA Tumor Viruses

Oncogenic RNA viruses are classified as retroviruses because they contain the enzyme reverse transcriptase (RNA-directed DNA polymerase) which directs reverse transcription of viral RNA into virus-specific cDNA. Although the human T cell leukemia or lymphocytotropic virus (HTLV-1) is the only retrovirus as-

Table 1.1 Animal Viruses Causing Tumors in Vivo (Natural Tumor) and/or in Vitro (Transformation)

RNA viruses	In vivo	In vitro
Avian leukemia virus	+	−
Avian sarcoma virus	+	+
Murine leukemia virus	+	−
Murine sarcoma virus	−	+
Murine mammary tumor virus	−	−
Feline leukemia virus	+	−
Feline sarcoma virus	+	+
Simian sarcoma virus	+	+

DNA viruses	In vivo	In vitro
Mouse polyoma virus	−	+
Monkey SV40 virus	−	+
Rabbit papilloma virus	+	−
Bovine papilloma virus	+	+
Simian adenovirus	−	−
Monkey herpes virus	−	−
Avian (Marek) herpes virus	+	−
Frog (Lucké) herpes virus	+	−
Woodchuck hepatitis virus	+	−
Monkey Yaba virus	+	−
Rabbit/deer fibroma-myxoma virus	+	−

sociated with human tumors, studies of oncogenic animal retroviruses have contributed much to the understanding of the basic genetic structure of these viruses. The standard leukemia virus contains three genes that are required for replication of the virus: *gag*, which codes for core proteins that are antigenic; *pol*, which codes for the enzyme reverse transcriptase; and *env*, which codes for glycoprotein structures protruding from the surface of the envelope of the virion. The above denotes the gene order from left to right with a 5′ at the left terminus and a 3′ at the right terminus, i.e., 5′-*gag-pol-env*-3′.

Human retroviruses, e.g., HTLV-1, have a fourth gene downstream from the *env* called *tat*. Its function is regulatory, and it codes for a nonstructural protein. This transactivating gene product alters the efficiency of transcription or translation of other viral genes. These two types of provirus structures are considered to be replication-competent but cannot transform tissue-culture cells in vitro because of the absence of the *onc* transforming gene. If they carry the *onc* gene in place of the *pol* gene through transduction of a proto-oncogene from normal cellular DNA into the retrovirus genome, the result is a replication-defective, transforming virus. This type is a direct transforming virus, as in defective acute leukemia

or sarcoma virus. Each of these virus genomes is bound on either side by repeated untranslated sequences called LTRs (long terminal repeats). These repeats contain promoter and enhancer sequences that regulate adjacent viral RNA synthesis. Replication-defective viruses can replicate only in the presence of a helper retrovirus which provides the deficient nucleotides through recombination. Rous avian sarcoma virus with inserted *src* oncogene is an exception, having both replication and transformation capabilities (49). Therefore, three types of retroviruses, determined by the structure of their genomes and their oncogenic potential for cellular transformation, will be described. They are: slow transforming viruses, acute transforming viruses, and human T cell leukemia viruses (HTLV).

SLOW TRANSFORMING VIRUSES

The slow transforming viruses cause neoplastic transformation by a mechanism called insertional mutagenesis, whereby proviral DNA is inserted near a proto-oncogene such as *c-myc* (31). The slow transforming viruses do not have oncogenes, are replication-competent, and eventually produce clonal tumors after a long period of latency. Their long latency period has also led them to be called chronic leukemia viruses. These viruses have the classic retroviral genomic structure of 5′-LTR-*gag-pol-env*-LTR-3′ and cause feline and murine leukemias, as well as avian lymphomas and leukosis (51, 52). It is interesting to note that an isolate of feline leukemia virus has recently been shown to produce an immunodeficiency disease in cats similar to AIDS (53). Insertion of the provirus upstream of the proto-oncogene may result in structural gene damage and/or promote and enhance expression of the proto-oncogene. These alterations of *c-myc* expression are consistent with modification changes leading to neoplastic transformation (31, 36).

Recently, two new proto-oncogenes, *int-1* and *int-2*, have been reported to exhibit temporary regulation within the first 10 days of mouse embryogenesis. They are not found in adult tissues except in the testis of sexually mature mice, but they are found in an activated state in mouse mammary carcinomas. This altered expression is believed to be due to insertion of mouse mammary tumor proviral DNA integrated near proto-oncogene *int-1* or *int-2.* Change of expression of *int-1* or *int-2* by insertion of the proviral DNA, which alters phenotype and growth characteristics of the cells involved, suggests that mouse mammary tumor proviral DNA plays a role in mouse mammary oncogenesis (54).

ACUTE TRANSFORMING VIRUSES

This group of retroviruses can rapidly induce tumors in animals following a short latent period or cause transformation of tissue culture systems. Although they are replication-defective, the lost genetic sequences are replaced by a cancer-causing gene called the viral oncogene or *v-onc*. These are host-derived proto-oncogenes that have been transduced following viral replication during viral infection. Carcinomas, leukemias, and sarcomas are tumor types which may be induced in animals by this group of oncogenic retrovirus and have been called acute leukemia viruses (55).

HUMAN T CELL LEUKEMIA VIRUSES

Human T cell lymphadenotropic, lymphocytotropic, or leukemia virus type 1 (HTLV-1) is a retrovirus which has an affinity for CD4+ cells. The virus was isolated in the laboratories of Dr. Robert Gallo from a T cell line, HUT 102, derived and cultured from a patient with a variant of cutaneous T cell lymphoma (56). Continuous T cell lines were established with the use of T cell growth factor, or interleukin-2 (IL-2), also discovered in the same laboratories. The HTLV-1 virus was designated as the cause of human adult T cell leukemia lymphoma (ATLL) when the proviral genome was found integrated in leukemic cell DNA (57). The proviral genomic order of 5'-LTR-*gag-pol-env-pX*-LTR-3' is characteristic of retroviruses except for a fourth noncellular gene that codes for a transactivating protein identified as p40^x and, in conjunction with unknown cellular factors and genes, regulates transcription from proviral LTRs. The HTLV-1 virus, therefore, differs significantly from the acute or slow transforming retroviruses, having a fourth genome called *pX* or *tat* which codes for a transactivating protein p40^x, a 40-kilodalton protein. This protein transactivates the HTLV-1 long terminal repeat, stimulating viral gene expression as well as regulating cellular genes and inducing production of IL-2 and IL-2R (IL-2 receptor). Growth and proliferation of the infected T cell occurs, and it is believed that this autocrine mechanism of leukemogenesis occurs in human adult T cell leukemia (58). This hypothesis was tested by using a transgenic mouse model in which an HTLV-*tat*-1 plasmid construct was injected into germ-line cells. Transgenic mouse *tat* gene then expressed *tat* protein under the control of the HTLV-1 5'-LTR regulatory region. Mesenchymal tumors developed under specific expression of *tat* protein, establishing HTLV-1 as a transforming virus and the gene product as an oncogenic protein (59).

Adult T cell leukemia/lymphoma is found in the southeastern United States, the Caribbean, Japan, and Africa. It is an aggressive T cell malignancy associated with hypercalcemia, lymphadenopathy, hepatosplenomegaly, skin nodules and erythroderma, bone marrow involvement, and lytic bone lesions. White blood cell counts vary from 7,000 to 190,000 per cubic millimeter. Anemia and thrombocytopenia are infrequently reported. HTLV-1-associated myelopathy, also known as tropical spastic paraparesis, is a neurologic disorder of the lower trunk and limbs presenting with mild paralysis and muscle spasticity. Transmission of HTLV-1 is only by infected cells, not by serum. It may be transmitted postnatally through infected lymphocytes in breast milk but will not be expressed till adulthood as adult T cell leukemia/lymphoma. Persons at risk are sex partners of seropositive persons, breast-feeding infants of seropositive mothers, IV drug abusers, and recipients of cellular blood products from seropositive donors. Serologic tests, e.g. HTLV-1 enzyme immunoassay, are preliminary and should be confirmed by a Western blot test which reveals antibodies to viral envelope, nucleic acid, and core proteins such as p24 and p19, radioimmunoprecipitation, or, ultimately, virus isolation. Because it has been indicated that HTLV-1 may be in our blood supply, donor screening is recommended. One must consider that, since the diseases caused by HTLV-1 can be insidious, crippling, or fatal and since the population of carriers is increasing, potential blood donors and transfusion recipients should not only be aware of HIV-1, the cause of AIDS, but should also be aware of HTLV-1, the cause of leukemia, lymphoma, spastic paraparesis, and myelopathy (60–65).

DNA Oncogenic Viruses

There are a large number of DNA animal tumor viruses (see Table 1.1), but this section will discuss only those DNA viruses that have been shown to be associated with tumors in humans. These include hepatitis B virus, human papilloma virus, Epstein-Barr virus, and herpes simplex virus. Adenovirus types 2, 5, and 12 have not been shown to cause tumors in humans (50), although they can cause tumors in laboratory animals.

Differences between RNA and DNA oncogenic viruses, as well as within the DNA oncogenic viruses themselves, are of paramount importance. Their mechanisms and/or involvement, directly or indirectly, regarding neoplastic transformation vary greatly. Hepatitis B virus is reported to lack transforming genes and, therefore, must be involved directly with target tissues in the neoplastic process, whereas human papilloma virus contains transforming sequences. Permissive target cells are usually not transformed but die following viral replication. Other cells may not permit viral replication but, instead, allow viral DNA to integrate into the host chromosome. The integration of oncogenic viral DNA into host chromosome may regulate the viral replication cycle by allowing early gene formation and, in some cases, interrupt or disallow formation of late viral genes prior to DNA replication. Transfection into susceptible cell cultures in vitro of constructs containing early viral genes (DNA) or cloned early viral gene DNA will result in transformation of those cells (66). Some of these early regions code for T and S proteins which express themselves as tumor antigens on the surface of the transformed cell; some of the T antigens will bind to the nuclear and/or plasma membrane of varied transformed cells, based on the cell system and the oncogenic virus.

Many of these findings relate to experiments using SV40, polyoma, and adenoviruses. SV40 virus with two T proteins (small and large) and polyoma virus with three T proteins (small, middle, and large) are papovaviruses found in monkey and mouse cells, respectively. Neither produce tumors in humans, but tumors result when either is inoculated into mouse cells or when SV40 is inoculated into neonatal hamster cells. It is interesting that, although SV40 virus contaminated early preparations of poliomyelitis virus vaccine that were grown in infected monkey kidney tissue culture cells, to date, no SV40-related tumors have occurred in the human population that was vaccinated. In polyoma virus, middle T antigen induces *c-src*

protein tyrosine kinase to increase over 50-fold when it complexes with normal cell membrane. This also occurs with Rous sarcoma virus, suggesting common regulatory pathways by different mechanisms for some DNA and RNA viruses (66). SV40 virus large T antigen binds to p53 nuclear protein of normal cells. This stimulates the p53 growth-promoting protein which up-regulates DNA synthesis, thereby contributing to the transformation process. This response can also counteract the activity of oncosuppressor or antioncogenes that produce growth inhibitory factors (43). Human papilloma virus is not unlike SV40 or polyoma virus that encode transforming genes involving these viruses in the neoplastic transformation process. Epstein-Barr virus is believed to require chromosomal translocation mutations to involve it in the multistep process of cell transformation. Recently, *ras* and *myc* oncogene products have been shown to be overexpressed in hepatitis B virus human hepatocellular carcinoma. Perhaps these new findings will help us understand some of the human tumor viruses as we address each virus and its mechanisms regarding tumorigenesis.

HUMAN PAPILLOMA VIRUS

The human papilloma virus (HPV) is a member of the Papovaviridae family, which includes papilloma, polyoma, and vacuolating viruses (Fig. 1.1). HPV is 55 nm in diameter, nonenveloped, and icosahedral, and contains circular double-stranded DNA with a genome of 8,000 nucleotides coding for nine proteins. Early genes are E1–7 and late genes are L1–2. To date, unlike with other papovaviruses, there is no system for in vitro cultivation; therefore, it is difficult to completely study HPV.

Papilloma viruses are classified by sequence homology using standard liquid-phase hybridization techniques. The type is determined by comparing the homology of the virus with other known HPV types; if the homology is less than 50%, a new type is established. There are presently over 62 types (67). A large number of these types are considered to be potentially oncogenic, whereas others, such as types 1, 2, and 4 that cause plantar warts (68), are considered benign. Types 6, 11, 16, 18, 31, 33, 35, 39, 42, 45, 49, 52, and 53–60 have been found in genital cancer (69), and types 5, 8, 9, 12, 14, 15, 17, 19–25, 36, and 40 have been found in epidermodysplasia verruciformis (70), a ge-

Figure 1.1. The human papilloma viruses are tumorigenic and measure 55 nm in diameter. They contain double-stranded DNA and have 42 capsomeres arranged in skew with icosahedral symmetry. *V,* virions; *N,* nucleus; *M,* fine granular material; *arrows,* extranuclear virions. Transmission electron microscopy (TEM) × 60,000. (From Lutzner MA. Viral diseases. In: Zelickson AS, ed. Ultrastructure of Normal and Abnormal Skin. Philadelphia: Lea and Febiger, 1967.)

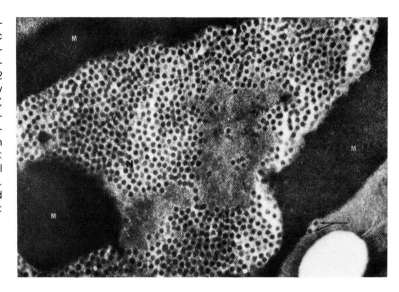

netic immunodeficiency disease that presents with flat warts. In AIDS patients, these warts may transform to squamous cell carcinoma. In other patients, up to 30% of these warts, when exposed to sunlight, will similarly transform (71). Types 6, 11, 30, and 40 are found in laryngeal condylomas, the incidence of which is increased by 30% in patients exposed to x-rays (72), and types 16, 18, 31, 33, 35, and 39 are associated with flat anogenital, intraepithelial neoplasia (73).

It is believed that the mechanism of papilloma virus benign infection involves establishment of the virus as a multicopy extrachromosomal episome or plasmid in the basal layer of the epithelium, whereas in malignant lesions it is integrated into the host genome. This is followed by expression of early proteins with basal and parabasal epithelial proliferation. Replication only occurs in differentiated cells of the upper epidermis. Cells mature and differentiate, becoming abundant and eosinophilic, as the cytoplasm shows indications of keratin synthesis. Using immunocytochemical methods, one can detect late gene expression of viral structural proteins by nuclear staining for HPV capsid antigens. Other methods for diagnosis and/or typing of HPV are filter in situ deoxyribonucleic acid hybridization, colposcopy, and cytologic or histopathologic procedures (74). A recent review (75) discusses the necessity for detection of HPV typing and the variety of techniques used for confirmation of the presence of the virus in primary skin or genital tumors. The authors conclude that typing at this time is a valuable research

tool, but therapy should not be totally based on whether low-risk or high-risk viruses are detected. They feel that too many variables still exist, the tests are too expensive, and that the Papanicolaou test is presently the best test to direct patient management.

As terminal differentiation of normal squamous epithelium of the cervix and skin occurs, involucrin, a component of the cellular protein envelope, is first observed in the parabasal cells, with intense progression and distribution in superficial layers. Therefore, involucrin is considered a marker of differentiation in nonneoplastic squamous epithelium when detected by immunocytochemical localization. In cervical dysplasias, HPV and an abnormal distribution of involucrin occur in differentiated squamous cell lesions. This altered expression of involucrin reflects one of the changes in cellular DNA synthesis and the differentiation of squamous epithelium imposed by the HPV virus infection. The evidence that HPV is the etiologic agent of cervical and anogenital cancer is compelling. Eighty percent or more of precancerous dysplastic cervical tissue contains HPV capsid protein and HPV DNA. HPV DNA is also found in 88% of all squamous cell carcinomas, 83% of all adenocarcinomas of the cervix, and in metastases from those tumors. It is believed that a spectrum of diseases exist based upon the type of tissue invaded, the type of HPV, environmental or iatrogenic carcinogens, and the immunologic profile of the host. It has been shown that HPV is a latent virus and may be activated in cases of severe cellular immunodeficient states (76, 77).

These criteria indicate infection alone is not sufficient to ensure the process of transformation and that several cofactors are probably necessary to continue the momentum. One such finding reports that perhaps HPV genomes code for transactivation factors that may activate proto-oncogenes such as *c-myc* in the host cell. These HPV sequences may act as insertional cis-acting promoter/enhancer mutagens leading directly or indirectly to neoplastic transformation. An HPV-18 integration site in HeLa cells was found to be closely 5′ of the *c-myc* locus (78). Another report indicates that viral transactivators, such as herpes simplex virus, which have been found in association with HPV in cervical carcinomas and tumor promotors such as 12-*O*-tetradecanoylphorbol-13-acetate (TPA), can activate and/or increase expression of HPV-18 in the development of cervical cancer. The authors of that report showed the HPV virus E2 gene protein product to be a strong transactivator-activating expression because it binds to sequence ACCG(N)TCGGT. HSV has a transinducing gene the product of which can activate the expression of the HPV-18 noncoding region in HeLa epithelial cell lines, as well as in a variety of other cell lines. They also found that HPV-18 promotor is activated by TPA and that transformed NIH-3T3 cell lines expressing integrated copies of HPV-18 E6–E7 regions from HPV-18 promoter increased expression when given TPA. Such increased expression resulted in morphologic changes of the NIH-3T3 cells. This work reinforced the thesis that malignant transformation is a multistep process and that many different kinds of events and/or criteria are involved in the conversion of the normal cell to the neoplastic state (79).

EPSTEIN-BARR VIRUS

The Epstein-Barr virus (EBV) belongs to the Herpesviridae family and is commonly known as the etiologic agent of infectious mononucleosis or "kissing disease." It is clear that most people experience a "silent" EBV infection or clinical infectious mononucleosis during their lifetimes because up to 90% of the population has antibodies to the EBV. A small percentage of people in the United States and a larger percentage of people in underdeveloped or third world countries experience lymphoprolif-erative disease in the form of B cell lymphomas (80) and, rarely, T cell lymphomas (81). Transplantation patients who are immuno-sup-pressed prior to surgery usually develop immune deficiency followed by activation of latent viruses such as human papilloma virus, herpesvirus, and/or Epstein-Barr virus. A large group of children in a general transplant program in a large eastern university hospital developed EBV infections that progressed to lymphoproliferative disease in the form of immunoblastic lymphoma (82). Although the children developed self-limiting infectious mononucleosis, it was followed by widespread visceral lymphoproliferation culminating in monoclonal B cell lymphoma. AIDS patients and their children have also been reported to develop EBV infection followed by uncontrolled lymphoproliferative disease or Burkitt's lymphoma leading to death due to a diffuse lymphoplasmic infiltrate involving multiple organs. The immune deficiency in these cases was attributable to activation of the latent EBV followed by lymphoproliferative disease (83, 84). Burkitt's lymphoma is commonly a childhood tumor which is endemic in New Guinea and Central Africa and presents as a B cell lymphoma. B lymphocytes are immortalized following infection by EBV; this is believed to be an initial step in the process of transformation. The virus infects the B cell following attachment to its C3d complement receptor. The infected cell produces an EBV nuclear-associated antigen 2 (EBNA-2) that is believed to initiate B cell transformation. At the same time, a second protein called the lymphocyte-detected membrane antigen is produced that is recognized by cytotoxic T cells. It kills the newly formed EBV-transformed cells, thereby controlling continued proliferation (85). It seems that these immunologic host-response controls do not operate efficiently in the areas of Africa where malaria is endemic. EBV infection induces a polyclonal B cell proliferation that is enhanced by mitogenic activity of the malarial parasite. This culminates in a severe immunosuppression resulting in continued proliferation of the EBV infected B lymphocytes. Driven by this biologic proliferation, random gene breaks within the B cells begin to occur, especially within the immunoglobulin gene locus in chromosomes 2, 14, or 22. Simultaneously, a break occurs at the locus for the *c-myc* proto-oncogene in chromosome 8. Translocation follows breakage of chromosomes 8 and 14 and the *c-myc* proto-oncogene is activated. This results in a monoclonal malignant population of EBV-containing B cells

Figure 1.2. Chromosomal abnormalities, which can be histologically identified, have been associated with human malignancy, including lymphoma. Selected G-banded chromosomes depicting specific chromosome defects preferentially found in various histologic subgroups of non-Hodgkin's lymphoma are seen here: A t(8;14)(q24.1;q32.3) in Burkitt's, non-Burkitt's, and immunoblastic lymphoma; a t(14;18)(q32;q21.3) in follicular lymphoma; a t(11;14)(q13;q32), a del(11)(q14.2q23), or a trisomy 12 in diffuse B small lymphocytic lymphoma; a t(12;14)(q13.1;q32.3) or an inv(14)(q11.2q32.3) in small T-lymphocytic lymphoma; a t(9;22)(q34;q11.2) in large cell lymphoblastic lymphoma; and del(6)(q21q25) in diffuse large cell lymphoma. (From Yunis JJ. Chromosomal rearrangements, genes, and fragile sites in cancer. In: DeVita VT, Hellman S, Rosenberg SA, eds. Important advances in oncology. Philadelphia: Lippincott, 1986.)

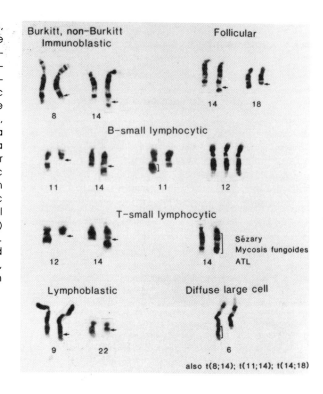

with the translocation t(8:14), which is consistent with Burkitt's lymphoma (Fig. 1.2). These cells are nonresistant to killing by the cytotoxic T cells as previously indicated. This translocation is found in tumors regardless of what part of the world Epstein-Barr viral lymphomas occur (86). Nasopharyngeal carcinoma is endemic in southern China, among Arctic Eskimos, and in Africa. Regardless of population or geographic source, the tumor is found to contain Epstein-Barr viral DNA. In endemic areas, patients are found to have high titers of IgA antibodies to EBV early antigen and viral capsid antigen, prior to tumor development. Following tumor appearance, patients develop high titers of antibodies to antiviral capsid antigen antibodies. The tumors aggressively metastasize through the cervical lymph nodes to the lungs, pleural cavities, and liver, and throughout the lymphatic system. Mapping of the genome from nasopharyngeal EBV-associated carcinoma cells has identified gene sequences responsible for the products of early antigen and transforming protein (87). The DNA viral genome is linear and composed of about 170,000 base pairs; and it exists in a circular form when in the latent state. The virus is 150–180 nm in diameter, has a central

core, a capsid layer of capsomeres in icosahedral form, and an outer envelope composed of lipoprotein.

HEPATITIS B VIRUS

Hepatitis B virus (HBV) particles contain partially double-stranded circularized DNA, with one strand longer than the other. There are four open reading frames coding for hepatitis B surface antigen (HB$_s$Ag) polypeptides, core and E antigens, endogenous DNA polymerase, and a basic polypeptide believed to direct transcriptional transactivation (88). The virion is 42 nm in diameter and is composed of an outer envelope containing HB$_s$Ag (composed of protein, carbohydrate, and lipid), a nucleocapsid representing the core antigen (HB$_c$Ag), and the core, which contains the circular double-stranded DNA and DNA polymerase.

Hepatocellular carcinoma (HCC), also called primary cancer of the liver or primary liver cancer, has been linked to HBV by compelling epidemiologic evidence. In 1981, Beasley et al. did a prospective study in Taiwan regarding relative risk of 22,707 men who were HB$_s$Ag-positive carriers. They found these men had a 217% higher risk of developing HCC than did

HB_sAg-negative men. Also, 51% of deaths in this group were due to cirrhosis of the liver and HCC (89). This suggested that the high incidence was somehow related to the HB_sAg-positive carrier. This was further substantiated by the Nobel laureate Dr. Baruch S. Blumberg who discovered the virus in 1963, originally calling it "Australia Antigen," but later labeling it hepatitis B surface antigen (90). One of the problems in identifying patients at risk is that no serologic markers can be found in up to 11% of HCC patients in developing countries and in up to 68% of those in industrialized areas. What is encouraging is that HBV-DNA sequences are found in HCC-DNA in 13–100% of these serologically negative patients. This, of course, points very strongly to the association of HBV with HCC, although some of the patients with non-A, non-B hepatitis have developed HCC. Other noted contributing factors or possible etiologies, carcinogens, or cocarcinogens are alcohol, cigarettes, oral contraceptives, and aflatoxin. Virus, viral products, chronic hepatitis, liver cirrhosis, and cocarcinogens all have been reported to be associated with increased risk in this multistep approach to HCC (91). In a recent study, HCC tissue and nonneoplastic liver tissue were sectioned and tested immunohistochemically using monoclonal antibodies to assess expression of *ras* and *myc* oncogene products (92). This study seemed plausible since oncogene expression has been reported innumerable times to be associated with a large variety of tumors. Immunoperoxidase and specific monoclonal antibodies to expressed *ras* p21 and *myc* p62 oncogene products in HCC were assayed using fibrotic, cholestatic, and nonneoplastic liver tissues as controls. All the controls were negative, and the HCC tested positive for increased *ras* p21 and *myc* p62. This just indicates another of the many similarities in human neoplasms: that activation of oncogenes in the potential tumor cell requires many pathways in the often confusing multistate process of neoplastic transformation.

RADIATION

Exposure to radiation is an important consideration when evaluating carcinogenic factors applicable to the lower extremities. It may be of ionizing or nonionizing types.

Nonionizing radiation is responsible for many basal cell and squamous cell carcinomas (93). Exposure to the ultraviolet component of sunlight is an actinic event which may be tumorigenic. Malignant melanoma is the most life-threatening of skin tumors resulting from sunlight exposure, but such neoplasia may also arise de novo or by malignant transformation of preexisting skin tumors such as nevi. Melanoma tumorigenesis may have an actinic component, but malignant transformation is clearly more involved and complicated than simple exposure to sunlight alone. The risk of actinically induced skin cancer depends on the type of skin involved (93): light-skinned individuals are at significantly greater risk than are dark-skinned individuals. Risk is dose-dependent, with tumors tending to occur on the sun-exposed parts of the body, although this is not universally true.

Exposure to ultraviolet radiation in Western society has increased in recent years. Travel to southern climates, lengthening life expectancy, and brief attire are among the factors which have enhanced encounters with environmental ultraviolet radiation. However, artificial sources of ultraviolet radiation may further increase the risk of actinically induced carcinogenesis (93). Recreational use of ultraviolet radiation for tanning is potentially hazardous (94), and psoralen phototherapies are associated with an element of skin cancer tumorigenesis. A risk-benefit ratio needs to be considered whenever intentional exposure to ultraviolet radiation is elected (95).

It is well-documented that ultraviolet tumors are antigenic. Presently known are tumor-specific antigens, identified as specific cytolytic and suppressor T cells, as well as antibody responses (96). Moreover, antigens arising from cross-reactive immune responses and gene area coding, although less well understood, are probable factors in actinic carcinogenesis. Appropriate immunotherapy of ultraviolet radiation-induced tumorigenesis constitutes a most viable treatment plan for this type of neoplasia (96).

Ionizing radiation, including roentgen or x-rays, α- and β- particles, and neutrons, may be carcinogenic in moderate and high dosages (97). Medical therapeutics, nuclear explosions, and occupational sources are implicated in most carcinogenic events involving ionizing radiation. The most common such events are lymphomas, leukemias, and carcinomas of the esophagus, stomach, and urinary bladder. Breast cancer, as well as tumors of the thymus, thyroid, and salivary glands have followed the therapeutic use of ionizing radiation as well. Direct exposure of a body part to x-rays may be carcinogenic. Radiation therapy for tinea capitis, for example, may result in brain tumors. Radiation therapy for benign skin lesions of the lower extremities, gynecologic procedures, contrast mediums, and radioisotopes used in the work place are similarly suspect (97). It is estimated that 40–45% of all ionizing radiation to which people are exposed is medically generated. Background radiation sources include earth elements such as radium, cosmic rays, and body emissions. About 1% of cancers involve exposure to various radiation sources (97).

It is possible that a threshold dose level of ionizing radiation needs to be reached before malignant transformation is initiated. Most ionizing radiation is cumulative in nature and this factor needs to be considered when establishing a threshold dose. The ability or failure of DNA to repair following cytotoxic doses of ionizing radiation is likely to be the determining factor in carcinogenesis.

HISTOLOGIC EVIDENCE FOR IMMUNOLOGIC INFLUENCES OF GERMINAL CENTER HYPERPLASIA

Malignant melanomas in humans, as well as in several experimental animal models, are used to correlate the occurrence of metastasis to lymph nodes and the relative degree of hyperplasia of germinal centers of nodes (98). Similar data is observed in prostatic and breast cancers (99). High statistical significance, along with impressive anatomic evidence, suggests a positive relationship between nodal metastasis and hyperplasia of the germinal centers of lymph nodes.

Poor patient survival is associated with germinal center hyperplasia, whereas sinus histiocytosis of lymph nodes is indicative of a more favorable prognosis. Indeed, nodes demonstrating germinal center hyperplasia appear to have inhibited sinus histiocytosis (98). Conversely, sinus histiocytosis exerts greater cytotoxic activity against tumor cells whenever germinal center hyperplastic is absent or limited. These data further indicate that there is a biologic competition between sinus histiocytosis and germinal center hyperplasia (100).

It would appear that small tumors stimulate sinus histiocytosis along with resistance to metastasis. However, as tumors enlarge, lymph nodes closest to the cancer progressively demonstrate germinal center hyperplasia and metastasis occurs in the relative absence of sinus histiocytosis.

PERIVASCULAR CUFFING

Delayed type hypersensitivity (DTH) is a type of immune response which is characterized by the infiltration of small lymphocytes around blood vessels (Fig. 1.3). These responses do not involve antibodies and are mediated by T type lymphocytes. Microvascular changes, characterized by severe disruption of small blood vessel circulation, have been observed in T cell lymphocyte-mediated DTH associated with

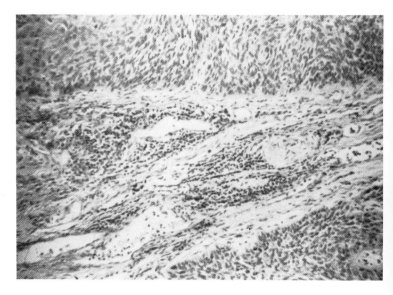

Figure 1.3. Delayed hypersensitivity damages endothelium of small blood vessels compromising the circulation through them. Infiltration of small lymphocytes around blood vessels is indicative of delayed type hypersensitivity. Perivascular cuffing is seen in this hematoxylin and eosin preparation. (From Hunter RL. Immunology and cancer. In: Moossa AR, Robson MC, Schimpff SC, eds. Comprehensive Textbook of Oncology. Baltimore: Williams and Wilkins, 1986.)

malignant tumors. Endothelial cell damage involves edema, degeneration, and necrosis in and about the intima of involved blood vessels. The microcirculation damage compromises blood flow and a local ischemia develops (101). Such changes effectively limit the growth and aggressive behavior of tumors as a result of local infarction. Appreciation of the phenomenon just discussed explains why some tumors undergo regression in the absence of evident immunologic attack. Significant infiltration of inflammatory cells, lymphocytes, and macrophages does not occur.

DTH induced by tuberculin is often associated with induration of the skin at the site of immunologic challenge (98). This induration is due to a deposition of fibrin that can be blocked by anticoagulants such as heparin. Fibrin meshwork associated with DTH reactions in the presence of tumors is in the form of a loosely formed gel (101). Cancers are, therefore, further isolated from contiguous normal tissues. Leakage of plasma and clot formation are not involved, as might be expected in trauma or in immune complex reactions.

SINUS HISTIOCYTOSIS

Sinus histiocytosis identifies that state of lymph nodes associated with cancer in which cords become distended by great numbers of small histiocytes (98). Histiocytes and activated macrophages crowd the lymph node sinuses at the same time (Fig. 1.4). As previously stated, the presence of sinus histiocytosis appears to be a positive indicator of survival in malignant disease (102). Recent studies also implicate sinus histiocytosis with massive lymphadenopathies (103–106). Activated macrophages seem to selectively kill malignant cells and these highly metabolic and phagocytic cells populate lymph node sinuses in great numbers. Macrophage activation occurs in the presence of lymphokines, which are produced by certain sensitized T lymphocytes. The ability of macrophages to block and destroy cancer cells relates to morphologically identifiable subcellular organelles such as cytoplasmic granules and lysosomal enzymes (98).

Arguments for the immunological basis of malignancy have been derived from cell culture experimentation. Malignant cells from cell cultures implanted into flexor surfaces of healthy individuals are met with a more or less immediate inflammatory response, and tumor regression is completed within a month. Conversely, patients with varying stages of coexistent malignancy exhibited varying degrees of implanted tumor cell growth and even metastasis (107). Clinical observations provide additional evidence for immunologic impairment as an etiology of cancer. Consider, for example, that immunologically compromised patients with kidney transplants demonstrate a significant rise in malignant diseases, including sarcomas, carcinomas, and lymphomas (108). Moreover, removal of transplanted organs with discontinuance of immunosuppressive drugs is frequently followed by regression of the cancer.

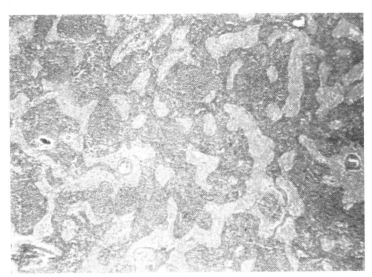

Figure 1.4. Sinus histiocytosis is indicative of improved prognosis in malignant and benign conditions. *Pale areas* are sinuses within lymph nodes packed and dilated by histiocytes. Such cells are probably macrophages capable of tumor destruction. (From Hunter RL. Immunology and cancer. In: Moossa AR, Robson MS, Schimpff SC, eds. Comprehensive Textbook of Oncology. Baltimore: Williams and Wilkins, 1986.)

The ability for host rejection of homografts is often impaired in patients with malignant disease (109). Such occurrences are attributed to immunologic phenomena, as are otherwise unexplainable regressions of tumors. Podiatrists are particularly interested in regression of primary and recurrent malignant melanomas on the lower extremities. Tumor cells at the epidermal-dermal junction of regressed lesions are absent in such cases. Other histologic findings include degenerate malignant melanocytes, interstitial edema, and vascular proliferation in the presence of an inflammatory skin infiltrate (110).

Evidence for an immunologic basis for malignant disease is based on scientific reports and anecdotal data. The use of immunologic testing as a monitor of cancer progression or regression gives additional credence to the concept. In general, most authorities agree that simpler tests are more reliable than complex ones (98). Recall antigens such as tuberculin and Candida give positive tests in cancer patients with good survival prognosis. Podiatrists are familiar with DNCB (dinitrochlorobenzene), which provides a strong immunologic challenge. Thus far, immune function tests are general and do not test for tumor-specific components. Tests measure secondary effects of tumors and it is necessary to understand how the immune system is reacting against the tumor in order to appreciate the test results (98). In addition, it is necessary to remember that malignancy alters the patient's general physiology and these changes can affect immune processes. Differential blood counts can provide valuable insight into the status of malignancy, but peripheral blood may not be an accurate indicator of what lymphocytes are doing about the tumor mass itself (98). However, the role of the killer lymphocytes and macrophages is indisputable evidence for an etiologic role of immune factors in human cancer.

INTERFERON

Interferon was first identified as a naturally occurring protein having antiviral properties (111). These substances are produced by most body cells and are biologic response modifiers with regulatory and defensive properties (112, 113). Apparently, interferon has a broad spectrum of activity against viruses but is not specific in its action. It is now determined that interferon could modulate cell growth, cell proliferation, and host responses to malignant diseases (113, 114). Antigenic, biologic, and physiochemical differences indicate that three classes of interferons exist: α, β, and δ (113, 115).

Two different types of interferons based on cellular origin are currently recognized. Type I interferon includes the α- and β- interferon classes derived from leukocytes and fibroblasts, respectively (116). A family of more than a dozen physiochemically related α-interferons has been identified (117). Type II interferon is a lymphokine derived of T lymphocytes and is a δ-class interferon. Cell structure and function are influenced at the cell surface and by biochemical actions which are distinctive to interferons.

Host defense mechanisms against cancer depend on an intact cellular immunity system. The general characteristics of the relationship of immunity with tumorigenesis have been generally discussed. However, the interferons present a special refinement of this system. Presumably, the absence of interferon production would be a carcinogenic defect. Several possibilities exist to explain the antitumor effects of interferon. The protein, in high concentrations, acts directly to inhibit the growth of malignant cells (111). Interferons very likely act to inhibit replication of oncogenic viruses. It is also clear that interferons stimulate macrophages and the reticuloendothelial system in bodily defenses against neoplasia. Interferon stimulates the activity of NK cells, a primary and nonspecific surveyor against malignant cells in the body.

Tumor regression, following the use of interferons, has been observed in carcinoma of the breast, established basal cell carcinoma (118), squamous cell carcinoma (118), malignant lymphoma (119), multiple myeloma (120), acute and chronic leukemia (121), AIDS-associated Kaposi's sarcoma (122), renal and bladder carcinomas (123), nasopharyngeal carcinoma (111), and malignant gliomas. Moreover, hematologic (124), neuroendocine (125), and ovarian, as well as solid and carcinoid tumors (126), respond favorably to interferons. Most important to those dealing with malignant melanomas of the lower extremities, interferons are shown to produce regression and to inhibit metastasis of these aggressive malignancies (108, 111, 119, 127). Premalignant lesions such as keratoacanthoma (118), condyloma acuminata, and viral warts

(128, 129) have been successfully treated with interferons. It is apparent that the interferons are useful in the treatment of premalignant and malignant conditions, some of which have podiatric relevance. Conversely, it is possible that defects in the body's ability to produce the interferons may permit carcinogenesis to proceed. The mobilization of the patient's own naturally occurring interferons is one area of study currently of interest in cancer therapy (127). It is important that side effects of cancer therapy that produce antibodies that neutralize the body's naturally occurring interferon be avoided (127).

Interferon is part of a generalized immune response active in the prevention of malignancy (113). Both natural and recombinant forms have proven useful (112, 113), although recombinant interferon-α is associated with a more narrow role in the control and treatment of malignancy. Topical, intramuscular, and subcutaneous routes are used in interferon therapy (115). Melanomas, and up to 80% of premalignant conditions such as papillomatosis and the condylomas, appear to be most responsive (115). The efficacy of interferon treatment is credited not only to enhanced immunologic activity but also to cell membrane effects, tumor antigen production, and the induction of certain enzymes which produce cytostatic effects that are antiproliferative.

Optimal use requires that improved accuracy of assay of the substances be achieved (114). Moreover, it is necessary to know the dose, route, schedule, duration, and the species of interferon best employed for any given malignant condition (113). Early intervention with interferon therapy improves the response rate (114), but interferons may also be useful when other treatment plans fail. Interferons may be useful in cancer therapies in combination with other modalities (127). Drugs with toxic effects may be combined with them in order that lower dosages of these substances can be employed with effective results. The efficacy of retinoids and synthetic analogues is enhanced by the use of interferons for primary neoadjuvant therapy in advanced malignancy (118). Combined therapies which employ interferon with lasers or podophyllin are shown to have more optimal use (115). The cost of interferon production was originally prohibitive, but large-scale production of human leukocyte interferon now promises to reduce costs to manageable levels. Therefore, greater use of the interferons alone or in combination is likely in the future.

NUTRITION

The role of nutrition in the etiology of human malignancy has been and continues to be a matter of controversy. While a great many references are available in support of nutrition in cancer therapeutics, articles to the contrary are equally forceful. Faddism and quackery are alleged and questions such as whether or not a change in diet can cure cancer are being raised (130, 131). Studies based on nutritional epidemiology are currently being conducted and observational methodologies emphasized (132). Fatty diets are best avoided in cancers of the colon (132, 133). Diets rich in fruits and vegetables appear to provide some protection against carcinoma of the lungs (132). Ethyl alcohol has a negative correlation to breast cancer, but this factor may be dose-dependent. Methionine and choline are lipotropic substances which may be considered carcinogenic (133). Calcium has been studied and may provide some protection against colon-rectal cancers. Zinc and selenium are also considered important in cancer protection (133–135). Selenium is often associated with retinol in anticancer activity, but studies are equivocal (136).

It is clear that cachexia occurs among cancer patients as a combined result of rigorous treatment plans and the effects of the malignant process itself. However, most feeding and metabolic problems can be anticipated and malnutrition can be prevented (134). Prompt intervention can and should save patients needless suffering and deterioration due to malnutrition. These facts are not at issue for purposes of this discussion. The use of macrobiotic diets for treatment and prevention, however, raises a question as to whether diet is actually etiologic in human cancer (136). Current wisdom suggests that dietary manipulation in terms of total calories and protein helps prevent carcinoma (133). Some studies seem to indicate that restrictions should be placed on the dietary intake of fat in breast cancer (137, 138). Other studies suggest a negative correlation (110). A rationale can be stated for modulation of iodine intake in thyroid cancers (139).

Malignancies demonstrated a 20% survival rate in 1930, but this percentage was improved to 50% by 1980 (132, 140). Further improvements of 33% can be achieved if patients choose to abstain from the use of tobacco. Judicious manipulations involving diet and nutritional supplements can save an additional 33% (132).

VITAMIN C

The question as to the benefit of vitamin C in cancer treatment and its possible use in preventing malignancy remains at issue. Linus Pauling, Ph.D., advocates the use of high dosages of ascorbic acid in malignancy. He argues that cancer deaths associated with high doses of vitamin C are not due to the prescription of the vitamin, but to the sudden termination of medication (140).

Contrary opinions from the medical community relative to the efficacy of vitamin C are based on institutional statistical data. In one study, patients treated with high doses of ascorbic acid were found to deteriorate more rapidly than those receiving sugar pills (141). Interference with vitamin C mechanisms because of cytotoxic drugs employed concurrently was eliminated in some hospital studies. Vitamin C was not viewed as helpful in cancer treatment in such a study at the Mayo Clinic (141).

Recent studies have provided additional credence as to the use of vitamin C in cancer prevention. Vitamin C is credited as preventative for esophageal cancer and inhibitory in carcinomas of skin, nerve, lung, and kidney tissues (142). The mechanism for the efficacy of vitamin C is associated with reactions against free radicals known to be toxic to gene loci as well as controls on polycyclic hydrocarbon metabolism (142). Vitamin C is said to provide a reduction of mutagenic activity and to protect against chemical carcinogenesis (142).

VITAMIN E

Vitamin E alone has not been shown to be definitively effective in mammary and colon cancers. Some benefits in terms of inhibitory activity are, however, associated with skin, liver, mouth, ear duct and forestomach involvements (142). Combinations of vitamins E and C are credited with inhibiting the formation of carcinogenic nitrosamines (142). Such synergism appears to inhibit tumor cell growth and to limit carcinogenically induced DNA damage (45).

VITAMIN A

Anecdotal and epidemiologic data suggest that vitamin A analogues have value in chemoprevention of cancers (143–146). Retinol is preformed vitamin A and its synthetic analogues. Carotenoids constitute a second class of the vitamin, produced when forms of provitamin A are converted as required by the body. Retinol and the other retinoids have potent hormone-like effects on cell growth and differentiation of epithelial tissues (147, 148). Epidemiologic studies tend to support the efficacy of carotene, while animal investigations find retinol to be involved in anticancer activities relative to neoplastic diseases of the integument (149).

Retinol is stored in the liver and transported to peripheral tissues as needed by binding to retinol-binding protein (RBP). Since long-term high intake of vitamin A may result in hypervitaminosis and hepatotoxicity, the widespread use of retinoids as a chemopreventive agent may be precluded, except among high-risk patients. Carotenoids may be directly absorbed from the intestine before conversion into retinol (149). They are stored principally in adipose tissue. β-Carotene has the ability to take certain free organic radicals and to deactivate excited molecules such as oxygen (150, 151). Carotene, therefore may have a direct protective effect against carcinogenesis by deactivating these molecules, which are generated during tissue metabolism.

Retinoid anticancer effects involve protein kinase C metabolism and ornithine decarboxylase induction (148). Epidermal growth factor receptor numbers are affected and intracellular polyamine levels are regulated by vitamin A. Synthetic derivatives of vitamin A appear to have higher therapeutic and preventative anticancer indices than does naturally occurring vitamin A (148).

Retinoids are useful in the treatment of actinic keratosis, keratoacanthoma, epidermolysis dysplasia verruciformis, leukoplakia, laryngeal papillomatosis, cervical dysplasia, and mycosis fungoides (149). Cutaneous malignancies, including refractory basal cell carcinoma, squamous cell carcinomas, and malignant melanoma, as well as leukemia and carcinomas of the bladder, are responsive to retinoid therapy. Vitamin A and its analogues are used in combined adjuvant therapy, and interferon is especially useful in this regard (148).

In summary, the use of carotene and retinoids (vitamins C and E) appears to be useful in cancer therapeutics in many types of malignant disease. The deprivation of these vitamins may leave patients at a disadvantage when carcinogenic activity is initiated. The cutaneous malignancies have a particular podiatric relevance in this regard.

PHENYLALANINE AND TYROSINE

The progression of malignant melanoma is associated with advancing levels of serum phenylalanine and tyrosinase. Conversely, restriction of the dietary intake of these substances is related to regression of this highly metastatic disease often found on the lower extremities (152). Active tyrosinase is present in comparatively large amounts in melanomas, and the enzyme is apparently active in intracellular respiratory activities necessary to tumorigenesis. Inhibition of cellular growth, therefore, might well be contained by limiting the required substrate tyrosine. The selective deprivation of energy should logically inhibit tumor growth, and this is found to be true (152).

Progression of malignant melanomas is directly correlated with serum phenylalanine and tyrosine levels. Metastatic disease occurred most commonly when dietary restrictions were not observed. This again relates directly to the availability of substrate provided. Additionally, it is possible that tyrosinase activity might well continue unsuppressed in melanoma tumor cells. Tyrosinase could, therefore, sequester in large amounts as melanin. Tyrosine and phenylalanine appear to have a causal relationship to tumorigenesis in malignant melanoma (152).

DIETARY FIBER

Recently, much has been made of the role of dietary fiber in the prevention of cancer. This line of evidence does not relate directly to the development of solid tumors of the lower extremities since the gastrointestinal tract is involved (153). But, pertinent factors involved in tumorigenesis of this type need to be understood in a discussion of this type. Anecdotal evidence suggests that the removal of dietary fiber in modern day life has resulted in significant increases in cancers of the colon and rectum (154).

Dietary fiber influences the physiology of the gastrointestinal tract in a variety of ways. The flow of saliva, with its several digestive enzymes, is stimulated in the mouth. The holding time of food in the stomach is extended and gastric secretions are diluted. Intestinal absorption is slowed and contents are further diluted. This is particularly significant relative to lipid absorption. In the large intestine, fiber serves as a bacterial substrate, binds certain ions, holds water, and reduces formation, concentration, and contact time of possible fecal mutagens (153). Fiber softens and enlarges the stool in the colon and reduces trauma and the need for straining during elimination. These factors argue for the dietary intake of fiber as preventative for colon-rectal cancers.

SUMMARY

Tumorigenesis and malignant transformation is a stepwise and multifactorial event. It is not likely, therefore, that human cancers will respond to a single therapeutic modality or approach. The cell cycle is materially changed in tumorigenesis. It is possible that normalizing the sequentially timed events of G_1, G_2, G_0, S, and M cell phases would tend to return diseased tissue to normal. Genetic abnormalities and oncogenes have important implications in tumor development and malignancy. Modifications can occur at the chromosomal or gene loci levels, and these factors might be modulated by principles of genetic engineering or manipulations of enzymes involved in histogenesis. Synergism and the processes of tumor initiation, promotion, and progression provide additional levels at which one may intervene in the process of tumor development. Interferon and interleukin II are proteins which are synthesized during cell metabolism that sometimes have remarkable anticancer properties. The development of cancer may be the result of a failure of cells to adequately produce these important substances. Vitamins such as retinoic acid and ascorbic acid, and proteins such as tyrosine and phenylalanine are thought to influence and control tumorigenesis. Viral and immunologic influences clearly have pivotal effects in initiating carcinogenesis and controls thereof. A knowledge of all the factors etiologic to cancer may provide the basis for the rational treatment of this feared malady.

REFERENCES

1. Spandidos DA, Anderson MLM. Oncogenes and oncosuppressor genes: their involvement in cancer. J Pathol 1989;157:1–10.
2. Weinberg RA. The genetic origins of human cancer. Cancer 1988;61:1963–1968.
3. Nowell PC. Molecular events in tumor development. N Engl J Med 1988;319:575–577.

4. Brosman SA, Brian C, Liu S. Oncogenes: their role in neoplasia. Virology 1987;30:1–10.

5. Huebner RM, Todaro GJ. Oncogenes or RNA tumor viruses as determinants of cancer. Proc Natl Acad Sci USA 1969;64:1087–1094.

6. Rous P. A sarcoma of the fowl transmissible by an agent separable from the tumor cells. J Exp Med 1910;12:696–705.

7. Hill M, Hillova J. Virus recovery in chicken cells tested with Rous sarcoma cell DNA. Nature 1972;237:35–39.

8. Stehelin D, Varmus HE, Bishop JM, Vogt PK. DNA related to the transforming gene(s) of avian sarcoma viruses is present in normal avian DNA. Nature 1976;260:170–173.

9. Bishop JM. Cellular oncogenes and retroviruses. Annu Rev Biochem 1983;52:301–354.

10. Bell JC. Oncogenes. Cancer Lett 1988;40:1–5.

11. Nishimura S, Sekiya T. Human cancer and cellular oncogenes. Biochem J. 1987;243:313–327.

12. Butturini A, Gale RP. Oncogenes and human leukemias. Int J Cell Cloning 1988;6:2–24.

13. Bos JL. The RAS gene family and human carcinogenesis. Mutat Res 1988;195:255–271.

14. Barbacid M. RAS genes. Annu Rev Biochem 1987;56:779–827.

15. Der JC. Cellular oncogenes and human carcinogenesis. Clin Chem 1987;33:641–646.

16. Hunter T, Cooper JA. Protein-tyrosine kinases. Annu Rev Biochem 1985;54:897–930.

17. Born P, Burger MM. The cytoskeletal protein vinculin contains transformation-sensitive covalently bound lipid. Science 1987;235:476–479.

18. Weinberg RA. The action of oncogenes in the cytoplasm and nucleus. Science 1985;230:770–776.

19. Dickson C, Peters G. Potential oncogene product related to growth factors. Nature 1987;326:833.

20. Doolittle RF, Hunkapiller MW, Hood LE, et al. Simian sarcoma virus onc gene, v-sis, is derived from the gene (or genes) encoding a platelet-derived growth factor. Science 1983;221:275–277.

21. Chiu I-M, Reddy EP, Givol D, et al. Nucleotide sequence analysis identifies the human c-sis proto-oncogene as a structural gene for platelet-derived growth factor. Cell 1984;37:123–129.

22. Stiles CD. The biologic role of oncogenes: insights from platelet derived growth factors. Cancer Res 1985;45:5215–5218.

23. Deuel TF. Polypeptide growth factors: roles in normal and abnormal cell growth. Annu Rev Cell Biol 1987;3:443–492.

24. Weinstein IB. Growth factors, oncogenes, and multistage carcinogenesis. J Cell Biochem 1987;33:213–224.

25. Sainsbury JRC, Farndon JR, Needham GK, et al. Epidermal growth factor receptor status as predictor of early recurrence of and death from breast cancer. Lancet 1987;1:1398–1402.

26. Clark SC, Kamen R. The human hematopoietic colony-stimulating factors. Science 1987;236(4806):1229–1237.

27. Cheers C, Haigh AM, Kelso A, et al. Production of colony-stimulating factors (CSFs) during infection: separate determinations of macrophage-, granulocyte-, granulocyte-macrophage-, and multi-CSFs. Infect Immun 1988;56:247–251.

28. Wheeler EF, Rettenmeier CW, Look AT, et al. The v-fms oncogene induces factor independence and tumorigenicity in CSF-1 dependent macrophage cell line. Nature 1986;324:377–380.

29. Williamson DJ, Begley CG. Colony-stimulating factors in the pathogenesis and treatment of disease. Postgrad Med J 1987;63:1061–1068.

30. Rodenhuis S, Van de Wetering ML, Mooi WJ, et al. Mutational activation of the K-ras oncogene. N Engl J Med 1987;317:929–935.

31. Alitalo K, Koskinen P, Makela TP, et al. Myc oncogenes: activation and amplification. Biochim Biophys Acta 1987;907:1–32.

32. Stam K, Heisterkamp N, Reynolds FH, Groffen J. Evidence that the phl gene encodes a 160,000-dalton phosphoprotein associated with kinase activity. J Mol Biol 1987;7:1955–1960.

33. Konopka JB, Watanase SM, Witte ON. An alteration of the human c-abl protein in K562 leukemia cells unmasks associated tyrosine kinase activity. Cell 1984;37:1035–1042.

34. Brodeur GM. Molecular correlates of cytogenetic abnormalities in human cancer cells: implication for oncogene activation. Prog Hematol 1986;16:229–256.

35. Seeger RC, Brodeur GM, Sather H, et al. Association of multiple copies of the n-myc oncogene with rapid progression of neuroblastomas. N Engl J Med 1984;313:1111–1116.

36. Cleveland JL, Morse HC, Rapp UR. Myc oncogenes and tumor induction. ISI Atlas of Science: Biochemistry 1988:93–100.

37. Slamon DJ, et al. Human breast cancer: correlation of relapse and survival with amplification of the HER-2/neu oncogene. Science 1987;235:177–182.

38. Sainsbury JRC, Farndon JR, Needham GK, et al. Epidermal growth factor receptor status as predictor of early recurrence of and death from breast cancer. Lancet 1987;1:1398–1402.

39. Friend SH, Dryia TP, Weinberg RA. Oncogenes and tumor-suppressing genes. N Engl J Med 1988;318:618–622.

40. Knudson AG. Hereditary cancer, oncogenes and anti-oncogenes. Cancer Res 1985;45:1437–1443.

41. Willman CL, Fenoglio-Preiser CM. Oncogenes, suppressor genes, and carcinogenesis. Hum Pathol 1987;18:895–902.

42. Friend SH, Bernards R, Rojelj S, et al. A human DNA segment with properties of the gene that predisposes to retinoblastoma and osteosarcoma. Nature 1986;323:643–646.

43. DeCaprio JA, Ludlow JW, Figge J, et al. SV40 large tumor antigen forms a specific complex with the product of the retinoblastoma susceptibility gene. Cell 1988;54:275–283.

44. Whyte P, Buchkovich KJ, Horowitz, JM, et al. Association between an oncogene and an antioncogene: the adenovirus E1A proteins

bind to the retinoblastoma gene product. Nature 1988;334:124–129.

45. Stowers SJ, Maronpot RR, Reynolds SH, et al. The role of oncogenes in chemical carcinogenesis. Environ Health Perspect 1987;75:81–86.

46. Scott JR. Oncogenes and cancer. Am J Reprod Immunol Microbiol 1987;15:24–28.

47. Hernandez AM. Repair, regeneration and fibrosis. In: Rubin E, Farber JL, eds. Pathology. Philadelphia: Lippincott, 1988:75–76.

48. Cotran SR, Kumar V, Robbins SL. Robbins pathologic basis of disease, 4th ed. Philadelphia: Saunders, 1989:251–253.

49. Svodoba J. Rous sarcoma virus. Intervirology 1986;26:1–60.

50. Green M, Wold WSM. Search for adenovirus genetic information in normal and malignant human tissues. In: Philips LA, ed. Viruses associated with human cancer. New York: Marcel Dekker, 1983:307–355.

51. Hsiung GD. Perspectives on retroviruses and the etiologic agent of AIDS. Yale J Biol Med 1987;60:505–514.

52. Rojko JL, Olsen RG. The immunobiology of the feline leukemia virus. Vet Immunol Immunopathol 1984;6:107–165.

53. Overbaugh J, Donahue PR, Quackenbush SL, et al. Molecular cloning of a feline leukemia virus that induces fatal immunodeficiency disease in cats. Science 1988;239:906–910.

54. Guerreo, I. Proto-oncogenes in pattern formation. Trends Genet 1987;3(10):269–271.

55. Bishop JM. The molecular genetics of cancer. Science 1987;235:305–311.

56. Poiesz BJ, Ruscetti FW, Gazdar AF, et al. Detection and isolation of type C retrovirus particles from fresh and cultured lymphocytes of a patient with cutaneous T-cell lymphoma. Proc Natl Acad Sci USA 1980;77:7415–7419.

57. Seiki M, Hattori S, Hirayma Y, et al. Human adult T-cell leukemia virus: complete nucleotide sequence of the provirus genome integrated in leukemia cell DNA. Proc Natl Acad Sci USA 1983;80:3618–3622.

58. Yoshida M, Seiki M. Recent advances in the molecular biology of HTLV-1: trans-activation of viral and cellular genes. Annu Rev Immunol 1987;5:541–559.

59. Nerenberg M, Hinrichs SH, Reynolds RK, et al. The tat gene of human T-lymphotropic virus type 1 induces mesenchymal tumors in transgenic mice. Science 1987;237:1324–1329.

60. Ehrlich GD, Poiesz BJ. Clinical and molecular parameters of HTLV-1 infection. Clin Lab Med 1988;8:65–84.

61. Roman GC. The neuroepidemiology of tropical spastic paraparesis. Ann Neurol 1988;23 suppl):S113–S120.

62. Toshiro H, Yasunobu T, Shunro S, et al. Human T-cell lymphotropic virus type 1 infection in neonates. Am J Dis Child 1987;141:764–765.

63. Kanner SB, Parks ES, Scott GB, et al. Simultaneous infections with human T-cell leukemia virus type 1 and the human immunodeficiency virus. J Infect Dis 1987;155:617–625.

64. Starkebaum G, Loughran TP, Kalyanaraman VS, et al. Serum reactivity to human T-cell leukemia/lymphoma virus type 1 proteins in patients with large granular lymphocytic leukemia. Lancet 1987;14:596–599.

65. Kin JH, Durack DT. Manifestations of human T-lymphotropic virus type 1 infection. Am J Med 1988;84:919–928.

66. Levine AJ. Oncogenes of DNA tumor viruses. Cancer Res 1988;48:493–496.

67. Howley PM, Schlegel R. The human papillomavirus: an overview. Am J Med 1988;85:155–158.

68. Abramson C, Fischman GJ. Purification and characterization of plantar human papillomavirus. J Am Podiatr Med Assoc 1987;77:123–133.

69. Meanwell CA. The epidemiology of human papilloma virus in relation to cervical cancer. Cancer Surv 1988;7:481–497.

70. Ostrow RS, Manias D, Mitchell AJ, et al. Epidermodysplasia verruciformis. Arch Dermatol 1987;123:1511–1516.

71. Milburn PB, Brandsma JL, Goldsman CI, et al. Disseminated warts and evolving squamous cell carcinoma in a patient with AIDS. J Am Acad Dermatol 1988;19:401–405.

72. Healy GB, Gelber RD, Trowbridge RN, et al. Treatment of recurrent respiratory papillomatosis with human leukocyte interferon. N Engl J Med 1988;319:401–407.

73. Ostrow RS, Faras AJ. The molecular biology of human papilloma viruses and the pathogenesis of genital papillomas and neoplasms. Cancer Metastasis Rev 1987;6:385–395.

74. McNichol PH, Guijon FB, Paraskevas M, et al. Comparison of filter in-situ deoxyribonucleic acid hybridization with cytologic, colposcopic, and histopathologic examination for detection of human papillomavirus infection in women with cervical intraepithelial neoplasia. Am J Obstet Gynecol 1989;160:265–270.

75. Roman A, Fife KH. Human papillomaviruses: are we ready to type? Clin Microbiol Rev 1989;2:166–190.

76. Ferenczy A, Mitae M, Nigari N, et al. Latent papillomavirus and recurring genital warts. N Engl J Med 1985;313:784–788.

77. ZurHausen H. Papillomaviruses in anogenital cancer as a model to understand the role of viruses in cancer. Cancer Res 1989;49:4677–4681.

78. Durst M, Croce CM, Gissman L, et al. Papillomavirus sequences integrate near cellular oncogenes in some cervical carcinomas. Proc Natl Acad Sci USA 1987;84:1070–1074.

79. Gius D, Laimins LA. Activation of human papillomavirus type 18 expression B herpes simplex virus type 1 viral transactivators and a phorbolester. J Virol 1989;63:555–563.

80. Brown NA, Liu C-R, Wang Y-F, et al. B-cell lymphoproliferation and lymphomagenesis are associated with clonotypic intracellular terminal regions of the Epstein-Barr virus. J Virol 1988;62:962–969.

81. Jones JF, Shurin S, Abramowsky C, et al. T-cell lymphomas containing Epstein-Barr

viral DNA in patients with chronic Epstein-Barr infections. N Engl J Med 1988;318: 733–741.

82. Jaffe R, Ho M, Miller G, et al. The frequency of Epstein-Barr virus infection and associated lymphoproliferative syndrome after transplantation and its manifestations in children. Transplantation 1988;45:719–727.

83. Beissner RS, Rappaport ES, Diaz JA. Fatal case of Epstein-Barr virus-induced lymphoproliferative disorder associated with AIDS infection. Arch Pathol Lab Med 1987;111: 250–253.

84. Kamani N, Kennedy J, Brandsma J. Burkitt lymphoma in a child with human immunodeficiency virus infection. J Pediatr 1988;112: 241–244.

85. Dillner J, Kallin B. The Epstein-Barr virus proteins. Adv Cancer Res 1988;50:95–158.

86. Purtilo DT. Epstein-Barr virus: the spectrum of its manifestations in human beings. South Med J 1987;80:943–947.

87. Sato H, Takimoto T, Hatano M, et al. Epstein-Barr virus with transforming and early antigen-inducing ability originating from nasopharyngeal carcinoma: mapping of the viral genome. J Gen Virol 1989;70:717–727.

88. Tiollais P, Pourcel C, Dejean A. The hepatitis B virus. Nature 1985;317:489–495.

89. Beasley RP, Hwang L, Lin C, et al. Hepatocellular carcinoma and hepatitis B virus: a prospective study of 22,707 men in Taiwan. Lancet 1981;2:1129–1133.

90. Blumberg BS, London WT. Hepatitis B virus and the prevention of primary cancer of the liver. J Natl Cancer Inst 1985;74:267–273.

91. Tabor E. Hepatocellular carcinoma: possible etiologies in patients without serologic evidence of hepatitis B infection. J Med Virol 1989;27:1–6.

92. Tiniakos D, Spandidos DA, Kakkanasa, et al. Expression of ras and myc oncogenes in human hepatocellular carcinoma and non-neoplastic liver tissues. Anticancer Res 1989; 9:715–722.

93. Morison WL. Skin cancer and artificial sources of UV radiation. J Dermatol Surg Oncol 1988;14:893–896.

94. Diffey BL. Use of AV-A sunbeds for cosmetic tanning. Br J Dermatol 1986;115:67–76.

95. Hensler T, Christophers E, Honigsmann H, et al. Skin tumors in the European PUVA study. J Am Acad Dermatol 1987;16:108–116.

96. Daynes RA, Burnham DK, DeWitt CW. The immunology of ultraviolet-radiation carcinogenesis. Cancer Surv 1985;4:51–99.

97. Thomas DB. Cancer epidemiology and prevention. In: Moossa AR, Robson MC, Schimpff SC, eds. Comprehensive textbook of oncology. Baltimore: Williams and Wilkins, 1986.

98. Hunter RL. Immunology and cancer. In: Moossa AR, Robson MC, Schimpff SC, eds. Comprehensive textbook of oncology. Baltimore: Williams and Wilkins, 1986.

99. Hunter RL, Ferguson DJ, Coppleson LW. Survival with mammary cancer related to the interaction of germinal center hyperplasia and sinus histiocytosis axillary and internal mammary lymph nodes. Cancer 1975;36:528–539.

100. Check IJ, Cobb M, Hunter RL. The relationships between cytotoxicity and prognostically significant histologic changes in lymph nodes from patients with cancer of the breast. Am J Pathol 1980;98:325–338.

101. Dvorak HF, Galli ST, Dvorak AM. Expression of cell mediated hypersensitivity in vivo—recent advances. Int Rev Exp Pathol 1980;21:120–145.

102. Berg JW. Morphologic evidence of immune response to breast cancer. Cancer 1971;28: 1453–1456.

103. Salmon JF, Duffield M. Sinus histiocytosis with massive lymphadenopathy. Am J Ophthalmol 1989;107:549–550.

104. Nawroz IM, Wilson-Storey D. Sinus histiocytosis with massive lymphadenopathy (Rosai-Dorfman disease). Histopathology 1989.

105. Foucar E, Rosai J, Dorfman RF. Sinus histiocytosis with massive lymphadenopathy. Current status and future directions. Arch Dermatol 1988;124:1211–1214.

106. Unni KK. Case report 457. Sinus histiocytosis with massive lymphadenopathy (Rosai-Dorfman disease) presenting as lesion in the sacrum. Skeletal Radiol 1988;17:129–132.

107. Southam CM, Moore AE, Rhoads CP. Homotransplantation of human cell lines. Science 1957;125:158–160.

108. Lee HM, Madge GE, Mendez-Picon G, et al. Surgical complications in renal transplant recipients. Surg Clin North Am 1978;58:285–304.

109. Green I, Corso PF. A study of skin homografting in patients with lymphomas. Blood 1959; 14:235–245.

110. Bodurtha AJ, Berkelhammer J, Kim YH, et al. A clinical histologic and immunologic study of a case of malignant melanoma undergoing spontaneous regression. Cancer 1976;37: 735–742.

111. Feinerman B. Tumor immunology and interferon. South Med J 1978;71:1409–1411.

112. Strander H. Clinical evaluation of treatment with interferon. Med Oncol Tumor Pharmacother 1989;6:87–91.

113. Figlin RA. Biotherapy with interferon—1988. Semin Oncol 1988;15(6 Suppl 6):3–9.

114. Gutterman JU. The role of interferons in the treatment of hematologic malignancies. Semin Hematol 1988;25(3 Suppl 3):3–8.

115. Weck PK, Buddin DA, Whisnant JK. Interferons in the treatment of genital human papillomavirus infections. Am J Med 1988;85: 159–164.

116. Nickoloff BJ, Basham TY, Merigan TC, et al. Immunomodulatory and antiproliferative effect of recombinant alpha, beta and gamma interferons on cultured human malignant squamous cell lines SCL-1 and SW 1271. J Invest Dermatol 1985;84:487–490.

117. Nagata S, Mantei N, Weissmann C. The structure of one of the eight or more distinct chromosomal genes for human interferon alpha. Nature 1980;287:401–408.

118. Lippman SM, Shimm DS, Meyskens FL. Non-

surgical treatments for skin cancer: retinoids and alpha-interferon. J Dermatol Surg Oncol 1988;14:862–869.

119. Cavalli F. Alpha-interferon in the treatment of malignant lymphoma. Br J Clin Pract Symp Suppl 1988;62:16–21.

120. Cooper MR. Interferons in the management of multiple myeloma. Semin Oncol 1988;15(5 Suppl 5):21–25.

121. Ozer H. Biotherapy of chronic myelogenous leukemia with interferon. Semin Oncol 1988; 15(5 Suppl 5):14–20.

122. Groopman JE, Scadden DT. Interferon therapy for Kaposi sarcoma associated with the acquired immunodeficiency syndrome (AIDS). Ann Intern Med 1989;1:335–337.

123. Muss HB. The role of biological response modifiers in metastatic renal cell carcinoma. Semin Oncol 1988;15(5 Suppl 5):30–34.

124. Gutterman JU. Clinical and biological activity of the interferons in hematologic malignancies. Prog Clin Biol Res 1988;288:337–348.

125. Oberg K. Treatment of neuroendocrine gut and pancreatic tumors with interferons. Acta Chir Scand Suppl 1989;549:56–62.

126. Kirkwood JM, Ernstoff MS. A clinical update: The role of interferon in the biotherapy of solid tumors. Oncol Nurs Forum 1988;15(Suppl 6):3–6.

127. Alm GV. Interferons. Acta Chir Scand Suppl 1989;549:35–39.

128. Tyring SK. Treatment of condyloma acuminatum with interferon. Semin Oncol 1988;15 (5 Suppl 5):35–40.

129. Gibson JR. The treatment of viral warts with interferons. J Antimicrob Chemother 1988; 21:391–393.

130. Herbert V. Faddism and quackery in cancer nutrition. Nutr Cancer, 1984;6:196–206.

131. Dickerson JW. Does diet cure cancer? J R Soc Health 1986;106:191–193.

132. Byers T. Diet and cancer. Any progress in the interim? Cancer 1988;62(8 Suppl):1713–1724.

133. Newberne PM, Conner MW. Dietary modifiers of cancer. Prog Clin Biol Res 1988;259: 105–129.

134. Buss CL. Nutritional support in cancer patients. Prim Care 1986;14:191–193.

135. Coates RJ, Weiss NS, Daling JR, Morris JS, Labbe RF. Serum levels of selenium and retinol and the subsequent risk of cancer. Am J Epidemiol 1988;128:515–523.

136. Bowman BB, Kushner RF, Dawson SC, et al. Macrobiotic diets for cancer treatment and prevention. J Clin Oncol 1984;2:702–711.

137. Lee-Han H, Cousins M, Beaton M, et al. Compliance in a randomized clinical trial of dietary

fat reduction in patients with breast dysplasia. Am J Clin Nutr 1988;48:575–586.

138. Boyd NF, Cousins M, Beaton M, et al. Methodological issues in clinical trials of dietary fat reduction in patients with breast dysplasia. Prog Clin Biol Res 1986;222:117–124.

139. Maxon HR, Thomas SR, Boehringer A, et al. Low iodine diet in I-131 ablation of thyroid remnants. Clin Nucl Med 1983;8:123–126.

140. Pauling L, Moertel C. Megadoses of vitamin C are valuable in the treatment of cancer. Nutr Rev 1986;44:28–32.

141. Hanck AB. Vitamin C and cancer. Prog Clin Biol Res 1988;259:307–320.

142. Shen LH, Boissonneault GS, Glauert HP. Vitamin C, vitamin E and cancer. Anticancer Res 1988;8:739–748.

143. Hennekens CH. Vitamin A analogues in cancer chemoprevention. In: DeVita VT, Hellman S, Rosenbery SA, eds. Important advances in oncology 1986. Philadelphia: Lippincott, 1986.

144. Basu TK, Temple NJ, Hodgson AM. Vitamin A, beta-carotene and cancer. Prog Clin Biol Res 1988;259:217–228.

145. Wolf G, Zerlauth G. Tumor promotion, vitamin A, and fibronectin. A review of recent work. Prog Clin Biol Res 1988;259:201–216.

146. Mettlin C. Levels of epidemiologic proof in studies of diet and cancer with special reference to dietary fat and vitamin A. Prog Clin Biol Res 1988;259:149–159.

147. Wolback SB, Howe PR. Tissue changes following deprivation of fat soluble vitamin A. J Exp Med 1925;42:753–777.

148. Lippman SM, Meyskens FL. Vitamin A derivatives in the prevention and treatment of human cancer. J Am Coll Nutr 1988;7: 269–284.

149. De Vet HC. The puzzling role of vitamin A in cancer prevention. Anticancer Res 1989; 9:145–151.

150. Krinsky NI, Deneke SM. Interaction of oxygen and oxy-radicals with carotenoids. J Natl Cancer Inst 1982;67:205–210.

151. Krinsky NI. Carotenoid protection against oxidation. Pure Appl Chem 1979;51:649–670.

152. Demopoulos JB. Effects of reducing phenylalanine-tyrosinase intake of patients with advanced malignant melanoma. Cancer 1966; 16:657–664.

153. Greenwald P, Lanze E. Role of dietary fiber in the prevention of cancer. In: DeVita VT, Hellman S, Rosenberg SA, eds. Important advances in oncology 1986. Philadelphia: Lippincott, 1986.

154. Burkitt DP. Related disease—related cause? Lancet 1969;2:1220–1231.

2

Epidemiology of Neoplasms of the Foot

—Roy E. Shore

Neoplasms of the foot have received little attention from epidemiologists, probably because malignancies are relatively uncommon, and, by and large, there are no unique tissues or types of cells in the foot which would define new forms of cancer of interest to researchers. In only a few cases was it even possible to locate incidence rates for particular types of cancers of the foot (where an incidence rate is defined as the number of persons developing a particular cancer per 100,000 population per year). So, in lieu of incidence rates, it will often be necessary to use the percent of tumors of a particular type which occur on the foot as opposed to other parts of the body.

Although incidence rates are low, neoplasms of the foot are seen with some frequency in podiatric practice. In 1973–1978, the American College of Foot Surgeons conducted a survey, based on a nationwide sample of podiatrists (1), of lesions occurring on the foot. Information was available on 2,720 foot lesions (excluding plantar warts and porokeratotic lesions), of which 84% were neoplastic in nature. Morton's neuroma (45% of neoplasms) and traumatic neuroma (15%) were by far the most common types of neoplasms. Others that constituted at least 2% of the neoplasms were fibromas/fibromatosis (6.5%), lipomas (4.3%), nevi (types unspecified) (3.7%), giant cell tumors (3.7%), and neurofibromas (2.1%). Of particular note is the fact that 3.3% of the neoplasms were malignant.

The study reported on the tissues of the foot in which the neoplasms occurred; a summary is shown in Table 2.1. The table shows that, while nerve tumors are the most frequent type of neoplasm, they very seldom are malignant. The majority of malignant neoplasms (75%) occurred on the skin. The skin cancers consisted of 32 melanomas, 14 squamous cell carcinomas (or variants thereof), 7 basal cell carcinomas, and 3 miscellaneous types. Eighteen of the remaining 19 cancers of the foot were various types of sarcomas, including 6 cases of Kaposi's sarcoma.

The clinical literature on various benign neoplasms that are characteristically found on the foot consists mainly of case series and provides little systematic information on the descriptive epidemiology of the neoplasms. Clinical reviews of many types of benign pedal tumors can be found; examples are intradermal nevi (2), eccrine poromas (3), various soft tissue tumors (4, 5), leiomyomas (6–9), hemangiomas (10), plasmacytomas (11), childhood fibrous tumors (12, 13), fibromas and fibromatoses (14–17), fibrohistiocytic tumors (18), giant cell tumors (19, 20), lipomas (21), osteomas (22, 23), enchondromas (24), schwannomas or neurilemomas (25–27), and neuromas (28–31). But these will not be considered here. The remainder of this review will concentrate on malignant neoplasms, covering some of the main types of malignant foot tumors plus others for which a selected amount of information is available.

Sarcomas occur in several types of tissues or organs, including bone, cartilage and joints, nerves, connective tissue, and blood vessels. The limited information available on several types of sarcomas of the foot will be reviewed.

MALIGNANCIES OF THE BONE

A population-based study by Price and Jeffree (32) in England showed that the annual whole-body incidence of all types of bone sarcoma was 7.4/1,000,000 population/year, which gives a lifetime probability (to age 85) of 68/100,000. The long bones of the leg are a common site for sarcomas, particularly for osteosarcoma, fibrosarcoma, and Paget's sarcoma. Sarcomas of the small bones of the hands or feet were uncommon, however, and accounted for only 4% of the bone sarcomas. Chondrosarcoma and Paget's sarcoma ac-

Table 2.1. Neoplasms of the Foot According to Type of Tissue Affected [a]

	Benign		Malignant	
Type of Tissue	Frequency	(%)	Frequency	(%)
Nerve	1413	(64)	1	(1)
Skin	339	(15)	56	(75)
Muscle, tendon, joint	108	(5)	2	(3)
Fatty or fibrous	215	(10)	6	(8)
Vascular	56	(3)	7	(9)
Bone	66	(3)	3	(4)
Total	2197	(100)	75	(100)

[a]From Berlin S. A review of 2,720 lesions of the foot. J Am Podiatr Med Assoc 1980;70:318–324.

counted for most of the foot sarcomas found in the study. Characteristics of a few types of sarcomas will be mentioned.

Osteosarcoma

Osteosarcoma, which arises from bone-forming cells (osteoblasts), accounts for about 28% of all bone cancer. It is the most common type of bone cancer in children and accounts for 50% of juvenile bone cancer (32, 33). It occurs with the greatest frequency between 15 and 24 years of age. Bones that grow rapidly are more prone to develop osteogenic sarcoma; hence the most common sites are near the epiphyses of the distal femur and the proximal tibia (33). Males are slightly more apt to develop osteosarcoma than females, and various studies have reported male/female ratios of 1.2–1.5 (34). Ewing's sarcoma also peaks in the same age range as osteosarcoma, but it seldom occurs in the bones of the foot.

Chondrosarcoma

Chondrosarcoma, which originates in the cartilage matrix-forming cells (chondroblasts), accounts for about 17% of bone sarcomas. It has the greatest propensity of occurring in the bones of the foot of any type of bone cancer. Chondrosarcoma occurs mostly after age 25, and the age-specific incidence shows little variation between ages 25 and 85. The age-adjusted annual incidence was 1.3 and 2.3/100,000 in two different population-based studies (32). The lifetime incidence is about 12–20/100,000. Preexisting bone disorders—Paget's disease, osteochondroma, or diaphyseal aclasis (improper formation of bone in the cartilage between the diaphysis and epiphysis)—may sometimes play a role in the develop-

ment of chondrosarcoma (34). Cases occasionally have histories of multiple enchondromas (Ollier's disease), enchondromas with hemangiomas (Maffucci's syndrome), or multiple hereditary exostoses (33).

Paget's Sarcoma

Paget's sarcoma, which accounts for about 18% of bone sarcomas, is a disease of old age. It occurs primarily after age 45, and the highest incidence by far is after age 85. Males and females develop Paget's sarcoma with equal frequency. In a population-based study in England, Paget's sarcoma contributed the second greatest number of cancer cases of bones of the foot, after chondrosarcoma (32).

Etiology of Bone Tumors

The only clearly documented environmental agent causing bone sarcomas is ionizing radiation, which primarily causes osteosarcoma, but also causes chondrosarcoma and fibrosarcoma (33). The classic study of radiation and bone cancer was a follow-up of women who in the 1920s had painted luminescent dials on clocks and watches using a paint containing radium. They used their tongues to produce fine tips on their paint brushes and thereby ingested substantial amounts of ^{226}Ra. Beginning within 10 yr of exposure, a number of them developed bone sarcomas; one report documented 63 among about 2,500 workers (35). The cancers were rather evenly distributed among many bones of the body, including several on the distal tibia (36). Studies of ^{224}Ra (37), which has been used in treating ankylosing spondylitis and tuberculosis, also showed high rates of bone sarcoma (53 among 900 patients). External irradiation (x-rays or gamma rays) causes bone sarcomas, but only rarely (38). Even though radiation exposure is clearly a cause of bone sarcomas, the percentage attributable to it is modest—estimated as 2% in one study (32)—because the risk per rad is relatively small and large radiation exposures are infrequent in the general population.

Although there is some evidence that viruses may be able to cause osteosarcoma in rodents, there is no evidence of a direct association in humans at this time (34). There is anecdotal evidence for cancer proneness among the families of bone sarcoma cases, but the percentage with familial factors appears to be small (33, 39).

Metastatic Bone Tumors

Libson et al. (40) recently reviewed metastatic cancer of the hand and foot. They found that such metastases are rare; less than 100 foot metastases have been reported in the literature. About half the foot metastases have been to the tarsus and a quarter to the calcaneus. In comparing metastases to the hands versus feet, they found that colorectal, renal, and bladder cancers more often metastasized to the foot. However, in no case was the hand or foot the major metastatic site for these cancers. About 50% of the foot metastases were from colorectal, kidney, and lung cancers.

SOFT-TISSUE MALIGNANCIES
Kaposi's Sarcoma

From the limited data available, Kaposi's sarcoma (KS) appears to be the most common malignancy of the foot other than skin cancers. It is a vascular neoplasm, often appearing on the skin. In terms of the epidemiology of KS, there are two distinct types (41–43). The classic type of KS is a disease of middle-to-old age. It occurs at an age of 60–65 yr on average and is 10–15 times as frequent in men as in women. It is most prevalent in central and southern Africa, with lesser concentrations in the Mediterranean and Eastern Europe. Various reports from African countries indicate that 4–13% of malignancies seen there are KS (43), whereas before the 1980s only 0.06% of United States cancers were KS. KS in Africa is seen primarily among Blacks, and is very uncommon among Caucasians or Asians dwelling in the same regions (42). Classic KS tends to be a rather indolent disease, often has little immune deficiency associated with it, and is more common in persons with the HLA-DR5 antigen.

By way of contrast, the epidemic type of KS associated with HIV infection and AIDS occurs at much younger ages (mean age of 35–40). It is most prevalent in the United States, Europe, and Haiti, and is an aggressive disease. The immune deficiency associated with the condition is often progressive and profound. It is of interest that people undergoing immunosuppressive therapy (e.g., kidney transplant patients) are also highly susceptible to KS, with one study showing a 50-fold increase among them (43). As with the classic type, it is more common among males, who constitute the large majority of AIDS cases.

Of particular interest is the fact that classic KS tends to occur on the skin of the lower extremities, with nodules on the foot being a common presentation. For instance, in an American series predating the HIV epidemic, 88% of cases initially presented with lesions distal to the knee (43). Examples of KS foot lesions, and their diagnosis and treatment, are found in reports by Rynkiewicz (44) and Richter (45). Early lesions in AIDS-associated KS, on the other hand, tend to be on the head, neck, and trunk (41), although they occur on the lower extremities as well. While classic KS nearly always presents with skin lesions, the primary lesion in AIDS-associated KS is frequently internal.

The percentage of AIDS patients with KS is greater among homosexuals than among intravenous drug users, but the reason for this is not well-understood. The evidence to date suggests that KS is associated, not with HIV infection per se, but with one or more of the opportunistic infections (e.g., cytomegalovirus) that are common to AIDS patients (43). Several studies have also shown suggestive associations between KS and the use of inhalant nitrates (amyl/butyl nitrate) by homosexuals (42).

Fibrosarcoma

Fibrosarcoma, which arises from the fibroblast-forming cells, was historically considered the most commonly occurring soft-tissue sarcoma. However, with advances in pathology and diagnosis, many of the cancers once considered fibrosarcoma are now recognized as synovial sarcoma, leiomyosarcoma, liposarcoma, malignant histiocytic tumors, or rhabdomyosarcoma (46). In one large series, 60% of the fibrosarcoma cases were between 40 and 70 yr of age, but appreciable numbers also occurred at ages 20–39 (46). Although the lower extremity accounted for 60% of the fibrosarcomas, most of these were malignancies of the thigh, and only 3% of fibrosarcomas were of the ankle or foot. Slightly more males than females develop fibrosarcomas (if fibrosarcoma of the breast is excluded), in a ratio of about 1.5:1.

In a study of soft-tissue sarcomas in childhood, fibrosarcoma was the most common type (46% of the total) (47). It accounts for 0.3% of cancer deaths below 15 yr of age, and 0.6% at ages 15–19 (48). There are slightly higher rates of juvenile fibrosarcoma among males than females, while rates among whites and nonwhites are virtually identical. Although a breakdown by anatomic site is not available for juvenile fibrosarcomas, about 26% of total juvenile sarcomas occur in the lower extremities (47). Most of the sarcomas of the extremities occur after puberty, which is consistent with the observation that soft tissues of the limbs proliferate rapidly at puberty and are, thereby, at higher risk for malignant transformation (47).

In searching for etiologic clues for fibrosarcomas, one study (46) noted that 19% of the patients had a positive family history of cancer, including one family in which the mother and all three children had sarcomas of various types. It is unclear whether trauma plays a role in the etiology. While 21% in the aforementioned series reported trauma before symptoms were noticed, it seems likely that in many cases the trauma merely served to alert the patient or doctor to the presence of a tumor (46). No correlation between blood group and fibrosarcoma has been found (46). Fibrosarcomas are known to be induced by ionizing radiation. Of 20 soft-tissue sarcomas found in irradiated tissues in one study, 70% were fibrosarcomas (49). Radium-226 is also known to induce fibrosarcomas (50).

Rhabdomyosarcoma

Two American studies show that rhabdomyosarcomas constitute 19% of all sarcomas. About 60% of cases are males, and there is a suggestion that Blacks are less susceptible than Whites (51). The embryonal type of rhabdomyosarcoma occurring in childhood is seldom found on the foot. However, the alveolar type, which occurs in adolescence and young adulthood and accounts for 10–20% of all rhabdomyosarcomas, tends to be found on the lower extremities, as does the pleomorphic type found at ages 30–70 (52, 53). Under age 15, about 10% of rhabdomyosarcomas occur in the lower extremities (54), while about 10% of adult pleomorphic rhabdomyosarcomas occur below the knee and 35% on the thigh. Rhabdomyosarcomas account for 2–3% of cancer deaths before age 20. Little is known about the etiology of rhabdomyosarcoma, except that there appears to be a familial-genetic component involving multiple familial sarcomas or involving breast cancer with diverse other cancers occurring at early ages in relatives (54).

Synovial Sarcoma

Another type of sarcoma with a predilection for the foot and ankle is the synovial sarcoma. Synovial sarcoma comprises 5–10% of soft-tissue malignancies and has a yearly incidence of about 3/100,000 population (51). It is most prevalent between the ages of 15 and 40. Approximately 55% of synovial sarcomas occur in males, and about 20% of synovial sarcomas occur on the foot or ankle (55, 56). The limited evidence available does not suggest a predilection for any racial group (51). Deaths from synovial sarcoma occur over an extended period of time; in one study the 5-yr survival rate was 74%, but the 10-yr survival rate was only 35% (57).

Other Soft-tissue Malignancies

Clinical discussions of a number of other types of soft-tissue sarcomas of the foot are available in the literature, e.g., epithelioid sarcoma (58, 59), leiomyosarcoma (60), clear cell sarcoma (5, 61), liposarcoma (57), and neurofibrosarcoma (47, 57). Discussions of other vascular malignancies are also available, e.g., hemangiopericytoma (62) and hemangioendothelioma (63). However, because these tumors are rare and the literature on them contains little epidemiologic information, they will not be reviewed here. A good clinical and pathologic summary is the volume by Enzinger and Weiss (51).

MALIGNANT MELANOMA

The first medical report of malignant melanoma in the United States, in 1837, described a case of malignant melanoma (MM) of the toe (64). MM accounts for about 2% of total cancer incidence in the United States (65) and causes more deaths than any other skin disease. It is the second or third most common malignancy of the foot. According to the common classification, there are three main types of MM: superficial spreading melanoma, malignant lentigo melanoma (which is the most benign form), and nodular melanoma (the most malignant form). Another type, which accounts for 3–4% of MMs, is acral lentiginous melanoma which is of interest because it has a predilection for the soles, palms, and nailbeds.

Population Rates

Since one cause of MM is ultraviolet exposure, it occurs most frequently among light-skinned groups (i.e., those with little protective melanin) with high solar exposure. Examples of rates among Whites (per 100,000/yr), which show a geographical gradient with amount of insolation, are: Australia, 15, United States, 8, and United Kingdom, 2 (65). Rates among darker ethnic groups are lower: American Blacks, 0.6, Nigerian Blacks, 0.5, South African Blacks, 0.8, South African Indians, 0.1, South African Coloureds, 0.5, Japanese, 0.4, United States Hispanics, 1.9, United States Chinese, 1.1 (65, 66). The incidence of MM has been increasing dramatically among White populations over the past several decades. The incidence is doubling about every 15 yr and the mortality every 20 yr (67). The increase is probably due in part to increases in recreational sun exposure and concomitant decreases in the amount of protective clothing. However, the changing patterns of sun exposure are unlikely to have a major impact upon MM of the foot, since it receives relatively little sun exposure.

MM of the Foot

A large and representative series of MM cases in the United States indicated that 16% of MMs in males and 37% in females occur on the lower extremities (68), and two reports have indicated that 10–12% of MMs occur on the foot (69, 70). However, the percentage on the foot differs greatly by racial group. About 3–8% of MM cases among Caucasians occur on the foot (71, 72). Contrastingly, several studies of African Blacks indicate that 62–77% of MMs occur on the foot (73–75), while studies of American Blacks showed 32–65% on the foot (76, 77). Seventy-three percent of MMs among Indians (78), 37% among Asians (72), and 24% among Texan Hispanics (77) were found on the foot. Thus, it is clear that the foot is a prime site of MM among more darkly pigmented ethnic groups.

The distribution of MM on the foot is about 50% dorsal, 40% plantar, and 11% subungual (67). The age distribution of MM on the lower extremities is similar to that on other parts of the body: about 20% occur before age 35, 55% between ages 35 and 64, and the remaining 25% after age 65.

MM Prognosis

In terms of prognosis, MM of the foot has two distinctions. First, as mentioned above, the acral lentiginous type of MM has a predilection for the foot, especially the plantar surface.

This type tends to occur at older ages and has a high incidence in Blacks and Japanese (67). Acral lentiginous melanoma frequently shows aggressive behavior, similar to nodular melanoma. Second, subungual MM, which is found on the hallux in 90% of cases, is a very malignant form. In one recent study, 25% of subungual MMs presented with metastases, and the 5-yr survival rate was only 33% (79). Thus, on average, pedal MMs tend to be rather malignant in behavior. In a large prognostic study, it was found that after subtype and stage of MM were taken into account, MM of the foot more frequently showed recurrence than did MM on other parts of the body (80). This was especially true if the initial MM lesion was ≥3 mm thick.

MM Etiology

The etiology of MM is diverse. Sunlight exposure has already been mentioned; it is generally agreed that sunlight plays a role in MM etiology, based on geographic gradients by latitude and on the high susceptibility of light-skinned subgroups who have little melanin to protect them from ultraviolet exposure. However, within populations, there seems to be little consistency in findings regarding the effects of the amount and patterning (i.e., chronic exposure versus occasional heavy exposure) of ultraviolet exposure upon MM risk (81). Familial factors play a role in about 10% of MM cases, and first-degree relatives of cases have a relative risk of about 1.7 for contracting MM themselves (67). The higher rates of MM among females than males have generated hypotheses that hormone factors may play a role in MM pathogenesis, but there is no indication that endogenous hormones are implicated, while the results regarding exogenous hormones are mixed (82).

It has been hypothesized that the high incidence of pedal MM among Blacks in Africa was due to foot trauma from going barefoot. This hypothesis was weakened, however, when it was observed that the incidence of pedal MM among them did not change remarkably with urbanization and shoe wearing (73). A second hypothesis concerning MM of the foot in Blacks was that nevi on the feet gave rise to MM. Although it is difficult to establish retrospectively a causal connection between a nevus and a MM lesion, there is some credence to this hypothesis. Different studies of Blacks have found nevi in 23–83% of foot MMs (69,

73), and an Indian study found that 40–50% of MMs appeared to have arisen from nevi (78). Unfortunately, none of these studies had a group without MM to serve as a comparison group. Nevertheless, their findings parallel other indications of the role of precursor lesions: (a) Hutchinson's melanotic freckle is a precursor of malignant lentigo melanoma; (b) congenital nevi >20 cm in diameter carry a 5–20% risk of melanotic malignancy (67); and (c) recently, the medical community has become aware of the dysplastic nevus syndrome as a major risk factor for MM (83).

NONMELANOTIC SKIN CANCER
Basal Cell Carcinoma (Epithelioma)

Among Whites in the United States, basal carcinoma (BCC) of the skin is by far the most common type of cancer, having an age-adjusted rate of 247/100,000/yr among males and 150 among females (84). The cumulative incidence among Whites by age 80 is about 26% in males and 16% in females. Among Blacks, on the other hand, BCC is less common than squamous cell carcinoma and has a rate <2/100,000/yr. In terms of etiology, BCC is known to be induced by ionizing radiation as well as by ultraviolet radiation (85, 86). Lightness of complexion, Celtic ancestry (87), nevoid basal cell carcinoma syndrome (88), xeroderma pigmentosum (33), and albinism (89) are strong susceptibility factors for BCC.

Although BCCs tend to occur on parts of the body with greater sun exposure, especially the face and neck, they nevertheless are found on the foot as well. A study in Denmark found that 2–4% of BCCs occurred on the lower extremities. In the survey conducted by the American College of Foot Surgeons (1), BCC was the third most common cancer of the foot, with half as many cases of BCC as of squamous cell carcinoma. Fortunately, BCC is quite easy to treat and is probably the single most benign type of cancer, with metastases occurring in only about one in 10,000 cases (90, 91). Its most negative features are the high recurrence rate and the frequent appearance of multiple lesions (92).

Squamous Cell Carcinoma

Rates of cutaneous squamous cell carcinoma (SCC) among Caucasians are about 65/100,000/yr for males and 24 for females, which gives a cumulative incidence by age 80 of about 8% in males and 3% in females (84). It is thus 4–6 times less common among Caucasians than BCC. From the available data, it appears that SCC incidence rates for Blacks are about 2/100,000/yr (84), which is at least as great as their rate of BCC. A report from the Sudan indicated that, among Blacks, 63% of skin cancers were SCCs (75).

Among United States Whites only 3–4% of SCCs occur on the lower extremities, and 0.4% on the foot (84). The incidence of SCC of the lower extremities among Whites was about 1/100,000/yr for both sexes (84). The picture is very different among Blacks. In a series of SCCs among United States Blacks, a third of the lesions occurred below the knee (93), and a quarter were reported on the lower extremities in an African series (75).

The fatality rate of SCC cases is not very precisely defined because of inadequate studies, but the three best studies to date have reported case-fatality rates of 1.4%, 0.6%, and 0.7% (94–96). Special note should be taken that SCCs associated with trauma, scars, burns, tropical ulcers, or radiation burns tend to metastasize much more frequently than do other SCC lesions (97–99).

SCC shares its etiologic agents and host-susceptibility factors with BCC (see above). Additional etiologic agents for SCC are burns, scars, and exposure to arsenic, polycyclic aromatic hydrocarbons, and lubricating oils (100–103). Two groups at very high risk of SCC are those who have been treated by oral 8-methoxypsoralen and ultraviolet-A radiation (PUVA) therapy for psoriasis (104, 105) and those receiving immunosuppressive therapy (106, 107).

CONCLUSION

Information on the epidemiology of foot neoplasms is sparse. Much of what is available is based on case series that are flawed because one cannot tell how representative the series is or what the rates occurring in the general population might be. It is clear, however, that benign neoplasms occur with high frequency and that malignant neoplasms, though not very common, are among the most serious of foot problems.

In conducting this survey of the epidemiology of foot neoplasms, two areas for further research became evident. A large systematic survey of malignancies encountered in podiatric practice, much along the lines of the American College of Foot Surgeons' general survey of foot lesions (1), could provide valuable information on the distributions of foot malignancies by type, and within type by age, sex, race, stage, prognosis, etc. Second, a relatively untapped area for investigation lies in documenting the epidemiologic and clinical aspects of foot malignancies associated with the AIDS epidemic. Finally, the field is in need of the "alert clinician" who will detect new clues to the etiology or other characteristics of neoplasms encountered in clinical practice. Many valuable insights in epidemiology, and medicine generally, have arisen in this way.

ACKNOWLEDGMENT

The author was supported in part by Center Grants from the National Institute of Environmental Health Sciences (ES00260) and the National Cancer Institute (CA13343).

REFERENCES

1. Berlin S. A review of 2,720 lesions of the foot. J Am Podiatr Med Assoc 1980;70:318–324.
2. McCarthy D. Podiatric implications of intradermal nevi. J Am Podiatr Med Assoc 1986;76:433–438.
3. Forman W, Streigold H. Eccrine poroma: review of the literature and case reports. J Foot Surg 1982;21:278–280.
4. Kirby E, Shereff, Lewis M. Soft-tissue tumors and tumor-like lesions of the foot. An analysis of eighty-three cases. J Bone Joint Surg (Am) 1989;71:621–626.
5. Seale K, Lange T, Monson D, Hackbarth D. Soft tissue tumors of the foot and ankle. Foot Ankle 1988;9:19–27.
6. Tsoutsouris G. Vascular leiomyoma. J Foot Surg 1982;21:37–41.
7. Hosey T, Jacob T, Kallet H. Vascular leiomyoma. A case report and review of the literature. J Am Podiatr Assoc 1984;74:93–95.
8. Genakos J, Wallace J, Napoli A, Pontarelli A, Terris A. Angioleiomyoma. A case report and literature review. J Am Podiatr Med Assoc 1987;77:101–102.
9. Galinski A, Aune C. Benign leiomyoma of the foot: a case report. Clin Podiatr Med Surg 1988;5:359–362.
10. Tubiolo A, Jones R, Chalker D. Cavernous hemangioma of the plantar forefoot. A literature review and case report. J Am Podiatr Med Assoc 1986;76:164–167.
11. Newcott E. A solitary plasmacytoma in the foot. J Am Podiatr Med Assoc 1987;77:187–190.
12. Mehregan A. Superficial fibrous tumors in childhood. J Cutan Pathol 1981;8:321–334.
13. Beckett J, Jacobs A. Recurring digital fibrous tumors of childhood: a review. Pediatrics 1977;59:401–406.
14. Bruns B, Hunter J, Yngve D. Plantar fibromatosis. Orthopedics 1986;9:755–756.
15. Bauder T, DiPrimio R. Neurofibromatosis of the feet. A review and case report. J Am Podiatr Assoc 1980;70:372–374.
16. Cohen M. Neurofibromatosis manifested in the foot. Literature review and case presentation. J Am Podiatr Assoc 1984;74:143–146.
17. Gill P, Rosenthal L, Wagreich C. Tenosynovial fibroma. A case report. J Am Podiatr Med Assoc 1988;78:368–369.
18. Freedman D, Luzzi A, Pellegrino P, Picciotti J. Benign and malignant fibrohistiocytic tumors. J Am Podiatr Med Assoc 1987;77:544–548.
19. Goldberg S, Feit J, McCarthy D. The podiatric implications of giant cell tumors. J Foot Surg 1986;25:208–216.
20. Milack G. Giant cell tumor of tendon sheath origin. A case report and literature review. J Am Podiatr Assoc 1983;73:643–645.
21. Cristofaro R, Maher JO. Digital lipoma of the foot in a child. A case report. J Bone Joint Surg (Am) 1988;70:128–130.
22. Hamilos D, Cervetti R. Osteoid osteoma of the hallux. J Foot Surg 1987;26:397–399.
23. Bakst R, Janigian J. Osteoid osteoma of the talus. A case report and literature review. J Am Podiatr Med Assoc 1987;77:512–516.
24. Perlman M, Gold M, Schor A. Enchondroma: a case report and literature review. J Foot Surg 1988;27:556–560.
25. Persing J, Nachbar J, Vollmer D. Tarsal tunnel syndrome caused by sciatic nerve schwannoma. Ann Plast Surg 1988;20:252–255.
26. Hennessee M, Walter JH, Wallace G, Lemont H, Quintavalle PR. Benign schwannoma. Clinical and histopathologic findings. J Am Podiatr Med Assoc 1985;75:310–314.
27. Bailey S, Williams J, Baerg R. Intraosseous neurilemmoma of the foot. A case report. J Am Podiatr Med Assoc 1987;77:294–297.
28. Alexander I, Johnson K, Parr J. Morton's neuroma: a review of recent concepts. Orthopedics 1987;10:103–106.
29. Addante J, Peicott P, Wong K, Brooks D. Interdigital neuromas. Results of surgical excision of 152 neuromas. J Am Podiatr Med Assoc 1986;76:493–495.
30. Kenzora J. Symptomatic incisional neuromas on the dorsum of the foot. Foot Ankle 1984;5:2–15.
31. Mann R, Reynolds J. Interdigital neuroma—a critical clinical analysis. Foot Ankle 1983;3:238–243.
32. Price C, Jeffree G. Incidence of bone sarcoma in SW England, 1946–74, in relation to age, sex, tumour site and histology. Br J Cancer 1977;36:511–522.
33. Glass A, Fraumeni J. Epidemiology of bone cancer in children. J Natl Cancer Inst 1970;44:187–199.
34. Kelsey J. Epidemiology of muscoloskeletal disorders. In: Lilienfeld AM, ed. Monographs in epidemiology and biostatistics, vol 3. New York: Oxford University Press, 1982.
35. Rowland R, Stehney A, Lucas H. Dose-response relationships for radium-induced bone sarcomas. Health Phys 1983;44 (Suppl):15–31.

36. Evans R. The effect of skeletally deposited alpha-ray emitters in man. Br J Radiol 1966;39:881–895.
37. Mays C, Spiess H, Chmelevsky D, Kellerer A. Bone sarcoma cumulative tumor rates in patients injected with 224-Ra. In: Gossner W, Gerber G, Hagen U, Luz A, eds. The radiobiology of radium and thorotrast. Munich: Urban & Schwarzenberg, 1985;27–31.
38. Brady L. Radiation-induced sarcomas of bone. Skeletal Radiol 1979;4:72–78.
39. Mulvihill J, Gralnick H, Whang-Peng J, Leventhal B. Multiple childhood osteosarcomas in an American Indian family with erythroid macrocytosis and skeletal anomalies. Cancer 1977; 40:3115–3122.
40. Libson E, Bloom R, Husband J, Stoker D. Metastatic tumours of bones of the hand and foot. A comparative review and report of 43 additional cases. Skeletal Radiol 1987;16:387–392.
41. Safai B. Kaposi's sarcoma: an overview of classical and epidemic forms. In: Broder S, ed. AIDS: modern concepts and therapeutic challenges. New York: Marcel Dekker, 1987; 205–218.
42. Friedman-Kien A, Ostreicher R. Overview of classical and epidemic Kaposi's sarcoma. In: Friedman-Kien A, Laubenstein L, eds. AIDS: the epidemic of Kaposi's sarcoma and opportunistic infections. New York: Masson, 1984; 23–34.
43. Gelmann E, Broder S. Kaposi's sarcoma in the setting of the AIDS pandemic. In: Broder S, ed. AIDS: modern concepts and therapeutic challenges. New York: Marcel Dekker, 1987; 219–232.
44. Rynkiewicz R, Sanders L. Kaposi's sarcoma. A report of two cases and literature review. J Am Podiatr Med Assoc 1986;76:137–141.
45. Richter P, Black J. Kaposi's sarcoma of the foot: case report and review. Milit Med 1984; 76:137–141.
46. Pritchard D, Soule E, Taylor W, Ivins J. Fibrosarcoma—a clinicopathologic and statistical study of 199 tumors of the soft tissues of the extremities and trunk. Cancer 1974;33:888–897.
47. Chabalko J, Creagan E, Fraumeni J. Epidemiology of selected sarcomas in children. J Natl Cancer Inst 1974;53:675–679.
48. Miller R. Fifty-two forms of childhood cancer: United States mortality experience, 1960–1966. J Pediatr 1969;75:685–689.
49. Kim J, Chu F, Woodard H, Melamed M, Huvos A, Cantin J. Radiation-induced soft-tissue and bone sarcoma. Radiology 1978;129:501–508.
50. Schlenker R, Keane A, Unnit K. Comparison of radium-induced and natural bone sarcomas by histological type, subject age and site of occurrence. In: Taylor D, Mays C, Gerber G, Thomas R, eds. Report 21, London: British Institute of Radiology, 1989;55–63.
51. Enzinger F, Weiss S. Soft tissue tumors. St. Louis: Mosby, 1983.
52. Miller RW, Dalager NA. Fatal rhabdomyosarcoma among children in the United States, 1960–69. Cancer. 1974;34:1897–1900.
53. Wu K. Rhabdomyosarcoma of the foot. J Foot Surg 1988;27:166–171.
54. Li F, Fraumeni J. Rhabdomyosarcoma in children: epidemiologic study and identification of a familial cancer syndrome. J Natl Cancer Inst 1969;43:1365–1373.
55. Mackenzie D. Synovial sarcoma: a review of 58 cases. Cancer 1966;19:169–180.
56. Cadman N, Soule E, Kelly P. Synovial sarcoma: an analysis of 134 tumors. Cancer 1965;18: 613–627.
57. Owens J, Shiu M, Smith R, Hajdu S. Soft tissue sarcomas of the hand and foot. Cancer 1985; 55:2010–2018.
58. Wu K. Epithelioid sarcoma of the foot. J Foot Surg 1988;27:472–477.
59. Fuselier C, Cachia V, Wong C, Rawlinson D, Myers W, Baker S, et al. Selected soft tissue malignancies of the foot: an in-depth study with case reports. J Foot Surg 1985;24:162–204.
60. Bernardone J, Scarlet J. Leiomyosarcoma: a case report and literature review. J Am Podiatr Med Assoc 1988;78:183–186.
61. Wu K. Clear cell sarcoma of the foot. J Foot Surg 1988;27:569–575.
62. Enzinger F, Smith B. Hemangiopericytoma: an analysis of 106 cases. Hum Pathol 1976;7: 61–82.
63. Chabalko J, Fraumeni J. Blood-vessel neoplasms in children: epidemiologic aspects. Med Pediat Oncol 1975;1:135–141.
64. Marmelzat W. The first case of malignant melanoma formally reported in America (1837) (case of melanosis by Issac Parrish, M.D.). J Dermatol Surg Oncol 1977;3:30–31.
65. Muir C, Waterhouse J, Mack T, Powell J, Whelan S. Cancer incidence in five continents, vol V, IARC Pub No 88. 1987;Lyon: International Agency for Research on Cancer.
66. Rippey J, Rippey E. Epidemiology of malignant melanoma of the skin in South Africa. S Afr Med J 1984;65:595–598.
67. Hutchinson B. Malignant melanoma in the lower extremity. A comprehensive overview. Clin Podiatr Med Surg 1986;3:533–550.
68. Axtell A, Cutler S, Myers M. Melanoma of skin. In: End results in cancer, NIH document 73-272. Washington, DC: United States Department of Health, Education and Welfare, 1972;148–152.
69. Haverkamp M, Rodman O. Malignant melanoma of the foot in black patients: a case report and literature survey. J Natl Med Assoc 1979;71:353–356.
70. Caputo W, Steinhart A. Malignant melanoma. Case study and review of the literature. J Am Podiatr Med Assoc 1988;78:29–33.
71. Iversen O, Larsen T, Grude T, Magnus K. Histological classification of malignant melanoma in relation to prognosis and cytogenesis. Excerpta Medica 1976;375:260–273.
72. Hinds M. Anatomic distribution of malignant melanoma of the skin among non-Caucasians in Hawaii. Br J Cancer 1979;40:497–499.
73. Lewis M. Malignant melanoma in Uganda. (The relationship between pigmentation and

malignant melanoma on the soles of the feet). Br J Cancer 1967;21:483–495.

74. Giraud R, Rippey E, Rippey J. Malignant melanoma of the skin in black Africans. S Afr Med J 1975;49:665–668.

75. Malik M, Hidaytalla A, Daoud E, El Hassan A. Superficial cancer in the Sudan. A study of 1225 primary malignant superficial tumours. Br J Cancer 1974;30:355–364.

76. Reintgen D, McCarty KM Jr, Cox E, Seigler H. Malignant melanoma in black American and white American populations. A comparative review. J Am Med Assoc 1982;248:1856–1859.

77. MacDonald E. Malignant melanoma among Negroes and Latin Americans in Texas. In: Gordon M, ed. Pigment cell biology: proceedings of the 4th Conference on the Biology of Normal and Atypical Pigment Cell Growth. New York: Academic Press, 1959;171–180.

78. Mulay D. Skin cancer in India. Natl Cancer Inst Monogr 1963;10:215–223.

79. Spinner S, Holberg S, Brook S. Malignant melanoma and podiatry—a review of the literature. J Foot Surg 1982;21:194–198.

80. Day CL Jr, Sober A, Kopf A, Lew R, Mihm M, Golomb F. A prognostic model for clinical stage I melanoma of the lower extremity. Location on foot as independent risk factor for recurrent disease. Surgery 1981;195:44–49.

81. Dubin N, Moseson M, Pasternack B. Sun exposure and malignant melanoma among susceptible individuals. Environ Health Perspect 1989;81:139–151.

82. Holman C, Armstrong B, Heenan P. Cutaneous malignant melanoma in women: exogenous sex hormones and reproductive factors. Br J Cancer 1984;50:673–680.

83. Greene M, Clark W, Tucker M, Elder D, Kraemer K, Guerry D, Witmer W, Thompson J, Matozzo I, Fraser M. Acquired precursors of cutaneous malignant melanoma. The familial dysplastic nevus syndrome. N Engl J Med 1985;312:91–97.

84. Scotto J, Fears T, Fraumeni J. Incidence of nonmelanoma skin cancer in the United States, NIH Publ. No. 83-2433. Washington, DC: United States Department of Health and Human Services, 1983. 113 p.

85. Shore R, Albert R, Reed M, Harley N, Pasternack B. Skin cancer incidence among children irradiated for ringworm of the scalp. Radiat Res 1984;100:192–204.

86. Van Daal W, Goslings B, Hermans J, Rutter D, Sepmeyer C, Vink M, Van Vloten W, Thomas P. Radiation-induced head and neck tumours: is the skin as sensitive as the thyroid gland? Eur J Cancer Clin Oncol 1983;19:1081–1086.

87. O'Beirn S, Judge P, Urbach F, MacCon C, Martin F. Skin cancer in County Galway, Ireland. Proc Natl Cancer Conf 1970;6:489–500.

88. Gorlin R. Nevoid basal-cell carcinoma syndrome. Medicine 1987;66:98–113.

89. Higginson J, Oettle A. Cancer incidence in the Bantu and "Cape Colored" races of South Africa: report of a cancer survey in the Transvaal (1953–55). J Natl Cancer Inst 1960;24:589–671.

90. Weedon D, Wall D. Metastatic basal cell carcinoma. Med J Aust 1975;2:177–179.

91. Kopf A. Computer analysis of 3531 basal-cell carcinomas of the skin. J Dermatol 1979;6:267–281.

92. Macdonald E. Some epidemiologic factors of skin cancer. J Am Med Wom Assoc 1967;22:235–240.

93. Fleming I, Barnawell J, Burlison P, Rankin J. Skin cancer in black patients. Cancer 1975;35:600–605.

94. Epstein E, Epstein N, Bragg K, Linden G. Metastases from squamous cell carcinomas of the skin. Arch Dermatol 1968;97:245–251.

95. Dunn J, Levin E, Linden G, Harzfeld L. Skin cancer as a cause of death. Calif Med 1965;102:361–363.

96. Giles G, Marks R, Foley P. Incidence of nonmelanocytic skin cancer treated in Australia. Br Med J 1988;296:13–17.

97. Ames F, Hickey R. Squamous cell carcinoma of the skin of the extremities. Intl Adv Surg Oncol 1980;3:179–199.

98. Conway H, Hugo N. Radiation dermatitis and malignancy. Plast Reconstruct Surg 1966;38:255–268.

99. Grier W. Squamous cell carcinoma of the body and extremities. In: Andrade R, Gumport S, Popkin G, Rees T, eds. Cancer of the skin, biology-diagnosis-management, vol I. Philadelphia: Saunders, 1976;916–932.

100. Oettle A. Skin cancer in Africa. Natl Cancer Inst Monogr 1963;10:197–214.

101. Isaacson C. Cancer of the skin in urban blacks of South Africa. Br J Dermatol 1979;100:347–350.

102. Everall J, Dowd P. Influence of environmental factors excluding ultraviolet radiation on the incidence of skin cancer. Bull Cancer (Paris) 1978;3:241–248.

103. Bourguet C, Checkoway H, Hulka B. A case-control study of skin cancer in the tire and rubber manufacturing industry. Am J Ind Med 1987;11:461–473.

104. Stern R, Laird N, Melski J, Parrish J, Fitzpatrick T, Bleich H. Cutaneous squamous-cell carcinoma in patients treated with PUVA. N Engl J Med 1984;310:1156–1161.

105. Stern R, Lange R. Non-melanoma skin cancer occurring in patients treated with PUVA five to ten years after first treatment. J Invest Dermatol 1988;91:120–124.

106. Walder B, Robertson M, Jeremy D. Skin cancer and immunosuppression. Lancet 1971;2:1282–1283.

107. Hoxtell E, Mandel J, Murray S, Schuman L, Goltz R. Incidence of skin carcinoma after renal transplantation. Arch Dermatol 1977;113:436–438.

3

Psychologic Aspects of Cancer

—Stephen A. Appelbaum

THE DOCTOR-PATIENT INTERACTION

Among the most moving, terrifying, and profound of life's experiences, for both patient and physician, is the diagnosis of cancer. The patient, for whom this is almost always a one-time event, reacts overtly and intensely (or, at least, does so after the numbness of the initial shock). The physician, with experience and practice, is thought to be insulated emotionally. He or she may not show, or even experience consciously, much emotion. But the physician, like everyone else, has at his or her core existential anxiety, or fear of death. Along with compassion, the physician may feel impotence at his or her inability to answer a patient's prayers, and to discharge perfectly the chosen duty of healer. He or she may also sense the dreary, draining process of treatments and side effects and the psychologic upheavals of the patient and the patient's relatives and friends. These are regular consequences of the cancer drama.

Such feelings take their tolls, even if unconsciously. Among these tolls can be a drop in efficiency of practice and in judgment, unwonted clumsiness of participation in the interpersonal aspects of the doctor-patient relationship, and emotional withdrawal from the patient (who now exacerbates the physician's difficulties). Conversely, some physicians may become grandiose in their self-expectations, claiming more than they can deliver; they may uncritically scratch around in esoterica, alternatives, or unproved methods for the magic that will not only cure the patient, but help the physician feel better about himself.

Among the lapses of judgment brought about by the stress of a cancer diagnosis is the most obvious—ignoring the question of whether the initial diagnosis is correct. Both patient and physician should know better than to believe blindly that diagnoses are 100% accurate. Yet they often behave as if that were true. The patient may have heard or read countless times about the value, if not necessity, of getting a second opinion, yet forgets that admonition. This lapse may be out of fear of hearing yet another terrifying opinion, or of offending the physician on whom life now literally seems to depend. On the physician's part, there may be an understandable reluctance to be contradicted by a colleague, of losing the image of omnipotence even though he or she knows the extent, for example, of laboratory errors, as well as differences of opinion among honorable and talented professionals. Not only second opinions, but the scheduling of ancillary, confirming, and staging examinations also may be influenced by the emotional reactions swirling through the cancer atmosphere. Such examinations may be overprescribed out of an anxious need on the part of the physician to be sure of or to disconfirm the awful reality, or conversely, the physician may neglect to prescribe examinations because of an unwillingness to confront his or her own fallibility or to question his or her sense of wholeness and competence.

Besides the question of the truth or falseness of diagnostic findings, there is the question of the communication of findings: technical ones to other professionals, and nontechnical ones to patients and relatives. Laboratory reports and informal conversations are not simply "reports," but implicit calls for action. The doctor and patient make important, sometimes life-and-death, decisions, according to a relative handful of words chosen to be put on a piece of paper or enunciated verbally. Yet as anyone attuned to the vagaries of language will attest, words may be treacherous things. They connote and denote, by their presence and absence. They may mean different things to different people. Yet well or poorly chosen, they bear an awesome responsibility. Take, for example, the diagnosis of cancer of the prostate as derived from a biopsy. This is a notoriously difficult judgment for a pathologist. Nonetheless, pathologists are trained to judge one way or another, no matter how ambiguous the evidence; it becomes a matter of professional honor. But reality does not necessarily conform to the requirement of certainty. If the reality is that a diagnosis is equivocal, additional pathology opinions outside the institution are required, in an atmosphere of scrutiny and exploration, rather than the pseudo-decisiveness dictated by rigid training and the emotional need to conform to it. Reality is savaged by stark, cold, "mildly differentiated carcinoma of the prostate" not followed by information reflecting the true picture of "judgment call" or "borderline decision," the scientific status of cell grading, if any, used, and the differences of opinion about these. Just a few words could make the difference between a person staggering through life with iatrogenic side effects of incorrect diagnosis, of radiation, and/or of chemotherapy, and a person who, on the basis of further study, is declared not to need treatment. The irony is staggering. A few different words in a phone call or hallway conversation from the pathologist to the attending physician could make the difference. But such communications may or may not be made. They are subject to the idiosyncrasies of individuals, how comfortable they are on the phone or in face-to-face conversation, how the participants get along, how busy they are, and on the psychologic dynamics of each department and discipline.

Empathy is much talked about, but its implications are often misunderstood. Basically, it refers to the ability to put one's self in the place of another in order to better understand and appreciate the other's experience and point of view. When dealing with sick people, this means being temporarily, and for the purposes of empathy, "sick." When giving a diagnosis of cancer, it means to temporarily and for the purposes of empathy, receive the diagnosis of cancer. Some physicians go into medicine in part to deal with their anxiety about becoming ill and confronting mortality. As physicians, they can be active and in control, rather than passive victims of inexorable events. To be empathic would undo the very defenses against anxiety on which they depend, to get into the situation they have designed themselves to

flee. How physicians handle this challenge influences their decisions as to how, where, when, and if to give their patients the diagnosis.

The "if" used to be a crucial, much debated, question. In Japan, patients still are ordinarily not told their cancer diagnoses. But, in the United States, the practice now is usually to do so. But accepted practice only helps somewhat with the underlying fears and discomforts that in the past usually dictated the decision not to tell (often rationalized as sparing the patient). In those underlying fears and discomforts, lay a minefield of possible errors. To defuse these, there are some guidelines. Do not give the diagnosis over the telephone. Do not swamp the patient with too much information about the next steps at a time when the patient needs to absorb the new reality and can hear only a limited amount of other information. Extend the possibility of hope, and indicate that there are things to do, if, indeed, there are. Have supportive people present or available: family members; a nurse; ideally, a recovered patient. Remember, cancer is a disease of patient, family, and friends. These are exemplary guidelines, but for full exploitation, they require that the physician more than dutifully follow them— that could be arranged by an administrative assistant or a robot. Full exploitation of these guidelines requires the interaction of one person with another. As Norman Cousins expressed it in *The Healing Heart* (1), it is not the distance from the hospital door to the bed that matters; it is the distance between the eyes of the physician and the eyes of the patient. At the time of diagnosis, as never before, the patient requires from the physician empathy, the participation of the physician in the inner experience of the patient, the anticipation of what the patient may be experiencing, the wisdom and patience to listen for cues and confirmation of that experience, and the projection of concern, compassion, and willingness (not just ability) to help and go the route.

Closely allied to diagnosis is prognosis; one implies the other. In the minds of many, the air of certainty surrounding things scientific suggests the future can be precisely predicted. Predictions are, of course, possible and supportable by general statistics in addition to the physician's personal experience. Yet, to the single patient who conceivably is the exception to the rule, his or her chances turn out to be 100%. Thus, never make a prediction that implies absolute certainty. "I give you six months to live," is inaccurate unless there is no, absolutely no, chance the patient will live a longer or shorter time, which is an empirical impossibility. The tone and formulation of such declamations are personally offensive, implying not a modest conveying of statistically based information, but a personal declaration of control over disease, the future, and fate. Better is "We may not be able to control the cancer beyond a half year or so, and you might want to make plans on that basis, but one can never be entirely sure about these things." Given that, the patient, like a soldier going into battle, can fortify himself with the feeling that he will be the exception. This maximizes whatever contribution hope makes for cure or comfort.

In many cancer situations, the physician is faced with a wrenching and complex choice between "doing everything" or "doing nothing." Doing everything has a seductive simplicity and conforms to the ingrained medical responsibility to save lives. Moreover, it protects against the real or fancied looming threat of malpractice suits. Yet, how humane is it to subject patients to the disfiguring, debilitating, painful, humiliating, or expensive accompaniments to doing every thing? Some patients might choose a shorter length of life to a dreadful quality of slightly prolonged, expensive, mutilated life. It is a decision hemmed in by legal, moral, personally idiosyncratic, and ethical considerations. These are best dealt with through awareness, frankness, and shared information with the patient and perhaps with colleagues. The worst way of dealing with it is through a mindless, impersonally bureaucratic, pseudo-certainty that excludes the reality and perspective of the patient.

What has been described here—compassion, sensitivity, empathy, and psychologic understanding of the patient that is often based on physician self-understanding and psychologic self-ease—can be subsumed under "bedside manner." That ancient, but apt, phrase is a reflection of what through the years has been known, subliminally or in conscious awareness: the physician is part of an ancient tradition of healing. That tradition began probably with the dawn of humanity and is embodied in a long line of witch doctors, shamans, and medicine men, eventually blooming into scientific medicine only a couple of hundred years ago. Indeed, even now, worldwide, more people are treated by nonscientific medical systems than by Western medicine. Such treatments include procedures as diverse as chanting, dancing, meditation, acupuncture, direct suggestion, and eating animal entrails. People are "healed" by all these means. Even healing by Western medicine is, in some instances, surpassed by placebos, inert substances that are 30–75% more effective than some medicines and capable even of producing side effects. Obviously, healing consists of a good deal more than the simple administration of scientifically tested interventions in a one-to-one correspondence with cure.

That healing can come about through wildly diverse means suggests that all methods of healing have some factor or factors in common. One such factor is the healing relationship, i.e., a person designated a patient with a disease enters into a contract with a person (or institution) designated as able to "make the patient better" by way of interventions sanctioned by the culture or subculture as ways of healing.

In pursuit of the essence of healing, I tested with psychologic tests (the Rorschach inkblots and Thematic Apperception Test cards) over 20 people who are nationally famous, in their circles, as laying-on-of-hands healers. Somewhat to my surprise, a rather homogeneous pattern emerged from the tests and my interviews. Included in this pattern were exhibitionism, grandiosity, and omnipotence (though usually cloaked with humility). In that sense, the laying-on-of-hands healers share with physicians, in conventional contemporary society, an exalted, highly visible position, and the attributes of being all-knowing and all-powerful.

Included also in the typical pattern of the healer was a psychologic commitment to the so-called oral stage of Freudian psychosexual development. This stage is prominent in approximately the first year of life, when the mother is all-powerful, and indeed can "make it better"; when cradling, touch, and soothing verbal expressions reassure the child of survival. Monkeys who fail to receive such reassurances prove to be unable to copulate in later life, and humans who are so deprived are subject to that and a wide range of psychologic and physical disabilities. It is plausible to assume that healing success in later life stems from proffering to patients, and summoning from them, the original healing paradigm based on a loving interaction between mother and child.

The strength of that paradigm and the ease with which it can be summoned may explain the perennial mystery of how it is that people vary so much in their responses to healing. That variability is inherent in the patient, the physician, and the match between them with regard to the strength and availability of the healing paradigm built into them early in life. We encounter here a paradox: those drawn to the physical sciences on which Western medicine largely depends, tend as a rule to be relatively distant from the mothering, loving, healing paradigm just described. They tend to be devoted more to facts than feelings, separateness more than symbiosis, numbers more than language, toughness more than tenderness. If they had wanted to go into the soft sciences that are more consonant with tender skills and values, they would have become psychologists, ministers, or English professors. And yet, with increasing peremptoriness, physicians are enjoined to be, in effect, psychologists. The paradox embodies a certain unfairness.

That "love equals healing" equation has implications for the selection and training of physician-lover-healers. It is generally accepted among psychotherapists that some disciplined self-examination contributes greatly to all psychologic interventions. These requirements and points of view are based on the idea that knowing and dealing with one's self helps one to know and deal with others. For psychologic sensitivity to be made a genuine part of medical interactions with its benefits maximized, rather than just being paid lip service, it follows that physicians, too, be vouchsafed the opportunity for systematic self-understanding. In the best of all possible worlds, such opportunities would be underwritten by the interested parties, namely the population served by physicians, the public, through government or other institutionalized auspices. In the less than perfect real world of expense and often limited number of trainers and psychotherapists, the problem could be dealt with, at least in part, by requiring medical students to participate in unstructured groups, for training and/or therapy. (In such groups, the line between the two is often hazy.) In England, particularly, graduate physicians have participated voluntarily in such groups for personal enhancement as well as to improve their practice with patients, with apparently salubrious results. Ultimately, what can be done about

making medical interventions more efficient by maximizing their psychologic aspects can only be known through recognizing the challenge to do so and meeting that challenge. All is certainly lost if physicians choose to withdraw behind numbers, facts, and emotional distance—to be victims of stunted "love."

PSYCHOLOGIC FACTORS IN THE ETIOLOGY AND COURSE OF CANCER

Many people now pay lip service to the idea of body-mind unity: the organism reacts as a whole, with bodily events having psychologic repercussions, and psychologic events having physiologic ones. However, many people find it extremely difficult to fully grasp that idea, and to behave accordingly. Most of us are still in thrall to the split between mind and body convincingly set forth by Descartes. That dualism stemmed from his religious need to separate what he took to be the unclean, unholy body from the sublime, holy soul or mind. It appealed to many others on that basis; it could also easily be understood that way. After all, one could touch, measure, and work concretely with the body, while the mind or soul seemed ineffable, indeed, of a different nature or substance. The industrial revolution spawned ways of working mechanically with the body, which led with dizzying rapidity to dramatic increases in knowledge about the body. The culture moved toward a faith that all problems could be solved technologically, a faith dramatically supported by the successes of modern medicine over the last 150 years.

During that same period, Freud grappled with the mind-body problem and solved it in ways that both decreased and increased the mind and body split. Trained as a physical and biologic scientist, yet having made startling discoveries about the mind, he first tried to unite the two ideas, and perhaps sides of himself, by conceiving of the mind in physical and neurologic terms, as in his tellingly named *Project for a Scientific Psychology* (2). But the core of his discoveries stubbornly refused to allow any such dismissal: ideas and feelings were regularly shown to influence bodily events. Freud settled for psychophysical parallelism. He never gave up his prediction that physicochemical events would one day be shown to underlie psychologic ones. But that was no longer his task. He thenceforth devoted his life to explorations of the psychologic. The popularity of his discoveries concretized the psychologic approach, giving rise to a high degree of professionalization of psychiatry and psychology. Thus, the mind-body split was carried forth by political, administrative, and economic forces. At the same time, Freudian practices increasingly revealed the falseness of that split. Those revelations resulted in "psychosomatic" medicine, the clumsy locution itself revealing the alien and uneasy juxtaposition of separateness. But, at least, the idea of unity was set forth, however gingerly.

In the last 25 years, overcoming the mind-body split has taken an enormous step forward with the rise of holistic medicine. That locution is apposite: the organism is a whole. It is separated into parts for practical reasons, not conceptual ones. Every psychologic event has a physical analogue, every physical event a psychologic one. Now, one can wonder how the perfectly obvious manifestations of that idea could have been overlooked. For example, one feels embarrassed, and the skin reddens; a mental image results in an erect penis or secretions from the vagina. Language reflects psychosomatic wisdom: he died of a broken heart, she worked or worried herself to death. Suddenly we notice that certain types of personalities are disposed to certain types of diseases, e.g., Type A personalities tend to experience cardiovascular problems, depressed patients tend toward cancer. Except for the influence of the mind-body split, we might have taken more seriously Galen's ancient observation of the connection between melancholia and breast cancer or Cannon's finding that emotions could stimulate the spleen to increase red blood cells (3).

I might have taken more seriously the implications of the ability of a psychologist to predict from the Rorschach inkblots whether a patient had a slow or fast-growing tumor (4). As it was, I was as incredulous as most people were when I encountered the idea that cancer could be brought about, and its course influenced, by psychologic factors. This occurred in the mid-1970s in the course of my experiences and studies of new therapies of the counterculture as reported in *Out in Inner Space: A Psychoanalyst Explores the New Therapies* (5). Alternative therapies are part of an alternative way of life which includes alternative views and practices of medicine.

The proximal cause of my interest in the relationship between psychology and cancer came about when a patient of mine developed cancer in the midst of two suicide attempts. I then remembered the story of a patient who had allegedly overcome cancer by means of psychologic treatment according to procedures developed and publicized by Carl Simonton, a radiologist, and Stephanie Simonton, a psychologist (6). Their ideas, partly because of their well-publicized work, have become virtually old-hat a mere 15 years later. Their basic position is that, by way of the immune system, stress allows for the growth of cancer cells, while the relative absence of stress, at least certain kinds, provides protection against cancer or helps the body deal with it. Treatment is in two parts. First is a meditation-visualization procedure. The alleged success of visualization in overcoming disease stems from the ancient Yogic belief that one creates reality with one's mind. Meditation is now scientifically documented as a means of changing such bodily functions as blood pressure and basal metabolism in preferred ways (7). It is plausible that thus quieting the system allows the body greater freedom to fight disease.

The second part of the Simonton approach is based on the belief that cancer is often a last-ditch despairing effort to solve life's problems and, thus, an expression of loss of alternatives, or of being trapped and hopeless. (These words are also used to describe the context of suicide.) To the extent that psychotherapy makes other solutions possible, it should work against the hopelessness that predisposes to cancer. In their work with cancer patients, the Simontons, not surprisingly to psychotherapists or other careful observers of the human condition, found seemingly insoluble problems. They reasoned backwards that these were implicated in the cancer. What was missing, of course, was a control group or a base rate such that one would know how many people with similar dilemmas did not develop cancer or any other physical manifestation.

Nonetheless, where there is smoke there may well be fire. Some more smoke, if not fire, is provided by an old literature—and a rapidly burgeoning new one gathered under the term "psychoneuroimmunology." Some samples from the old literature: LeShan (8) notes that cancer patients tend to have difficult early relationships, find substitutes for them in later life, then lose the substitutes. Rorschach test findings from Thomas' 30-yr longitudinal study of medical students (9) reveals that the psychologically best-adjusted subjects had the lowest proportion of cancer, only 3%, while the two least well-adjusted groups had 12 and 13% occurrences. Schmale and Iker (10) interviewed subjects before biopsies for cervical cancer, and, on the basis of subjects' feelings of hopelessness, were able to predict which ones would have positive biopsies. Personality characteristics have been related to particular kinds of cancers; breast cancer with sex-role difficulty (11), lung cancer with poor outlets for discharge of emotions (12), leukemia and lymphoma with grief over the loss of a mother (13), and cervical cancer with childhood deprivation (14). The association of cancer with grieving is supported by the finding that people who have lost a significant love object are at increased risk for cancer for 1–2 yr afterward. In support of this observation, men whose wives had died of breast cancer had poorer lymphocyte proliferation than before their wives' deaths (15).

Psychoneuroimmunologists are concerned with the effect of mental attitudes on the body's resistance to disease by way of mind, brain, and immune system (16). More specifically, they deal with the transmission of information by way of the limbic-hypothalamic modulation of the autonomic, endocrine, immune, and neuropeptide systems. In the few years since it became conceptualized and studied, psychoneuroimmunology has developed a sizeable literature. Study after study demonstrate the effects on the body of emotional states: on blood pressure, immunoglobin A, catecholamine surges, virus-related diseases, and tumor development, among others. Further studies delineate the factors that bring about the more global effects, for example, distress and loneliness are related to reduced levels of γ-interferon, lessened numbers and responsiveness of NK cells and T lymphocytes, and increased antibody titers to latent viruses. This latest spate of research decisively moves the hypothesis from the province of dreamers, (or at least those who fail adequately to test their dreams) to the arena of hard science.

For most people, nothing is more persuasive than their own experiences. For that reason I saw in psychotherapy, and tested with psychologic tests, 24 cancer patients (17). This was hardly an outcome study because of, among other reasons, a great variability in the numbers of times patients were seen, widely diverse kinds of cancer and points in its course,

no control group or base rate, and one therapist who may or may not be representative. For what it is worth, any rosy expectations (that I, at least secretly, harbored) that patients would be cured were unsupported. That is not to say the psychotherapy had no effect in prolonging length or quality of life. The patients said that it did, which, of course, in turn is difficult to evaluate.

Apart from outcome, however, my experiences support a major, reiterated hypothesis about the cancer-disposed and maintaining state of mind: cancer patients have considerable difficulty acknowledging, expressing, and contending with aggression, particularly as it arises within themselves. That is hardly an unusual state of affairs, among psychiatric patients or nonpsychiatric citizens. But these cancer patients had the difficulty to an unusual degree. With 14 of the 24, I am satisfied that their fear of the fantasized repercussions of their anger resulted in submissiveness, excessive sweetness, hyperconcern for the needs of others, and difficulties realizing and asserting their rights, as well as others of the behaviors that characteristically stem from fear that other people, and often themselves, will know of their anger. As an example, when instructed to visualize, during meditation, cancer cells being attacked and destroyed, a patient instead had her white cells "washing over" the cancer cells. I called attention to her use of a soothing rather than an attacking image. At her next session, she reported that she had visualized the white corpuscles using knives to cut and dice the cancer cells. When I asked her to draw the image that she had visualized, the knives were absent. "I just left the knives off," she lamely explained. Another patient described destroying his cancer cells by way of poisoning, but inadvertently substituted "fertilization," for "poisoning."

The hypothesis of inhibited aggression being related to cancer has for years been implicitly confirmed by the oft-repeated observation by hospital personnel: the difficult, contentious, fighting cancer patients do better physically than the submissive, compliant, "good" patients. As measured by extensor and flexor drawings of human figures, those who directed anger outward were disposed toward hypertension, while those who directed it inward were disposed toward cancer (18).

Rorschach inkblots, among many other

things, yield a measure of the extent to which people discharge tension by way of ideas or affect. I gave the test to nine of the cancer patients, and all showed a marked propensity to discharge through affect rather than through ideas. Such discharge could be expressed in labile, tempestuous moods, in impulsive large-muscle actions—or somatization. Thus, one can speculate that these cancer patients, inhibited in discharging through thought, feelings, or overt behavior, "took it out" on their bodies. Insight-oriented psychotherapy, by way of lifting repressions, could make ideas more available as a means of discharge and processing. Plausibly, this would lessen the propensity to respond somatically, and, thus, help prevent or ameliorate cancer.

One has to save good ideas from people. To establish a link between ideas and feelings and cancer should not dispose us toward the belief that all disease comes about and can be cured through psychologic means as is sometimes implied, consciously or unconsciously, but some of the adherents of the psychologic point of view. One accounts far better for the data, not only on the cancer-personality link, but on inheritance, smoking, air pollution, exercise, and diet links, through thinking in terms of multifactors rather than in terms of simple cause and effect or single-cause models. A reasonable model is that cancer is caused by or related to numerous interacting factors which are in ratios to one another. That is, the more of one that is present, the less of another is needed to reach the critical point. For example, an otherwise healthy person who has practiced a generally salubrious style of life would require considerable psychologic stress to develop cancer, and vice versa.

There is now developing an understandable, in some ways needed, backlash against the holistic point of view. Some physicians argue that patients come to them for the expertise in which they are trained and expected to be proficient. They deride exchanging medical expertise for psychology or for bedside manner. They have a point, but then so does everybody involved. That is the point. The reality of the whole organism does not yield to conventions of training, titles, and styles of practice. The challenge is to integrate all aspects of the cancer reality, in proportion appropriate to each particular situation. A daunting task? Certainly. But one which is, in principle, accomplishable—beginning with awareness.

REFERENCES

1. Cousins N. The healing heart. New York: Avon Books, 1983:115.
2. Freud S. Project for a scientific psychology. In: Standard Edition I. London: Hogarth, 1966: 283–344.
3. Cannon WB. The emergency function of the adrenal medulla in pain and the major emotions. J Physiol 1926;33:356–372.
4. Klopfer B. Psychological variables in human cancer. J Projective Techniques 1957;21:331–340.
5. Appelbaum SA. Out in inner space—a psychoanalyst explores the new therapies. New York: Doubleday/Anchor, 1979.
6. Simonton C, Simonton SM, Creighton J. Getting well again. Los Angeles: Jeremy Tarcher, Inc, 1978.
7. Benson H. The relaxation response. New York: William Morrow, 1975.
8. LeShan L. An emotional life-history pattern associated with neoplastic disease. Ann N Y Acad Sci 1966;125:780–793.
9. Graves PL, Mead LA, Pearson TA. The Rorschach interaction scale as a potential predictor of cancer. Psychosomatic Med 1986;48:544–563.
10. Schmale AH, Iker H. Hopelessness as a predictor of cervical cancer. Soc Sci Med 1971;5:95–100.
11. Bacon CL, Renneker R, Cutler M. A psychosomatic survey of cancer of the breast. Psychosomatic Med 1952;14:453–460.
12. Kissen DM. Lung cancer, inhalation, and personality. In: Kissen DM, LeShan L, eds. Psychosomatic aspects of neoplastic disease. Philadelphia: Lippincott, 1963:3–11.
13. Greene WA Jr. The psychosocial setting of the development of leukemia and lymphoma. Ann NY Acad Sci 1966;125:794–801.
14. Wheeler JI, Caldwell BM. Psychological evaluation of women with cancer of the breast and of the cervix. Psychosomatic Med 1955;17:256–268.
15. Schleifer S, Keller S, Camerino M, Thornton J, Stein M. Suppression of lymphocyte stimulation following bereavement. J Am Med Assoc 1977;250:374–377.
16. Rossi EL. From mind to molecule: a state dependent memory, learning, and behavior theory of mind-body healing. Advances 1987;4:46–60.
17. Appelbaum SA. Exploring the relationship between personality and cancer. In: Goldberg J, ed. Psychotherapeutic treatment of cancer patients. New York: Free Press, 1981:116–128.
18. Harrower M, Thomas CB, Altman A. Human figure drawings in a prospective study of six disorders: hypertension, coronary heart disease, malignant tumor, suicide, mental illness, and emotional disturbance. J Nerv Ment Dis 1975; 101:191–199.

4

Differentiation between Benign and Malignant Neoplasia: Primary and Secondary

—Donald R. Cole

CELLULAR BASIS OF NEOPLASIA

A single aberrant cell is all that is required to produce a malignancy. This is actually a rare event when one considers the billions of cells that compose our organs (7).

Current thinking is that, through clonal growth, a single transformed cell may eventually arrive at a clinically detectable neoplasm (2). The available information suggests that cancer is a many-faceted process involving initiating and promoting factors. The initiators transform a normal cell into a malignant cell. The promoters provide selection advantages for growth of the transformed malignant cell. Almost all plant and animal cells have four major properties: (*a*) growth in size (hypertrophy), (*b*) maturation or differentiation, (*c*) normal function, and (*d*) reproduction. In the transformed condition, the cell appears to lose the ability to function normally and to differentiate.

The consensus is that (5), when this happens, transformation from a normal cellular state to a neoplastic one has occurred. It may be that the cell, no longer involved with the demands of maturing and/or normal functioning, now devotes more time to growing and reproducing.

By definition, a tumor is an abnormal swelling that can also represent the initial state of a clinically detectable neoplasm. The neoplasm is a new tissue growth without physiologic function. The neoplastic process may start out as a benign tumor, ultimately progressing to a malignant one (cancer).

The principal features of cancer are multifaceted: (*a*) local invasion, (*b*) local destruction, (*c*) metastasis, (*d*) tissue atypia (anaplasia), (*e*) pleomorphism, (*f*) increased mitosis, and (*g*) aneuploidy (abnormal DNA content). The biologic behavior of neoplasms varies tremendously from benign to malignant. There is the so-called preinvasive "in situ" cancer. These lesions have most of the morphologic features of cancer but lack invasiveness. They seem to represent an early stage in cancer development in which the tumor is confined to the epithelium. The microscopic appearance may vary throughout a given neoplasm; some neoplasms appear microscopically malignant but act biologically benign. Some identical microscopic patterns may represent totally different diseases.

Since there are hundreds of different types of neoplasms with different degrees of the above-mentioned factors, the accurate diagnosis can only be made by an expert pathologist with adequate information regarding the tissue source and history of the patient, and an adequate tumor specimen to examine.

EXAMINATION OF THE TUMOR

Since podiatrists are frequently the first line of defense in the early and, therefore, most critical phase of diagnosis, they serve a major role in avoiding mutilation and preserving life (5). Their determination of what to biopsy, how to biopsy, what to do with the biopsy, and where ultimately to refer the patient are vital. Performing a complete physical examination and obtaining a proper history are essential. *Clinical Methods in Surgery* (3), provides an excellent summary of the major components a proper history should include. They are:

I. History
1. *Duration*—When was the tumor first noted? Was it present since birth or did it appear subsequently? If it is of short duration, especially if associated with pain, it is more likely to be inflammatory in nature. The longer the dura-

PODIATRIC NEOPLASIA FLOW CHART

1. HISTORY · · · · 2. → PHYSICAL EXAMINATION · · ·> 1. General
    ↓   2. Local

  1. Duration   a. Inspection
  2. Site and shape   b. Palpation
  3. Onset   c. Ausculation
  4. Progress   d. Measurement
  5. Pain   e. Lymph drains
  6. Numbers of
     swellings
  7. Complications
  8. Cachexia
  9. Recurrence
     (postexcision)

                 ∨

  3. BIOPSY PRINCIPLES AND PROCEDURES
    1. Incisional or excisional
    2. Selecting a pathologist—
       handling the biopsy
    3. Ancillary diagnostic techniques

             ∨

  4. STAGING
    1. TNM (Tumor Nodes Metastasis)

             ∨

  5. ONCOLOGICAL REFERRAL

tion, with little change, the more likely the possibility of benignity. However, in certain highly malignant and rapidly growing cancers, duration may be short—or long in some uncommon, chronic inflammations. A painless tumor, present for a long time, is likely to be neoplastic and may be missed by the patient. This is not likely in the leg and/or foot.

2. *Site and Shape*—This may afford a clue as to the anatomic origin of the lesion.

3. *Onset*—Did the tumor begin with trauma? Did it grow rapidly, steadily, or very slowly?

4. *Progress*—Has growth been slow or seemingly stationary for a long period (benignity)? Has it regrown after a quiescent period of months or years (ma-

lignant transformation from a benign status)? Or, has it been continually increasing (malignancy and/or inflammation)? If the tumor gets smaller, this suggests an inflammatory element in the lesion.

5. *Pain*—Is it localized or referred? Is it throbbing or dull? The latter is suggestive of inflammation. Did the pain appear before the swelling or after it? Swelling before pain suggests neoplasia, whereas pain before swelling suggests inflammation. Pain is usually absent in benign situations and early cancer. It frequently connotes complications in cancer, such as ulceration, deep infiltration, and involvement of nerves and/or deep structures.

6. *Similar Swellings*—Are there similar swellings elsewhere in the body? This

can be seen in multiple benign tumor diseases or in advanced metastatic cancer.

7. *Complications*—If ulceration, bleeding, fungation, and/or softening are present, when did they first appear?

8. *Loss of Body Weight or Cachexia*—Is the patient losing weight since the appearance of the swelling? How much weight has the patient lost? The loss of body weight is a cardinal sign of cancer.

9. *Recurrence of Lesion after Excision*—This is a general sign of malignancy, even if the original diagnosis was a benign tumor.

II. Physical Examination

1. *General*—Observe the entire patient. Note any signs of anemia, cachexia, tumefaction, or fever.

2. *Local*

   a. *Inspection.* Observe the tumor. note the following:

      1) Single or multiple

      2) Location and extent (horizontal and vertical)

      3) Color

      4) Size and shape

      5) Surface

      6) Edge—Is it pedunculated or sessile?

      7) Pulsation—Does it pulsate with each pulse beat?

      8) Any pressure effects—Is there any evidence of pressure effects in the limb distal to the swelling, as edema, due to interference with venous or lymphatic flow or muscle wasting due to nerve involvement?

   b. *Palpation*

      1) Local temperature—This is best felt with the back of the fingers. Compare with the normal skin nearby. Elevation in local temperature is usually present in acute inflammatory conditions, but also in certain cancerous situations due to increased vascularity.

      2) Tenderness—This is more marked in inflammatory conditions than in neoplasia.

      3) Surface—Note whether it is smooth, lobular, nodular, or rough and irregular.

4) Edge or margin—Determine whether it is well-defined and clean-cut, as in benign tumors, or ill-defined as in some inflammations and cancers.

5) Consistency—It may be soft, cystic, firm, stony hard (cancer), or bony hard (cartilaginous tumors). Pitting upon pressure usually indicates edematous tissue.

6) Fluctuation—This indicates the presence of fluid or gas.

7) Anatomical Plane and Fixity—Determine whether the swelling is attached, adherent, or fixed to the skin, subcutaneous tissue, deep fascia, muscle, tendon, vessel, nerve, or bone. Test the fixity with the muscle contracting. One observes whether the swelling diminishes in size when it lies under the muscle, remains unaltered when incorporated in the muscle, or becomes prominent when pushed forward by the underlying taut muscle. While the muscle is still contracting, test the mobility of the swelling. A tumor adherent to the muscle becomes immobile with muscle contraction. Mobility is best tested in the direction of the muscle fibers. When the muscle or tendon is torn, contraction of the muscle will cause a circumscribed swelling to appear.

   a) Fixity to tendon—A swelling in connection with a tendon becomes fixed when its muscle contracts against resistance.

   b) Fixity to vessels and nerves—Tumors in connection with vessels and nerves can be moved at right angles to their axes, but not along the direction of the axes.

   c) Fixity to bone—Swellings fixed to bones cannot be moved apart from the bone.

8) Pulsation—Note whether the tumor is pulsating. If so, it may be an aneurysm (expansile pulsation). It may also be a swelling over an artery in which the pul-

sation is transmitted, or it may be a vascular neoplasm.

9) Thrill—Commonly found in an arteriovenous communication.

10) Percussion—Gaseous swellings are resonant. Fluid or solid swellings are dull.

11) Movements of the neighboring joints should be tested and any impairment noted.

c. *Auscultation*—All pulsatile swellings should be examined with a stethoscope for murmurs. A continuous buzzing sound is heard in an aneurysmal varix.

d. *Measurements*—Ascertain the size of the tumor to determine its rate of growth by taking measurements at intervals.

e. *Lymph drainage*—The tumor area must always be examined. Malignant neoplasms frequently will drain into nearby lymph nodes, manifesting themselves as metastatic deposits (4).

III. Biopsy Principles and Procedures

The 1986 edition of the *Cancer Manual* of the American Cancer Society (5), includes an excellent section on biopsy principles and procedures.

Incisional or Excisional

Open biopsies may be either incisional or excisional, depending on size, location of tumor, and potential surgical treatment options available. For small, easily accessible tumors, excisional biopsy under local anesthesia is the procedure of choice. The pathologist has the entire lesion to examine, the tumor is completely excised, and the therapy may be complete.

Incisional biopsy must be used when the lesion is too large to excise on an ambulatory basis or when the initial therapy may involve another modality. Punch biopsy of cutaneous lesions and incisional biopsy of larger neoplastic masses are examples where incisional biopsies can be utilized. All biopsies should be planned so that they do not interfere with the ultimate treatment of the lesion.

Selecting a Pathologist—Handling the Biopsy

It is the responsibility of the physician performing the biopsy to see that tissue is properly and expeditiously handled. With the advent of specialized diagnostic techniques, biopsies can no longer be placed routinely in fixatives and sent to pathologists. It may be necessary to perform immunohistochemical or ultrastructural evaluations to make an accurate diagnosis or to characterize a given malignancy. These techniques require either fresh tissue or tissue prepared in a specific manner. If there is a question as to specific studies to be performed, the biopsy specimen should be submitted in the fresh state, in saline solution, to the pathologist as quickly as possible. Notify the pathologist in advance of the specimen's arrival. The surgeon must be aware that small samples of tissue may be subject to the trauma of crushing, dehydration, and other physical changes that make it difficult for a pathologist to render an accurate diagnosis. Thus, the smaller the sample, the greater the likelihood of obtaining nondiagnostic material. The morphologic diagnosis of cancer is not always clear-cut; therefore the pathologist should be informed fully of the patient's presenting syndrome and the clinical impression of the diagnosis.

Previous histologic studies of the same patient are most valuable in rendering diagnosis and prognosis. Likewise, any therapy rendered to the patient may be important since some therapies may alter pathologic appearance.

Frozen sections provide a rapid diagnosis at the expense of cellular detail. Therefore, they are less reliable, and staging and therapeutic procedures should be deferred until permanent sections have been interpreted by a pathologist. If a frozen section is taken, additional material from the same site must be submitted for a permanent section.

Ancillary Diagnostic Techniques

A number of ancillary diagnostic techniques are available to the pathologist in addition to routine light microscopy. Their value is primarily in classifying tumors by cell of origin. The most widely used of these techniques is special staining, using mucicarmine stain, periodic acid-Schiff stain, silver stain, and other stains that demonstrate the presence of particular chemical constituents in tumor cells that may define their histologic origins.

In addition, there is the electron microscope for greater resolution at the histologic level. Ultrastructural studies combined with enzyme staining may confirm the presence of a specific enzyme characteristic of a given cell line. A most promising technique is immunohistologic staining in which the development of monoclonal antibodies enable the production of purified antibodies specific to antigenic components of given tumor cells.

IV. Staging

According to Neiman and Smith (5), the staging system most commonly used for involved organs is that of the American Joint Committee for Cancer Staging and End-results Reporting, the TNM system. T refers to extent of primary tumor, including size, depth, and invasion of adjacent structures. Increasing extent of local spread is designated by numerical subsets T1, T2, T3, and T4. N refers to regional lymph node metastasis. Subsets again depend upon extent (e.g., N0, N1, and N2). M refers to distant metastasis. Once a stage is assigned, it remains the same throughout the course of the disease for recording purposes.

Primary neoplasms refer to the site of the original tumor; secondary neoplasms refer to the metastatic site. One can often diagnose the primary neoplasm site from the appearance and location of the secondary neoplasm.

The state of the art in diagnostic examination for neoplasms of the lower extremities is magnetic resonance imaging (MRI). The human body is made up of trillions of atoms. When it is placed in the strong magnetic field of the MRI, the cores of its hydrogen atoms line up with the magnetic field like small magnets. The information generated is fed into a computer that analyzes and creates the images. This examination should frequently be done in addition to standard x-ray views, since MRI does not show calcium well.

REFERENCES

1. Buchner T, Hiddeman W, Wormann B, et al. Differential pattern of DNA—aneuploidy in human malignancies. Pathol Res Pract 1985;179: 310–317.
2. Costanza ME. Cancer prevention and detection. In: Cady B, ed. Cancer manual. 7th ed. Boston: American Cancer Society Massachusetts Division, Inc., 1986:14–35.
3. Das K. Clinical methods in surgery, 8th ed. Calcutta: 1968.
4. Nicholson GL. Organ specificity of tumor metastasis: role of preferential adhesion, invasion and growth of malignant cells at specific secondary sites. Cancer Metastasis Rev 1988;7:143–188.
5. Neiman RS, Smith TJ. Biopsy principles, pathologic evaluation of specimens, and staging of cases. In: Cady B, ed. Cancer manual. 7th ed. Boston: American Cancer Society Massachusetts Division, Inc., 1986:36–44.
6. Nowell PC. Molecular events in tumor development [editorial]. N Engl J Med 1988;319: 575–576.
7. Pack GT, ed. Tumors of hands and feet. St. Louis: Mosby, 1939:9.

Soft-tissue Neoplasia

Part A/ **Vascular Neoplasia**

—Mark A. Kosinski

The pediatric physician encounters, almost daily, neoplasia of vascular origin. However, one's index of suspicion must always be high. Vascular neoplasms tend to look alike. A lesion which may appear to be nothing more than a bruise or patch of cellulitis may actually be a low-grade angiosarcoma. One may be surprised when the specimen, thought sure to be a solitary pyogenic granuloma, returns from the pathologist with a microscopic diagnosis of Kaposi's sarcoma. It is important, therefore, that one is aware of the types, characteristics, and treatments of neoplasia that may be encountered.

CLINICAL DIAGNOSIS

Perhaps the most distinguishing feature of a vascular neoplasm is its color. Superficial lesions usually appear red, violaceous, or blue; deeper ones may be somewhat more difficult to detect. A faint hue may be the only indication that it is an underlying vascular tumor. Occasionally, the lesion may be colorless, as in the case of hemangiopericytoma (1).

The temperature of skin overlying a hypervascular neoplasm may be elevated. If large enough, soft bruits, characterizing turbulent flow, may be identified on Doppler or stethoscopic examination. A positive Branham's test may signify arteriovenous shunting (2). Needle aspiration of blood or blood-tinged fluid is a strong indicator that it is a vascular lesion. Diascopy may be of value in determining whether the red color of a cutaneous lesion is due to capillary dilatation or extravasation of red blood cells (3).

Pain may be a diagnostic feature of the lesion itself or the result of compression of adjacent structures. Diminished pulse and a cool extremity may be due to tumor thrombus, aneurysmal dilatation of proximal vessels, or compression (4). Vascular obstruction may account for edema or thrombophlebitis (5). Unilateral varicosities can occur secondary to compression of venous structures or by arteriovenous shunting within the tumor itself (6).

One must obtain a detailed history of the suspect lesion including onset, duration, antecedent trauma, and changes in size and appearance. A newly arisen lesion which shows a recent alteration in character should arouse considerably more suspicion than one that has remained unchanged since birth.

History must be carefully correlated with physical examination, radiographic analysis, and biopsy. Taken alone, a history of trauma may be of questionable value. A mass which has arisen following trauma may simply signify a muscle rupture with organized hematoma. Conversely, trauma has been implicated in the development of hemangioma and has been reported to have occurred antecedent to some cases of angiosarcoma (7).

DIAGNOSTIC PROCEDURES

Many vascular neoplasms demand a rigorous evaluation to determine their extent of involvement. A patient may present with a single cutaneous nodule of Kaposi's sarcoma, yet harbor widespread visceral dissemination. Arnn et al. (8), report a case of systemic angioendotheliomatosis presenting with hemolytic anemia (8). Widespread hemangioma may result in a consumption coagulopathy characterized by thrombocytopenia (9, 10). Of course, in those patients diagnosed with malignant neoplasia, an exhaustive search for metastatic lesions must be carried out.

Immunohistochemical Evaluation

Factor VIII-related antigen (factor VIII-Ag) has been widely used as a marker for endothelial cells in both normal and neoplastic tissue (11). The presence of factor VIII-Ag can aid the pathologist in determining whether a particular neoplasm is of endothelial, and hence, vascular origin. Variation in staining of normal endothelial cells and an inconsistency in reacting with malignant tumors of endothelial cell origin have been noted as limitations of factor VIII-Ag staining (12).

Ulex europaeus I lectin (UEA I), a plant protein derived from the seeds of the leguminous shrub *Ulex europaeus,* has likewise been found to bind to endothelial cells (13). While it appears to possess greater sensitivity than factor VIII-Ag, it is less specific and is reported to recognize antigens in various types of epithelium (12). UEA I may have its greatest value in studying vascular tumors in those cases of weak or questionable reactivity to factor VIII-Ag.

Plain Film Radiography

Often, the vascular neoplasm will appear as nothing more than a nonspecific soft-tissue density on plain film x-ray. Occasionally however, one may detect tell-tale calcifications within the lesion itself.

The presence of phleboliths in hemangiomas has been well-documented (14, 15). Jones and Roberts (15) have noted these calcifications consist of concentric rings of increased density, interspersed with rings of decreased density, thus imparting a classic "mother of pearl appearance." Calcifications occurring in a speckled pattern are reported in cases of hemangiopericytomas (4, 16, 17).

In the case of aggressive or malignant lesions, plain film radiography and radionuclide scans may be useful in screening for the presence of bone involvement or metastases. Should the size and nature warrant, the physician has at his disposal several more specific imaging techniques, including angiography, computerized tomography, and magnetic resonance imaging.

Angiography

Although nonspecific for tissue type, angiography can be a powerful diagnostic tool, particularly with respect to vascular neoplasia. Arteriography can aid the physician in planning his surgical approach, giving information as to size, location of feeder vessels, and relation of the lesion to surrounding soft-tissue and osseous structures.

Malignant neoplasms are frequently heterogenous, containing avascular areas of necrosis and organized hematoma. Biopsy from such areas may result in a fatal misdiagnosis. Angiosarcomas, in particular, exhibit a high degree of heterogeneity. In a series of soft-tissue neoplasms studied by Levin et al. (18), 10% of biopsies taken from malignant tumors were interpreted as benign due to poor biopsy location.

Since areas of increased vascularity correspond to the most malignant areas of the tumor, angiography can guide the surgeon to the most vascular and, hence, most aggressive section.

Although one is able to confirm the existence of a vascular neoplasm and to visualize previously undetected satellite or metastatic lesions, clear distinction between malignant and benign tumors on the basis of angiography is not always possible. Nevertheless, certain generalizations can be made to aid the physician in his assessment of the neoplasm.

Lesions that are malignant, or benign with malignant clinical behavior, tend to be those with vessels that pursue a random, purposeless course. The vessel walls are coarse, ragged, and end abruptly at the tumor border. Tumor staining, which represents the filling of numerous small vessels with contrast material, may be seen. Arteriovenous shunting within the lesion may also be present (16, 18, 19). Malignant hemangioendothelioma (18), Kaposi's sarcoma (18, 19) and hemangiopericytoma (16, 18) are reported to exhibit these features.

The presence of small vessels around an avascular area, the presence of straight veins running at right angles to the normal flow of venous blood, and the presence of vascular pools during the venous phase have additionally been noted by Hoeffel et al. (16), to suggest malignancy. In the case of hemangiopericytoma, Sutton and Pratt et al. (20), suggest a positive correlation between degree of vascularity and degree of malignancy.

In contrast, lesions may exhibit a hypervascular pattern in which orderly, smooth-walled vessels taper to a fine caliber (18). In this category, it is more uncertain whether the lesion is neoplastic or inflammatory.

Levin et al. (18), suggest that, while sharply demarcated masses are most likely neoplastic, poorly delineated lesions may be either neoplastic or inflammatory. Lesions rich in small, regular vessels without the presence of tumor stain are most indicative of benign lesions such as vascular hematomas (21).

A muscle rupture with organized hematoma may mimic a vascular neoplasm clinically, but is difficult to distinguish angiographically. The accumulation of contrast material in streaks corresponding to muscle striations, and the abundance of capillary vessels secondary to the formation of granulation tissue around the hematoma, suggest the lesion is of traumatic rather than neoplastic origin (22).

Computerized Tomography

Compared to angiography, computerized tomography (CT) can better define the relationship of tumor to specific muscle groups and fascial planes (23), and can better detect lobulations, cystic spaces, and calcifications within the lesion itself (17).

Contrast enhancement is useful in indicating the vascular nature of a tumor. Rauch et al. (23), recommend a series of unenhanced CT images first be performed, followed by contrast studies. Bolus injection of contrast material is recommended over drip infusion in producing optimal vascular enhancement (23). Reverse contrast enhancement may prove useful in indicating the presence of necrosis (24).

Although CT scanning can distinguish local processes from frankly invasive lesions, differentiation between malignant and benign neoplasms on this basis alone may not be possible (24). However, as with angiography, the presence of hemorrhagic or necrotic areas is highly suggestive of a malignant process.

Due to CT scanning's ability to detect small nodules often missed on conventional radiographs, patients diagnosed as having vascular neoplasms with metastatic potential should undergo a CT scan of the chest to rule out pulmonary involvement (25).

Magnetic Resonance Imaging

Complications resulting from ionizing radiation and the administration of contrast material can be avoided with magnetic resonance imaging (MRI). The advantage of MRI over CT scanning or angiography is the marked increased in contrast between tumor and surrounding tissue (26). The relationship to specific muscle groups, bones, and vascular structures can be accurately determined (11). As such, it has the greatest potential in evaluating the success of treatment and the detection of recurrence (26, 27).

Despite the high-contrast potential of MRI, there is little diagnostic specificity for the majority of soft-tissue tumors (28). The exact arteries and veins draining and feeding a neoplasm cannot be accurately determined, and phleboliths, a feature of many vascular neoplasms, are rarely visible. The optimal, noninvasive approach, therefore, may be complementary MRI and angiographic studies.

DIFFERENTIAL DIAGNOSIS, TREATMENT, AND PROGNOSIS
Hemangiomas

These common lesions, composed of dilated vascular spaces, are almost always benign. Trauma is the suggested etiology of some (14), although the vast majority are congenital in origin. Predilection for the female, together with the reported fluctuation in size during puberty, pregnancy, and menopause, suggest a possible hormonal influence (14, 29).

Phleboliths, often seen on radiographic examination, are thought to result from the calcification of organized thrombi within vessel walls (30, 31). Occlusion of vascular channels with phleboliths may occasionally cause the hemangioma to undergo spontaneous regression (14).

Hemangiomas can occur in any living tissue and are well-documented in the lower extremity (30, 32–34). Depending on morphology, they can be divided into capillary and cavernous types. Distinction between the two is not always clear-cut. Many capillary hemangiomas contain cavernous areas and vice versa. Classification can vary depending on the author.

Sequestration of large amounts of blood and platelets within extensive hemangiomas may lead to a consumption coagulopathy known as the Kasabach-Merritt syndrome. Characterized by thrombocytopenia, purpuric skin lesions, and disseminated intravascular coagulation, it is reported to occur with both capillary and cavernous hemangiomas (9, 10).

Capillary Hemangioma

Composed of a fine network of dilated capillaries and capillary buds and lined with flattened endothelial cells, capillary hemangiomas represent the most common blood vessel lesion (14).

Capillary hemangiomas are usually flat, although they may be elevated or pedunculated. They may be either deep-seated or confined to the skin and superficial soft tissue. Phlebolith formation is reported (30). Bleeding may occur in superficial lesions, where the epithelial covering is thin. Size can range from the tiny cherry angioma to the large, disfiguring strawberry nevus.

CHERRY ANGIOMA

These small (2–3 mm), plump, bright-red papules are commonly found on the extremities. They may occur from young adulthood through old age. Their histology is that of a capillary hemangioma, with vascular spaces progressively dilating as the lesion matures. Since these lesions follow a benign course, treatment is necessary only for cosmesis. Electrocautery is usually curative (35).

PYOGENIC GRANULOMA

Pyogenic granulomas are benign vascular neoplasms, histologically resembling capillary hemangiomas. Although they may be of any size, they are usually small, between 5 mm and 2 cm. The lesions may appear anywhere on the body and show no predilection for age or sex (36).

Pyogenic granulomas typically appear as bright red to purple, pedunculated papules. They are friable and bleed easily with minor trauma. Secondary infection and ulceration may occur. Although usually solitary, multiple satellite lesions have been reported (37, 38). Although cutaneous lesions are most common, Cooper et al. (39) report 18 cases of pyogenic granuloma occurring intravenously.

Trauma appears to be the most common etiologic factor, although these neoplasms are reported to occur spontaneously on normal skin without inciting incident. On the lower extremity, pyogenic granulomas are commonly seen in conjunction with paronychias, where they appear as singular, red, cherry-like papules adjacent to the offending nail spicule (Fig. 5.1). Subungual lesions may occur in patients with a history of direct trauma to the nail plate.

These pedunculated lesions receive their blood supply through comparatively large feeder vessels which originate deep in the dermis and reach upward through the stalk. Treatment, therefore, must include excision and cautery of the feeder vessel as well. Electrocoagulation or application of silver nitrate to the base, after excision, is suggested. Even so, recurrence still occurs, and may also include the appearance of satellite lesions. In the absence of treatment, some lesions may simply involute spontaneously whereas others persist indefinitely as capillary hemangiomas (35).

Pyogenic granulomas bear a striking resemblance to solitary, pedunculated lesions of Kaposi's sarcoma. Excision and biopsy of all lesions is, therefore, imperative.

JUVENILE HEMANGIOMA (STRAWBERRY NEVUS)

Juvenile hemangiomas are usually noticed shortly after birth when they may first appear as a flat, erythematous macule. The lesion continues to grow with the child, often becoming raised and polypoid. The maximum size is usually reached by age 6 mo (7). Although primarily classified as a capillary hemangioma, cavernous elements may also be found. The tumor's predilection is for the head and neck and it is only rarely found on the lower extremity.

The course of these lesions is quite predictable. Juvenile hemangiomas characteristically involute, leaving behind a small, lightly pigmented scar. Regression usually begins by age 2 or 3 yr. Those still present by age 7 do not usually undergo further change (35, 36).

The best course of action is to simply observe the lesion through its stages. Cosmetic surgery is best reserved for adulthood after the lesion has "run its course." Extensive, disfiguring hemangiomas may frequently regress to a point where surgery is unnecessary. In those cases where early intervention is warranted, systemic steroids may be employed to hasten involution (40).

Cavernous Hemangioma

The appearance of cavernous hemangiomas on the lower extremity is well-documented (16, 32, 34, 41, 42). Although primarily involving the skin and subcutaneous tissue, cavernous hemangiomas may also be found in deeper structures and internal organs (42). Shallow et al. (43) and Jenkins et al. (44) report the quadriceps muscle to be the most frequent lower extremity site of occurrence.

Blood vessels in this type of hemangioma exhibit significantly more dilatation than do those in the capillary type. Pools and cavernous sinuses may develop, with circulation within the lesion sluggish. As are capillary hemangiomas, cavernous hemangiomas are of endothelial origin.

Cavernous hemangiomas are usually soft and spongy, having a "bag of worms" or "spaghetti-like" consistency (14, 34). In a study of 73 cases of discrete hemangiomas of the lower extremity, Johnson et al. (14) reported pain and the presence of a tissue mass to be the most common symptom, whereas a palpable tissue mass was the most common physical finding.

Depending on their depth, cavernous hemangiomas may appear either red, blue, or dark

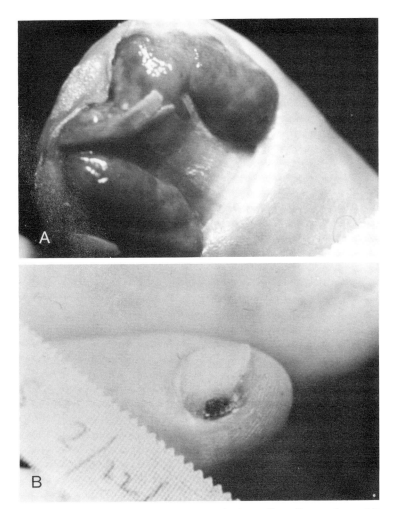

Figure 5.1. Pyogenic granuloma secondary to paronychia formation. (**A,** courtesy of Howard Fox DPM.)

blue in color. Although slow-growing, they have the potential to reach enormous size.

VERRUCOUS HEMANGIOMA

It can safely be said that verrucous hemangiomas occur more frequently than they are diagnosed. They are true vascular malformations, bearing no relation to verruca vulgaris, a lesion for which they are commonly mistaken.

Verrucous hemangiomas are benign and confined to the skin and subcutaneous tissue. Reactive epidermal acanthosis, papillomatosis, and hyperkeratosis are characteristic findings. Features of both capillary and cavernous hemangiomas may be seen within a single lesion (45).

Verrucous hemangiomas occur at any age, although they appear most frequently from infancy through adolescence. Immature lesions present as soft, smooth, well-demarcated red to blue papules. As they mature, their color may change to brown, dark blue, or black. Older lesions develop a characteristic warty, hyperkeratotic appearance. Trauma may incite transition into the verrucous phase. Verrucous hemangiomas exhibit slow, superficial spread and vary in size from a few millimeters to several centimeters. Satellite lesions are sometimes seen (45).

Since enlargement is inevitable, treatment of early lesions is advisable. Excision and biopsy with electrocautery of the base is recommended. Local recurrence is possible following incomplete excision (45, 46).

BLUE RUBBER BLEB NEVUS

Blue rubber bleb nevi are present at birth, often increasing in size and number with the age of the patient. True to their name, these cavernous hemangiomas may appear as small

(1–3 cm), compressible dark-blue nodules, primarily affecting the dermis and subcutaneous tissue. Localized sweating has been reported to occur directly over the tumor site (35).

Occasionally, visceral lesions may occur, in which case the term "blue rubber bleb nevus syndrome" is applied. Ulceration of internal neoplasms may cause chronic gastrointestinal bleeding and anemia. Patients suspected of this syndrome should be evaluated accordingly (9, 47).

NEVUS FLAMMEUS (PORT-WINE STAIN)

Variously classified as an angioma or telangiectasia, nevus flammeus is characterized by well-circumscribed pink to deep-purple macules. Usually present at birth, they may show some regression as the patient progresses toward adulthood. Small nodular lesions representing capillary or cavernous hemangiomas may be found interspersed throughout.

When seen on the back, nevus flammeus may signify an underlying arteriovenous malformation of the spinal cord (35). A comprehensive physical examination is, therefore, warranted in all patients. The carbon dioxide and argon laser are effective in treating cutaneous manifestations of selected port-wine stains.

KLIPPEL-TRENAUNAY SYNDROME (OSTEOHYPERTROPHIC NEVUS FLAMMEUS)

Klippel-Trenaunay syndrome is characterized by the unmistakable triad of varicosities, limb hypertrophy (bone and soft tissue), and extensive nevus flammeus. Although most often affecting a single limb, the syndrome may be so severe as to include one entire side of the body. When it occurs, it is always present at birth.

Associated malformations are reported and include spina bifida occulta, neurofibromatosis, atrial septal defects, pelvic nonfusion, gigantism of the digits, syndactyly, and compensatory equinus deformities secondary to limb-length discrepancy (48). Cutaneous ulcers, hemorrhage from ruptured varices, deep vein thrombophlebitis, and pulmonary emboli may occur as a result of venous and lymphatic abnormalities.

Plain radiographs show bone hypertrophy and osteoporosis. Angiography underscores the vascularity of these lesions. If encountered, arteriovenous fistulas are more representative of the Parkes-Weber syndrome, of which they are a distinguishing feature (2).

Treatment is aimed at normalizing the size of the limb and preventing the sequela of venous insufficiency. Surgical intervention, including venous ligation and stripping, evacuation of hematomas, and debulking procedures are suggested (48, 49). Amputation is an option in severe cases and is performed so that the patient may lead a normal life. Pressure-gradient stockings are recommended for those not amenable to invasive therapy (48, 49). Regardless of the chosen plan of treatment, the physician must be aware of the increased risk of deep vein thrombophlebitis and pulmonary embolus among these patients.

MAFFUCCI'S SYNDROME

Multiple cavernous hemangiomas, osteochondromas, and defects in ossification compose the characteristic triad of Maffucci's syndrome. Pathologic fractures are common. It has been estimated that 20% of patients with Maffucci's syndrome will eventually develop chondrosarcoma (36, 50).

Hemangioma of Deep Tissue

SYNOVIAL HEMANGIOMA

Synovial hemangiomas are extremely rare lesions that typically appear during childhood or adolescence. Presentation is uniarticular, with the knee being the most common site of involvement. Symptoms include pain and sensitivity to minor trauma, a progressive decrease in range of motion, and muscle atrophy of the involved limb. A spongy, tender mass may be palpated, occasionally associated with an overlying cutaneous hemangioma. Limb-length discrepancy secondary to premature maturation of the epiphyses of the involved extremity may be seen (51, 52).

Joint aspiration yields blood or blood-stained fluid. Plain radiographs may reveal characteristic phleboliths (30). Angiography and arthrography can aid in the differentiation of synovial hemangioma from joint effusion. Due to the periarticular location, they may be confused clinically with other neoplasms of synovial origin.

HEMANGIOMA OF MUSCLE

Hemangiomas may occur in any striated muscle, although they are most commonly described in the quadriceps (43, 44). They are often first noticed during childhood and adolescence and may be antecedent to trauma. Swelling and impairment of function are common symptoms. If present, pain may occur either on palpation or with contraction of the affected muscle.

Plain radiographs may show phlebolith formation, estimated to occur in 50% of these neoplasms (15). Intramuscular hemangiomas may grow and expand between muscle fibers (53). Angiography may reveal vessels oriented in a characteristic striated pattern, formed by their parallel entry between muscle fascicles (18, 36). Surgery aims at complete excision.

HEMANGIOMA OF NERVE

Hemangiomas have been described involving the peroneal and posterior tibial nerves (36). Unlike those of muscle and synovium, there appears to be no characteristic age of onset. Symptoms are related to the nerves affected. Since these are benign lesions, the benefits of excision should be weighed carefully and excision attempted only by an experienced microsurgeon.

Glomus Tumors

Glomus tumors are small (3 mm to 1 cm) slow-growing nodules representing benign hyperplasia of normal glomus structures. Red, blue, or normal in color, they may occur as solitary, multiple, or multiple painless lesions (54).

Glomus tumors may be found anywhere but favor the fingers, toes, and nail beds (50). They have been described in skin and subcutaneous tissue as well as in deeper structures (e.g., muscle, bone, and joints) (55–58). They may occur as a result of trauma.

Glomus tumors are generally characterized by both exquisite pain evoked by light touch and extreme sensitivity to heat and cold. The size has little bearing on the severity of symptoms. Excruciating pain may be elicited by a lesion no larger than the head of a pin.

Pain may be of such intensity as to cause splinting or guarding of the affected part. Melancholia, neuroses, insomnia, and requests for amputation are reported to occur in extreme cases (58).

DIAGNOSTIC TESTS

Love's Pin Test

The pain of a glomus tumor is often quite specific and localizable by the patient. The point of a sharp object (such as an ordinary pin) may be used to carefully examine the area surrounding the suspected lesion. Characteristic pain is elicited when the point is lightly brushed across the skin overlying the tumor. Accurate to within 1 cm, this test is especially useful when the lesion is of such small size and at a depth sufficient to render it clinically invisible (60). In the case of subungual lesions, compression of the nail plate will usually reproduce the symptoms.

Hildreth's Ischemia Test

As described by Hildreth (61), occlusion of blood flow to an affected extremity by a blood pressure cuff will prevent the characteristic pain response of a glomus tumor to light touch. The cuff must be inflated either before or immediately following the administration of a light touch for the test to be valid.

ROENTGENOGRAPHIC EVALUATION

Arteriography may reveal star-shaped telangiectatic zones surrounding the lesion (62). Osteolytic defects with sclerotic borders may be seen on plain film x-ray in those tumors which erode into adjacent bone (63). Thermography, infrared photography, transillumination and digital plethysmography are nonspecific and of limited value in establishing a diagnosis.

DIFFERENTIAL DIAGNOSIS

Owing to its sensitivity to temperature, its frequent occurrence in the digits, and the bluish hue often taken on during an attack of pain, a glomus tumor may be confused with Raynaud's phenomenon. Glomus tumors may erode into bone, giving the appearance of a Brodie's abscess on x-ray. The dark-blue to black color of some glomus tumors may cause this lesion to be mistaken for a melanoma, especially when it occurs in the nail bed. Other differentials have been reported to include epidermal inclusion cyst (64), neurofibroma (60), neuroma, and factitious illness (65).

TREATMENT

Local injections, chemical or surgical sympathectomy, analgesics, and soaks are ineffective in affording permanent relief. Surgical excision of well-encapsulated lesions is curative, although complete resolution of symptoms may not ensue immediately (60).

Failure of surgery to permanently alleviate symptoms of a histologically proven glomus tumor may be due to missed multiple lesions or the formation of new ones. Since glomus tumors have been reported to infiltrate locally, meticulous dissection and preservation of vital structures is imperative.

Metastatic potential is suggested (66) but evidence is inconclusive. Critics postulate reported cases may actually be hemangiopericytomas, which are close histologic analogues of the glomus tumor (54, 57).

Glomangiosarcoma

Enzinger and Weiss (67) report four cases of this extremely rare tumor, three of which appeared on the lower extremity. The lesions contained areas of benign glomus tumor interspersed with areas resembling an immature form of fibrosarcoma or leiosarcoma. Since these sarcomatous changes arose in the midst of a benign glomus tumor, it is imperative that the physician routinely examine several sections of a suspect lesion before a final diagnosis is made.

Hemangiopericytoma

Hemangiopericytomas are rare, deep-seated mesenchymal tumors arising from pericytes of Zimmerman. Since pericytes are found in capillaries and venules, hemangiopericytomas may occur in all types of tissue and be found anywhere in the body. They are usually small, reaching an average size of 6 cm, although lesions as large as 1000 g are reported (6).

Favoring the musculoskeletal system, they are most commonly found in the anterior thigh. Although the median age of occurrence is 45, hemangiopericytomas have been described in patients from birth through age 92 (4, 6).

There is a high degree of variability. Approximately half are malignant (1, 6) with the remainder being either borderline malignant or benign. Stout (68) notes the thigh has more malignant lesions than any other site.

Histology cannot reliably differentiate malignant from benign forms nor predict the possibility of future metastases (6). However, increased cellularity, prominent mitotic activity and foci of hemorrhage and necrosis are noted to be highly suggestive of malignancy (4, 6).

Sites of metastases include the liver, bone, lungs, and lymph nodes (1, 4, 6, 50). In a group studied by McMasters et al. (4), metastases were observed in 64.5% of patients with malignant or potentially malignant tumors.

CLINICAL FEATURES

Patients usually present with a painless, slowly enlarging mass (4, 6). The lack of coloration may be explained by the compression of capillary lumina by proliferating pericytes (1). Pain is usually a late symptom, resulting from compression of adjacent structures (4). The pain of the hemangiopericytoma is dull and continuous, distinct from the lancinating paroxysms of the glomus tumor. Local elevation of skin temperature, telangiectasias overlying the lesion, and the auscultation of bruits secondary to arteriovenous shunting within the tumor are additionally reported as clinical findings (1, 4, 6). Histologically, extraskeletal mesenchymal chondrosarcoma, infantile fibrosarcoma, malignant fibrous histiocytoma, malignant schwannoma, and liposarcoma are reported to exhibit a hemangiopericytoma-like pattern (69).

COURSE

Clinical course is variable and depends upon the malignant potential of the tumor. Growth is often slow and insidious. Rapid growth with death taking place within a matter of months is reported in extreme cases (1).

DIAGNOSIS

Plain film radiographs exhibit nonspecific soft-tissue density. Speckled calcification and bone erosion may occur but are considered rare findings (6). Primary hemangiopericytomas of bone are reported (70). CT scans of the chest should be taken in all suspected cases to rule out pulmonary metastases.

Angiography frequently depicts a highly vascular lesion comprised of tortuous vessels. Correlation between degree of vascularity and degree of malignancy has been suggested (16, 20). Angiography cannot differentiate conclusively between hemangiopericytoma and similarly appearing hypervascular neoplasms (e.g. fibrosarcoma, hemangioma, and muscular hematoma). Biopsy alone is diagnostic. As noted by Alpern et al. (17), CT scans may reveal a large, lobulated, soft-tissue mass with cystic attenuation zones, septations, and speckled areas of calcification.

TREATMENT

Although hemangiopericytomas are relatively radioresistant, adjunctive radiotherapy is used for treatment of metastatic lesions with some success (6). Results of chemotherapy are disappointing (4, 6, 71). Wide surgical excision is the treatment of choice. Amputation may be necessary if size or location dictate (1, 4, 6, 16, 20, 71).

As reported by Backwinkel and Diddams (1), hemangiopericytomas are highly malignant over a lifetime in over 50% of all cases, with a recurrence rate of 80% for lesions of the nervous system and 50.5% for those of the musculoskeletal system. Recurrence preceded metastases in two-thirds of the patients studied by Enzinger and Smith (5).

Since recurrence with metastases is reported up to 16 yr after initial excision, lifetime followup is mandatory (1, 4, 17).

Proliferating Angioendotheliomatosis

First described by Pfleger and Tappeiner (72) in 1959, proliferating angioendotheliomatosis may occur in either malignant or benign forms. Although similar in appearance, each pursues a dramatically different course.

MALIGNANT PROLIFERATING ANGIOENDOTHELIOMATOSIS

Malignant proliferating angioendotheliomatosis may be described as the diffuse, malignant proliferation of vascular endothelium, resulting in complete or partial obstruction of the vascular lumen (73, 74).

Autopsy reveals the multifocal nature of this disease. Blood vessels of the skin, subcutaneous tissue, and virtually every internal organ may be affected. Noncohesive, neoplastic endothelial cells may be seen to fill the lumen of all tissues involved (8). Many of the endothelial cells are atypical in appearance and may be distinguished by hyperchromatic nuclei, often in mitosis (75, 76). The disease may originate internally, or begin cutaneously, rapidly progressing to viscera (77). Extravascular extension may also be seen (73, 75).

Most commonly found on the legs and trunk, cutaneous lesions may appear either as widespread erythematous patches or intercutaneous and subcutaneous nodules varying in size from one to several centimeters (73, 76). Tortuous superficial vessels may be seen to overly the lesions (73).

This disease's presentation and course are highly variable. The formation of new, cutaneous lesions may be painful (76). Mature lesions may decrease in size, leaving behind a red to brown scar (76). Visceral involvement may be heralded by vague constitutional symptoms or reflect specific organ dysfunction.

The cell of origin remains a point of conjecture. Arnn et al. (8), think this condition represents a truly neoplastic process of vascular endothelium. Although neoplastic cells contain the presence of factor VIII-Ag strongly suggesting endothelial origin (8, 73), Dominguez et al. (77) argue that tumor cells may be the manifestation of bidirectional lymphoid and endothelial differentiation. Scott et al. (78) think this tumor may actually represent an unusual form of lymphoma.

The course of this disease is rapidly fatal. Treatment is supportive. The administration of systemic steroids is found to have no effect on either cutaneous or visceral lesions (76).

REACTIVE PROLIFERATING ANGIOENDOTHELIOMATOSIS

Cutaneous lesions of this benign variant resemble that of its malignant counterpart, making a distinction between the two on clinical examination difficult. There is marked endothelial cell proliferation within the capillaries of the dermis and subcutaneous tissue, leading to full or partial obstruction of the vessel lumen. Proliferating endothelial cells may appear normal or show varying degrees of atypicality (75). Therefore, definitive differentiation of malignant from benign forms, even on microscopic examination, may not always be possible.

The course of the disease is self-limited. The dermatoses is usually clear within 6–12 months, although lesions lasting up to several years are reported (72, 75, 78). Unlike its malignant counterpart, there is no reported systemic involvement.

Angiosarcoma

These rapidly growing, aggressive, malignant neoplasms account for approximately 1% of all soft-tissue sarcomas (79, 80). Although favoring skin and superficial soft tissue, they are found in every organ including bone.

Angiosarcomas may arise from the endothelial cells of blood vessels of any internal organ but are most commonly reported in bone and striated muscle (7). Metastases is primarily hematogenous and favors, but is not limited to, the lung, liver, and regional lymph nodes (81). Occasionally, metastases occur via the lymphatic system (7).

The outlook for patients is poor. Disease mortality is due either to direct extension or metastases. In a retrospective study of forty-four cases of angiosarcoma of the skin and soft tissue, Maddox et al. (81), notes the median survival time is 20 months.

Soft-tissue sarcomas may be assigned a grade of 1 to 3. Low-grade (grade 1) sarcomas may be locally invasive and virtually never metastasize. High-grade sarcomas (grade 2 or 3) are more aggressive and present the problem of metastasis and widespread dissemination (79).

With respect to its appearance on the lower extremity, angiosarcomas may be classified as cutaneous angiosarcomas without lymphedema, cutaneous angiosarcomas associated with lymphedema (lymphangiosarcoma), postirradiation angiosarcomas, or angiosarcomas of deep soft tissue and bone.

CUTANEOUS ANGIOSARCOMA WITHOUT LYMPHEDEMA

Although favoring the head, neck, and scalp, cutaneous angiosarcoma unassociated with lymphedema does appear on the lower extremity. Of 101 cases of cutaneous angiosarcoma studied at the Armed Forces Institute of Pathology, Enzinger and Weiss (79) report 13 on the leg.

The precise etiology is unknown. Antecedent trauma has been reported in some patients (7), although the significance of trauma in stimulating the sarcomatous degeneration of blood vessel endothelium is unclear.

Clinical appearance is variable and may be correlated to the degree of histologic differentiation. Low-grade lesions may appear as firm red to purple nodules reminiscent of Kaposi's sarcoma (81, 82). They may be moderately painful or totally asymptomatic. Smaller satellite lesions may be seen (7).

Early lesions may be mistaken by the patient or physician for a common blood blister or a simple bruise. Often, it is their innocuous appearance that leads to misdiagnosis and a critical delay in treatment.

More undifferentiated tumors may present as focal areas of reddening with indurated borders. With time, these lesions may darken and become raised, nodular, or ulcerated (7, 83).

ANGIOSARCOMA ASSOCIATED WITH LYMPHEDEMA (LYMPHANGIOSARCOMA)

In 1948, Stewart and Treves (84) described six cases of angiosarcoma arising in the lymphedematous upper extremities of postmastectomy patients. Since then, the occurrence of this neoplasm is similarly documented in the leg.

Lymphangiosarcomas are histologically identical to angiosarcomas (83, 85). The presence of factor VIII-Ag in neoplastic endothelial cells suggests a vascular rather than lymphatic origin (86). Chronic lower extremity lymphedema, regardless of etiology, has the potential to give rise to angiosarcoma (80, 87).

Since the podiatric physician is confronted with lower extremity edema on a routine basis, he/she must constantly be aware of the possibility of malignant change. Latency periods of 6 months (87) to 46 yr (88) are reported. The likelihood of such sarcomatous degeneration is estimated to be less than 1% (86). Although the pathogenesis is unclear, it has been suggested that chronic lymphatic obstruction may result in a defect in cellular immunity at a local level, creating an "immunologically privileged site" in which malignant degeneration may proceed unchecked (89).

Patients may present early with an innocuous-appearing lesion resembling a bruise or patch of cellulitis. Blue, black, or purple nodules and plaques may subsequently appear within the ecchymotic area (90, 91). The lesion may ulcerate later.

Chronic leg ulcers associated with lymphedema may also give rise to angiosarcoma, with firm, hemorrhagic nodules appearing in or around the ulcer itself (80, 92). Long-standing ulcers must be biopsied to rule out malignant transformation.

Of all forms of angiosarcoma, that secondary to vascular stasis appears to have the poorest prognosis and shortest survival time (81). The need for regular inspection and treatment of chronically lymphedematous extremities is, therefore, imperative.

POSTIRRADIATION ANGIOSARCOMA

The physician must always be aware of the possibility of sarcomatous degeneration occurring within the treatment field of patients who have undergone radiotherapy for soft-tissue and osseous neoplasms (75, 81, 93).

Before long-term consequences were known, radiation was accepted treatment for many lower extremity dermatologic conditions including tinea pedis, verruca plantaris, and psoriasis. Elderly patients, in particular, may present with a history of such therapy and must be considered at high risk for developing radiation-induced malignancy.

ANGIOSARCOMA OF DEEP SOFT TISSUE

Angiosarcoma arising in deep soft tissue represents a rare clinical entity. Of 366 cases studied at the Armed Forces Institute of Pathology between 1966 and 1976, Enzinger and Weiss (79) noted 86 neoplasms restricted to deep soft tissue, with 38% of those occurring on the lower extremity.

The tumors may occur at any age, with a male to female predominance of 2:1. Presentation is usually that of a large hemorrhagic mass. Arteriovenous shunting within the lesion is reported (79).

ANGIOSARCOMA OF BONE

Intraosseous angiosarcoma represents a malignant tumor of the vascular precursor cells of bone vessels (94). Angiosarcoma of bone is reported in individuals from age 3 through 74, with a male to female predominance of 2:1 (94).

Favoring the lower extremity, these tumors typically involve the metaphyseal region of long bones (95). Pain and swelling are common presenting symptoms. A history of antecedent trauma may be elicited.

Although periosteal reaction is often absent, plain film radiographs show expansile, osteolytic lesions often described as "soap bubble" in appearance (94, 96, 97, 98). Single or multiple bones may be involved. Nuclear imaging reveals increased uptake at the tumor site. Profuse bleeding can be expected on biopsy (96).

Angiosarcoma of bone shares the uniformly poor prognosis of its soft-tissue counterparts. As with other forms of angiosarcoma, the existence and extent of metastases must be determined at the time of diagnosis.

Diagnosis

Angiosarcomas are frequently heterogenous. Varying degrees of differentiation are noted to occur within the same tumor, with diagnostic features being found only in deeper portions (80, 87). Incisional, shave, or punch biopsies may be misleading. It is imperative, therefore, that suspect neoplasms be excised and biopsied in toto. If size precludes total resection, the surgeon may utilize angiography, CT scanning, or MRI to guide him to the most vascular and, hence, most malignant area of the tumor.

The results of factor VIII-Ag in angiosarcomas are variable and may be related to histologic differentiation and heterogeneity within the tumor. UEA I may be useful in this regard. In a study of 27 angiosarcomas, Ordonez and Batsakis (12) report that, while only 20 specimens showed positive staining with factor VIII-Ag, all stained with UEA I.

Treatment

Local recurrence and early metastases are common (79, 81, 83, 93). Size is suggested as a prognostic indicator, with lesions smaller than 5 cm having a slightly better outlook (79, 81). Ablative surgery, radiation therapy, and chemotherapy are useful in the control of this highly aggressive neoplasm. Reports of success with either one or a combination of modalities, however, are variable and underscore the unpredictability of the disease (70, 83, 93, 95, 96).

Pseudoangiosarcoma

Masson's intravascular hemangioendothelioma (pseudoangiosarcoma) is a benign vascular neoplasm that may be easily mistaken for an angiosarcoma. Clinical and histologic features are strikingly similar. Distinction can be made only on microscopic examination by one who is experienced with both entities. Diagnostic features include papillary growth of hyperplastic endothelial cells supported by delicate fibrous stalks, confined within the vessel lumen (99).

As opposed to the often fatal course of angiosarcoma, pseudoangiosarcoma is invariably benign. Before embarking on a treatment plan, it is, therefore, imperative that a correct diagnosis be made.

Kaposi's Sarcoma

Over the past several years, Kaposi's sarcoma (KS) has achieved the dubious distinction of becoming the single most common malignant vascular neoplasm of the lower extremity (42). Although most often perceived as a manifestation of the human immunodeficiency virus (HIV) infection, four clinical types are recognized: (a) classic (Mediterranean) KS, (b) African KS, (c) KS associated with immunosuppression (other than AIDS), and (d) epidemic (AIDS-related) KS. Although uncertainty exists regarding the cell of origin, endothelial and mesenchymal cells are strongly implicated (100–103).

The occurrence of this malignant, vascular neoplasm is well-documented on the lower extremity (104–109). Lesions of Kaposi's sarcoma are characteristically violaceous in appearance, and generally progress through macular, plaque, and nodular stages. Patients with KS may be at increased risk for developing secondary lymphoreticular malignancies (110). Some studies have noted a high percentage of KS patients with diabetes mellitus and anemia (111). Regression is reported (100, 112–114) and has been ascribed to thrombotic and immunologic factors (100, 112).

CLASSIC KS

First described by Moritz Kaposi in 1972, classic KS favors individuals of Mediterranean and Ashkenazic Jewish heritage (115). Median age of occurrence is 63 yr (50–80 yr old), although there are two reported cases appearing in children of Italian ancestry, unrelated to the acquired immune deficiency syndrome (116, 117). Although there is strong male predominance (15:1), classic KS is reported to occur in females (118).

Lesions often present as firm, violaceous, pea-shaped nodules favoring the foot or lower leg. Increasing in size and number, they may gradually coalesce into large plaques which may later ulcerate.

Patients may complain of pain or feelings of "tightness" in the affected extremity (115). Venous stasis and brawny edema often precede or accompany the lesions and signify infiltration into lymphatics and veins (100, 101). Early lesions may spread along superficial veins and be mistaken for thrombophlebitis (101). Pruritus is also reported (100).

The course of classic KS is usually indolent, although late, widespread cutaneous and visceral involvement may occur (119). Average survival is 13 yr but is comparable to age-matched controls without KS (101, 119). Rarely is the neoplasm solely responsible for death (120).

Of the four clinical types, the nodular form is the most common. Florid, infiltrative, and lymphadenopathic variants, frequently seen in African KS, are less common in European and North American patients (121).

AFRICAN KS

When compared to its Mediterranean counterpart, African KS represents a significantly more aggressive form of the disease. Endemic to much of the continent, it is estimated to account for 9% of all soft-tissue tumors in Kenya and Uganda (122). Blacks are affected more often than non-Blacks (112). Although a male predominance is noted (13:1), a reversal of sex ratios in White populations of South Africa and Nigeria is reported (119).

African KS may present in either nodular, florid, infiltrative or lymphadenopathic forms. Visceral involvement is reported in 10–70% of cases, with the most common site being the bowel (119).

Initial nodules almost always involve the lower extremity. Lesions may undergo spontaneous regression. The disease can remain indolent for years before eventually progressing to the florid stage (123).

Occurring predominantly in patients over 50 yr of age, the florid stage is characterized by fungating, exophytic skin lesions. Infiltration into deep tissue and bone, with spreading to regional lymph nodes, may occur (100, 112, 119, 123, 124). Periods of quiescence may be fol-

lowed by explosive acceleration (100, 119). Function of the affected limb is almost always compromised (123).

The infiltrative form is by far the most aggressive. Tumors penetrate into deep fascia and bone and may even arise within bone and periosteum (124). The affected limb exhibits a characteristic "woody edema" (123). Tumors are large and ulcerative, often becoming secondarily infected. Infiltrative lesions are the most resistant to treatment and carry the poorest prognoses.

The lymphadenopathic form most commonly presents in children and adolescents, with female children and adolescents accounting for 25% of all cases (119). Generalized lymphadenopathy is common and is often the presenting symptom. Visceral involvement may also occur, although cutaneous lesions are rare (112, 119).

Thought to arise from lymphatic endothelium, the lymphadenopathic variant occurs in the same endemic region as Burkitt's lymphoma and may present features indistinguishable from lymphosarcoma (123, 125). Prognosis is poor, with survival estimated at only 2–3 yr (112).

EPIDEMIC KAPOSI'S (EKS)

It is estimated that 30% of patients with AIDS will develop Kaposi's sarcoma (126). Lesions of EKS (AIDS-related Kaposi's) differ markedly in appearance and distribution from those of Mediterranean or African types. Lesions may occur anywhere on the body surface (127), although they have been observed to frequently follow the lines of cleavage as seen in pityriasis rosea (128).

Lesions may arise internally either with or without cutaneous involvement, and are described in all organs except the brain (129). Forty to fifty percent of EKS patients are found to have gastrointestinal involvement and 35% have hepatic involvement at autopsy (130, 131). Pulmonary lesions are reported in 30–40% of EKS cases (130, 131). Symptoms of organ involvement include fever, anorexia, gastrointestinal hemorrhage and diarrhea (119), but since patients with EKS may have these symptoms secondary to other manifestations of AIDS, they are of little diagnostic value.

Cutaneous lesions usually begin as small, flat, pink patches, becoming raised and violaceous later. Size ranges from a few millimeters to several centimeters. Patients may present with either single or multiple lesions.

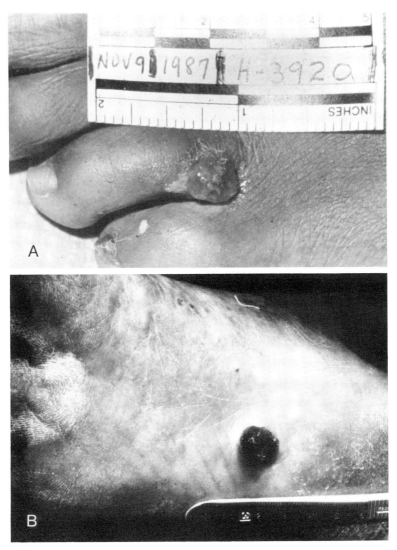

Figure 5.2.   A, solitary lesion of Kaposi's sarcoma in a young homosexual male. The patient was otherwise asymptomatic and unaware of his positive HIV status. (Courtesy of Donnamarie Stewart DPM). **B,** 60-year-old White male with friable violaceous nodule of Kaposi's sarcoma on the plantar aspect of the right foot. History of blood transfusion 6 yr prior; the patient refused HIV testing. (From Cohen EJ, Cole D, Stewart DM, Weiss G, Kosinski M, Giorgini R. Kaposi's sarcoma of the lower extremity as the first sign of AIDS. J Am Podiatr Med Assoc 1990;80:127–134.)

Lesions may also appear pedunculated and friable, giving the appearance of a pyogenic granuloma. Cohen et al. (105), report 4 cases of primary EKS appearing as solitary granulomatous lesions on the foot as the first clinical manifestation of HIV infection (105) (Fig. 5.2).

The course of EKS is variable, dependent largely upon the extent of the tumor, organ system involved, and the degree of impairment of the immune system. Spontaneous regression of EKS lesions has been reported (113–114).

Lowenthal et al. (129) notes that, while some patients undergo an indolent course, others may experience explosive, fulminant disease with multisystem involvement. The mean survival for patients with EKS has been reported to be 18–22 months (129). The patient with AIDS, however, is more likely to succumb to diseases other than Kaposi's sarcoma (119).

KS IN IATROGENICALLY IMMUNOSUPPRESSED INDIVIDUALS

KS developing in iatrogenically immunosuppressed individuals has been well-documented. Most commonly described in renal transplant recipients, it has also been reported in patients with systemic lupus erythematosus, lymphoid malignancies, and autoimmune diseases (101, 132, 133).

Discontinuance of immunosuppressive therapy has been reported to result in spontaneous regression of KS lesions (133). The occurrence of KS in this patient population strengthens the hypothesis that the disease may be immunologically linked.

ETIOLOGY

The precise etiology of Kaposi's sarcoma is unknown. Safai (119) suggests the cause to be multifactorial, occurring as a result of one or a combination of genetic factors, environmental factors, infectious agents, and immune suppression. Marmor et al. (134), suggest that patients with a genetic predisposition to KS require less immunodeficiency to express the disease than patients without. Studies of histocompatibility antigens suggest an increased frequency of HLA-DR5 among classic, African, and EKS patients (120, 135).

A serologic association between cytomegalovirus infection and KS is seen in American, African, and European patients (128, 136, 137). Renal transplant recipients also appear to have high incidences of cytomegalovirus infection. As suggested by Safai and Anhalt, persistent infection with a retrovirus in genetically susceptible patients with abnormal immune function may also play a role in the development of KS (120).

DIAGNOSIS

Lesions of KS may mimic other vascular and nonvascular neoplasms. Biopsy alone is diagnostic. Interweaving bands of spindle cells and vascular structures, encased in a reticular and collagen fiber framework, characterize this vascular neoplasm. Extravasated red blood cells and hemosiderin deposits may be seen between spindle cells. The histopathology of Kaposi's sarcoma in viscera and lymph nodes is similar to that seen in the skin (100, 101).

Factor VIII-Ag is noted to be present in KS specimens (138), although some reports state the contrary (139). Angiographic findings for KS consist of fine, interwoven vascular channels with arteriovenous shunting and an accelerated venous phase (19).

TREATMENT

Patients with small, stable, asymptomatic lesions of the lower extremity require no specific treatment (129). Local excision may be performed for cosmesis. However in EKS, where lesions tend to be multifocal, excision for reasons other than biopsy may be impractical. Clinicians should observe the disease for progression and be aware that, particularly in EKS, patients presenting with one or two cutaneous lesions may have extensive internal involvement.

In those patients with significant lower extremity involvement, or in whom lesions are painful or disfiguring or interfere with function, several effective treatment modalities exist.

Radiotherapy is the treatment of choice for localized, nodular KS (101, 123). However, side effects of radiation in an already immuno-compromised patient, as well as the possibility of recurrence, must be considered. Lesions of Kaposi's sarcoma are highly radiosensitive. Patients with nonepidemic KS have shown complete remission in 93–100% of cases (129).

For patients with invasive or disseminated forms of the disease, and for widespread EKS, chemotherapy is recommended (123, 129). Response rates of up to 25% in EKS patients and up to 80% in non-EKS patients are reported with single-agent vinca alkaloid therapy (129, 140, 141).

Combination chemotherapy has been tried with the aim of reducing side effects while maintaining efficacy. Vinblastine-vincristine regimens are successful in this regard. Combination chemotherapy in advanced EKS patients, however, is found to result in an extremely high rate of opportunistic infections (129). Optimal chemotherapy has yet to be defined.

Although still experimental, administration of biologic response modifiers, (e.g., interleukin or recombinant α-interferon) shows promising results.

Mitsuyasu (132) notes that while tumor stage has no prognostic significance in terms of response to interferon therapy, patients with fever, weight loss and opportunistic infection exhibit a poorer response to therapy. Other investigators (132, 142) likewise suggest that response to interferon therapy may depend on the state of the immune system at the time of treatment. Response of EKS to interferon is reported to be approximately 20–40% (79, 101, 129).

Pseudo-Kaposi's Sarcoma

Known also as acroangiodermatitis of Mali (143) or acroangiodermatitis of Bluefarb (144), pseudo-Kaposi's sarcoma may present in a form clinically indistinguishable from Kaposi's sarcoma itself. It is however, totally benign.

Pseudo-Kaposi's sarcoma favors the lower leg, ankle, and dorsum of the foot. The lesions are violaceous, and characteristically resemble the patch stage of KS. They may coalesce to form plaques and nodules. The etiology is an underlying arteriovenous malformation of either congenital or traumatic origin. As such, pain, warmth, edema, stasis changes, bruits and a palpable thrill may accompany cutaneous lesions. Angiography will establish the presence of an arteriovenous malformation (145). Very occasionally, pseudo-Kaposi's sarcoma is described in association with the Klippel-Trenaunay syndrome (146).

Definitive diagnosis is by histologic examination. Both KS and pseudo-Kaposi's sarcoma have vascular spaces lined by increased numbers of oval and spindle cells. Ackerman et al. (147) notes that pseudo-Kaposi's sarcoma exhibits thick-walled vessels lined by plump endothelial cells, with vascular spaces being round to oval.

In an age where one may be quick to assign a diagnosis of Kaposi's sarcoma on the basis of history and appearance alone, the physician must be aware of the existence of more innocuous differentials.

REFERENCES

1. Backwinkel K, Diddams J. Hemangiopericytoma, report of a case and comprehensive review of the literature. Cancer 1970;25:896–901.
2. Branham HH. Aneurysmal varix of the femoral artery and vein. Int J Surg 1890;3:250–255.
3. Fitzpatrick TB. Fundamentals of dermatologic diagnosis. In: Fitzpatrick TB, ed. Dermatology in general medicine. New York: McGraw-Hill, 1979:10–37.
4. McMasters M, Soule E, Ivins J. Hemangiopericytoma, a clinicopathologic study and long term followup of 60 patients. Cancer 1975;36:2232–2244.
5. Enzinger FM, Weiss SW. Hemangioendothelioma: vascular tumors of intermediate malignancy. In: Enzinger FM, Weiss SW, eds. Soft tissue tumors. St Louis: Mosby, 1988:533–544.
6. Enzinger FM, Smith BH. Hemangiopericytoma, an analysis of 106 cases. Hum Pathol 1976;7:61–82.
7. Girard C, Johnson WC, Graham JH. Cutaneous angiosarcoma. Cancer 1970;26:868–883.
8. Arnn ET, Yam LT, Li CY. Systemic angioendotheliomatosis presenting with hemolytic anemia. Am J Clin Pathol 1983;80:246–251.
9. Kwan TH, Mihm MC. The skin. In: Robbins SL, Cotran RS, eds. Pathologic basis of disease. Philadelphia: Saunders, 1979:1417–1461.
10. Straub PW, Kessler S, Schreiber A, Frick PG. Chronic intravascular coagulation in Kasabach-Merritt syndrome. Arch Intern Med 1972;129:475–478.
11. Enzinger FM, Weiss SW. Immunohistochemistry of soft tissue lesions. In: Enzinger FM, Weiss SW, eds. Soft tissue tumors. St Louis: Mosby, 1988:83–100.
12. Ordonez N, Batsakis J. Comparison of Ulex europaeus I lectin and factor VIII-related antigen in vascular lesions. Arch Pathol Lab Med 1984;108:129–132.
13. Holthofer H, Virtanen I, Kariniemi L, Hormia M, Linder E, Miettinen A. Ulex europaeus I lectin as a marker for human vascular endothelium in human tissues. Lab Invest 1982;47:60–66.
14. Johnson EW, Ghormley RK, Dockerty MB. Hemangiomas of the extremities. Surg Gynecol Obstet 1956;102:531–538.
15. Jones RW, Roberts RE. Calcification, decalcification and deossification. Br J Surg 1934;21:461–499.
16. Hoeffel JC, Chardot C, Parache R, Brauer B, Delagoutte J, Henry M. Radiologic patterns of hemangiopericytoma of the leg. Am J Surg 1972;123:591–593.
17. Alpern MB, Thorsen MK, Kellman GM, Pojunas K, Lawson TL. CT appearance of hemangiopericytoma. J Comput Assist Tomogr 1986;10:264–267.
18. Levin DC, Watson RC, Baltaxe HA. Arteriography in diagnosis and management of peripheral soft tissue masses. Radiology 1972;103:53–58.
19. Wechsler HL. Kaposi's sarcoma, angiographic findings before and after orthovoltage treatment. Arch Dermatol 1967;96:69–70.
20. Sutton D, Pratt AE. Angiography of hemangiopericytoma. Clin Radiol 1967;18:324–329.
21. Margulis A, Murphy TO. Arteriography in neoplasms of the extremities. AJR 1958;80:330–339.
22. Sterner B, Wickbom I. Angiography in 3 cases of muscle rupture with organizing haematoma. Acta Radiol 1966;4:169–178.
23. Rauch R, Silverman P, Korobkin M, Dunnick NR, Moore AV, Wertman D, et al. Computed tomography of benign angiomatous lesions of the extremities. J Comput Assist Tomogr 1984;8:1143–1146.
24. Hermann GH, Rose JS. Computed tomography in bone and soft tissue pathology of the extremities. J Comput Assist Tomogr 1979;3:58–66.
25. Chang AE, Rosenberg SA. Clinical evaluation and treatment of soft tissue tumors. In: En-

zinger FM, Weiss SW, eds. Soft tissue tumors. St. Louis: Mosby, 1988:19–42.

26. Kaplan PA, Williams SM. Mucocutaneous and peripheral soft tissue hemangiomas: MR imaging. Radiology 1987;163:163–166.

27. Cohen JM, Weinreb JC, Redman HC. Arteriovenous malformations of the extremities: MR imaging. Radiology 1986;158:475–479.

28. Madewell JE, Moser RP. Radiologic evaluation of soft tissue tumors. In: Enzinger FM, Weiss SW, eds. Soft tissue tumors. St. Louis: Mosby, 1988:43–82.

29. Enzinger FM, Weiss SW. Benign tumors and tumorlike lesions of blood vessels. In: Enzinger FM, Weiss SW, eds. Soft tissue tumors. St. Louis: Mosby, 1988:489–532.

30. Miller SJ, Patton GW, Xenos D, Wulf MR. Multiple capillary hemangiomas of the foot with associated phleboliths, a case report. J Am Podiatr Med Assoc 1980;70:364–369.

31. Fulton MN, Sosman MC. Venous angiomas of skeletal muscle, report of four cases. J Am Med Assoc 1942;119:319–324.

32. Cortese CJ. Cavernous hemangioma of the foot. J Foot Surg 1976;15:72–76.

33. Simon M. Benign hemangioma: a case report. J Foot Surg 1977;16:157–161.

34. Borden JI, Shea TP. Cavernous hemangioma of the foot, a case report and review. J Am Podiatr Assoc 1976;66:484–490.

35. From L. Vascular neoplasms, pseudoneoplasms and hyperplasias. In: Fitzpatrick TB, ed. Dermatology in general medicine. New York: McGraw-Hill, 1979;725–742.

36. Rowe L. Granuloma pyogenicum, differential diagnosis. Arch Dermatol 1958;78:341–347.

37. Zaynoun ST, Juljulian HH, Kurban AK. Pyogenic granuloma with multiple satellites. Arch Dermatol 1974;109:689–691.

38. Coskey RJ, Mehregan AH. Granuloma pyogenicum with multiple satellite recurrences. Arch Dermatol 1967;96:71–73.

39. Cooper PH, McAllister HA, Helwig EB. Intravenous pyogenic granuloma, a study of 18 cases. Am J Surg Pathol 1979;3:221–228.

40. Esterly NB. Hemangiomas. In: Madden S, ed. Current dermatologic therapy. Philadelphia: Saunders, 1982:206–208.

41. Berlin SJ. A laboratory review of 67,000 foot tumors and lesions. J Am Podiatr Assoc 1984;74:341–347.

42. Pack GT, Miller TR. Hemangiomas: classification, diagnosis and treatment. Angiology 1950;1:406–426.

43. Shallow TA, Eger SA, Wagner FB Jr. Primary hemangiomatous tumors of skeletal muscle. Ann Surg 1944;119:700–740.

44. Jenkins HP, Delaney PA. Benign angiomatous tumors of skeletal muscles. Surg Gynecol Obstet 1932;55:464–480.

45. Imperial R, Helwig EB. Verrucous hemangioma, a clinicopathologic study of 21 cases. Arch Dermatol 1967;96:247–253.

46. Lynch PJ. Localized cutaneous angiokeratomas. In: Madden S, ed. Current dermatologic therapy. Philadelphia: Saunders, 1982:33–34.

47. Fretzin DF, Potter B. Blue rubber bleb nevus.

48. Baskerville PA, Ackroyd JS, Thomas ML, Browse NL. The Klippel-Trenaunay syndrome: clinical, radiological and hemodynamic features and management. Br J Surg 1985;72:232–236.

49. Baskerville PA, Ackroyd JS, Browse NL. The etiology of the Klippel-Trenaunay syndrome. Ann Surg 1985;202:624–627.

50. Robbins SL, Cotran RS. Blood vessels. In: Robbins SL, Cotran RS, eds. Pathologic basis of disease. Philadelphia: Saunders, 1979:393–642.

51. Forrest J, Staple TW. Synovial hemangioma of the knee, demonstration by arthrography and arteriography. AJR 1978;112:512–516.

52. Larsen IJ, Landry RM. Hemangioma of the synovial membrane. J Bone Joint Surg (Am) 1969;51:1210–1212.

53. Hajdu SI. Tumors of vessels. In: Hajdu SI, ed. Pathology of soft tissue tumors. Philadelphia: Lea & Febiger, 1979:367–425.

54. Huestron JT. Multiple painless glomus tumors. Br Med J 1961;1:1210–1212.

55. Heifitz NM. Surgical excision and discussion of rearfoot glomangioma, a case report. J Am Podiatr Med Assoc 1977;67:427–428.

56. Lumley JSP, Stansfeld AG. Infiltrating glomus tumor of the lower limb. Br Med J 1972;1:484–485.

57. Murray MR, Stout AP. The glomus tumor, investigation of its behavior, and the identity of its "epitheloid" cell. Am J Pathol 1942;18:183–195.

58. Alberts DF. Glomus tumor, a case report. J Am Podiatr Assoc 1971;61:23.

59. Smyth M. Glomus-cell tumors in the lower extremity, report of two cases. J Bone Joint Surg (Am) 1971;53:157–159.

60. Love JG. Glomus tumors; diagnosis and treatment. Proc Staff Meet Mayo Clin 1944;19:113–116.

61. Hildreth DH. The ischemia test for glomus tumor: a new diagnostic test. Rev Surg 1970;27:147–148.

62. Brenner MA, Kalish SR. Glomus tumors with special reference to children's feet. J Am Podiatr Assoc 1978;68:715–720.

63. Harris WR. Erosion of bone produced by glomus tumor. Can Med Assoc J 1954;70:684–685.

64. Galinski AW, Vlahos M. Glomus tumor or glomangioma in podiatric medicine. J Am Podiatr Med Assoc 1975;65:167–170.

65. Quigley JT. A glomus tumor of the heel pad, a case report. J Bone Joint Surg (Am) 1979;61:443–444.

66. Symmers W. Glomus tumors. Br Med J 1973;2:50–51.

67. Enzinger FM, Weiss SW. Glomus tumors. In: Enzinger FM, Weiss SW, eds. Soft tissue tumors. St. Louis: Mosby, 1988;581–595.

68. Stout AP. Tumors featuring pericytes: glomus tumor and hemangiopericytoma. Lab Invest 1956;5:217–233.

69. Tsuneyoshi M, Daimaru Y, Enjoji M. Malignant hemangiopericytoma and other sarcomas with hemangiopericytoma-like pattern. Pathol Res Pract 1984;178:446–453.

Arch Intern Med 1965;116:924–929.

70. Dorfman HD, Steiner GC, Jaffee HL. Vascular tumors of bone. Hum Pathol 1971;2:349–376.

71. Aguste LJ, Razack MS, Sako K. Hemangiopericytoma. J Surg Oncol 1982;20:260–264.

72. Pfleger L, Tappeiner J. Zur Kenntnis der systemisierten Endotheliomatose der cutanen Blutgefasse (Reticuloendotheliosen?). Hautarzt 1959;10:359–363.

73. Braverman IM, Lerner AB. Diffuse malignant proliferation of vascular endothelium, a possible new clinical and pathological entity. Arch Dermatol 1961;84:22–30.

74. Kauh YC, McFarland JP, Carnabuci GG, Luscombe HA. Malignant proliferating angioendotheliomatosis. Arch Dermatol 1980;116:803–806.

75. Lever WF, Schaumburg-Lever G. Tumors of vascular tissue. In: Lever WF, Schaumburg-Lever G, eds. Histopathology of the skin. Philadelphia: Lippincott, 1983:623–651.

76. Fievez M, Fievez C, Hustin J. Proliferating systematized angioendotheliomatosis. Arch Dermatol 1971;104:320–324.

77. Dominguez FE, Rosen LB, Kramer HC. Malignant angioendotheliomatosis proliferans, report of an autopsied case studied with immunoperoxidase. Am J Dermatopathol 1986;8:419–425.

78. Scott PW, Silvers DN, Helwig EB. Proliferating angioendotheliomatosis. Arch Pathol 1975;99:323–326.

79. Enzinger FM, Weiss SW. Malignant vascular tumors. In: Enzinger FM, Weiss SW, eds. Soft tissue tumors. St. Louis: Mosby, 1988:545–580.

80. Kofler H, Pichler E, Romani N, Philadelphy H, Fritsch P. Hemangiosarcoma in chronic leg ulcers. Arch Dermatol 1988;124:1080–1082.

81. Maddox JC, Evans HL. Angiosarcoma of skin and soft tissue, a study of forty-four cases. Cancer 1981;48:1907–1921.

82. Capo V, Ozzello L, Fenoglio CM, Lombardi L, Rilke F. Angiosarcomas arising in edematous extremities: immunostaining for factor VIII-related antigen and ultrastructural features. Hum Pathol 1985;16:144–150.

83. Morales PH, Lindberg RD, Barkley HT. Soft tissue angiosarcomas. J Radiat Oncol Biol Physiol 1981;7:1655–1659.

84. Stewart FW, Treves N. Lymphangiosarcoma in post mastectomy lymphedema. Cancer 1948;1:64–81.

85. Hodgkinson DJ, Soule EH, Woods JE. Cutaneous angiosarcomas of the head and neck. Cancer 1979;44:1106–1113.

86. Schmitz-Rixen T, Horsch S, Arnold G, Peters PE. Angiosarcoma in primary lymphedema of the lower extremity: Stewart-Treves syndrome. Lymphology 1984;17:50–53.

87. Martorell F. Tumorigenic lymphedema. Angiology 1951;2:386–392.

88. Kettle EH. Tumors arising from endothelium. Proc R Soc Med 1918;11:19–34.

89. Schreiber H, Barry FM, Russell WC, Mason W., Ponsky J, Pories W. Stewart-Treves syndrome, a lethal complication of post mastectomy lymphedema and regional immune deficiency. Arch Surg 1979;114:82–85.

90. McBride CM, Reeder JW, Smith JL. Angiosarcoma in the lymphedematous limb. South Med J 1969;62:378–380.

91. Gajraj H, Barker SG. Lymphangiosarcoma complicating chronic primary lymphoedema. Br J Surg 1987;74:1190.

92. Halkier-Sorensen L, Kjeldsen H, Foged E, Sogaard H. Angiosarcoma of the leg, a case report. Acta Derm Venereol (Stockh) 1986;120(suppl):93–95.

93. Rosai J, Sumner HW, Kostianovsky M, Perez-Mesa C. Angiosarcoma of the skin, a clinicopathologic and fine structural study. Hum Pathol 1976;7:83–109.

94. Salmassi S, Zarabi MZ, Navato C. Multicentric angiosarcoma of the tarsal and metatarsal bones, a case report and literature review. Mo Med 1985;82:304–307.

95. Campanacci M, Boriani S, Giunti A. Hemangioendothelioma of bone, a study of 29 cases. Cancer 1980;46:804–814.

96. Bundens WD, Brighton CT. Malignant hemangioendothelioma of bone, report of two cases and review of the literature. J Bone Joint Surg (Am) 1965;47:762–772.

97. Bohn LE. Diagnosis: multicentric angiosarcoma of bone involving the right lower extremity. Skeletal Radiol 1982;8:303–305.

98. Cohen M, Polakof S, Vivas W. Angiosarcoma affecting the bones of the lower extremities, a case report. J Am Podiatr Assoc 1987;77:297–302.

99. Kuo T, Sayers C, Sayers P, Rosai J. Masson's "vegetant intravascular hemangioendothelioma": a lesion often mistaken for angiosarcoma. Cancer 1976;38:1227–1236.

100. Safai B, Good RA. Kaposi's sarcoma: a review and recent developments. Clin Bull (Mem Sloan-Kettering Cancer Cent) 1980;10:62–68.

101. Mitsuyasu RT, Groopman JE. Biology and therapy of Kaposi's sarcoma. Semin Oncol 1984;11:53–59.

102. Mustakallio KK, Levonen E, Raekallio J. Histochemistry of Kaposi's sarcoma. I. Hydrolases and phosphorylase. Exp Mol Pathol 1963;2:303–316.

103. Loring WE, Wolman SR. Idiopathic multiple hemorrhagic sarcoma of the lung (Kaposi's sarcoma). NY State J Med 1965;65:668–676.

104. Shilling GA, Black JR. Kaposi's sarcoma of the lower extremity, a case report. J Am Podiatr Med Assoc 1987;77:89–92.

105. Cohen EJ, Cole D, Stewart DM, Weiss G, Kosinski M, Giorgini R. Kaposi's sarcoma of the lower extremity as the first sign of AIDS. J Am Podiatr Med Assoc 1990;80:127–134.

106. Footer R. Kaposi's sarcoma. J Am Podiatr Assoc 1978;68:712–714.

107. David D, Glaser PR. Kaposi's sarcoma of the foot, a six year followup. J Am Podiatr Assoc 1983;4:214–216.

108. Stern D, Jacobs C. Kaposi's sarcoma, a digital case and literature review. J Am Podiatr Assoc 1981;71:694–697.

109. Richter PA, Black JR. Recurring Kaposi's sarcoma of the foot, a case report. J Am Podiatr Assoc 1985;75:162–165.

110. Ulbright TM, Santa Cruz DJ. Kaposi's sarcoma: relationship with hematologic, lymphoid, and thymic neoplasia. Cancer 1981;47:963–973.

111. Hurlbut WB, Lincoln CS Jr. Multiple hemorrhagic sarcoma and diabetes mellitus. Arch Intern Med 1949;84:738–750.

112. Safai B, Weiss H. Clinical manifestations of Kaposi's sarcoma. In: Pearl MA, Armstrong D, eds. The acquired immune deficiency syndrome, and infections of homosexual men. New York: York Medical Books, 1984:210–224.

113. Janier M, Vignon MD, Cottenot F. Spontaneously healing Kaposi's sarcoma in AIDS; correspondence. N Engl J Med 1985;312: 1638–1639.

114. Real FX, Krown SE. Spontaneous regression of Kaposi's sarcoma in patients with AIDS; correspondence. N Engl J Med 1985;313:1659.

115. Kaposi M. Idiopathic multiple pigmented sarcoma of the skin. Arch Dermatol Syphillis 1872; 4:265–273. Translated from the German for C-A Cancer Journal for Clinicians, vol. 32 no. 6, p. 342–347, 1982, and reprinted from Archiv Für Dermatologie Und Syphillis 4:265–273, 1872.

116. Bisceglia M, Amini M, Borman C. Primary Kaposi's sarcoma of the lymph node in children. Cancer 1988;61:1715–1718.

117. Dutz W, Stout AP. Kaposi's sarcoma in infants and children. Cancer 1960;13:684–694.

118. Laor Y, Schwartz RA. Epidemiologic aspects of American Kaposi's sarcoma. J Surg Oncol 1979;12:299–303.

119. Safai B. Pathophysiology and epidemiology of epidemic Kaposi's sarcoma. Semin Oncol 1987;14:7–12.

120. Safai B, Anhalt TS. Kaposi's sarcoma. Semin Dermatol 1984;3:69–77.

121. Rothman S. Some clinical aspects of Kaposi's sarcoma in the European and North American populations. Acta Un Int Cancer 1962;18: 364–371.

122. Dorfman RF. Kaposi's sarcoma revisited. Hum Pathol 1984;15:1013–1017.

123. Ziegler JL, Tempelton AC, Vogel CL. Kaposi's sarcoma: a comparison of classical, endemic and epidemic forms. Semin Oncol 1984;11: 47–52.

124. Tempelton A. Kaposi's sarcoma. Pathol Annu 1981;16:315–336.

125. Olweny CLM, Kaddumukasa A, Atine I, Owor R, Magrath I, Ziegler JL. Childhood Kaposi's sarcoma, clinical features and therapy. Br J Cancer 1976;33:555–563.

126. Giraldo G, Beth E, Buonaqurao FM. Kaposi's sarcoma: a natural model of interrelationships between viruses, immunologic responses, genetics, and oncogenesis. Antibiot Chemother 1984;32:1–11.

127. Laurence J. Dermatologic manifestations of HIV infection. Infect Surg 1987;6:488–496.

128. Myskowski PL, Romano JF, Safai B. Kaposi's sarcoma in young homosexual men. Cutis 1983;29:31–34.

129. Lowenthal DA, Safai B, Koziner B. Malignant neoplasia in AIDS. Infect Surg 1987;6: 413–420.

130. Niedt G, Schinella RA. Acquired immunodeficiency syndrome: clinicopathologic study of 56 autopsies. Arch Pathol Lab Med 1985;109: 727–734.

131. Hui AN, Koss MN, Meyer PR. Necropsy findings in acquired immunodeficiency syndrome: a comparison of premortem diagnosis with postmortem findings. Hum Pathol 1984;15: 670–676.

132. Mitsuyasu RT. Clinical variants and staging of Kaposi's sarcoma. Semin Oncol 1987;14(suppl 3):13–18.

133. Harwood AR, Osoba D, Hofstader SL, Goldstein MB, Cardella CJ, Holecek MJ, et al. Kaposi's sarcoma in recipients of renal transplants. Am J Med 1979;67:759–765.

134. Marmor M, Friedman-Kiev A, Zoller-Pazner S, Stahl R, Rubinstein P, Lauberstein L, et al. Kaposi's sarcoma in homosexual men. Ann Intern Med 1984;100:809–815.

135. Pollack MS, Safai B, Myskowski PL, Gold JW, Pandey JW, Dupont B. Frequency of HLA and Gm immunogenic markers in Kaposi's sarcoma. Tissue Antigens 1983;21:1–8.

136. Giraldo G, Beth E, Henle W, Kourilsky F, Henle G, Niké V, et al. Antibody patterns to herpes viruses in Kaposi's sarcoma: serological association of European Kaposi's sarcoma with cytomegalovirus. Int J Cancer 1975;15: 839–848.

137. Giraldo G, Beth E, Henle W, et al. Antibody patterns to herpes viruses in Kaposi's sarcoma. II. Serological association of American Kaposi's sarcoma with cytomegalovirus. Int J Cancer 1979;22:126–131.

138. Guarda LG, Silva EG, Ordonez NG, Smith JL. Factor VIII in Kaposi's sarcoma. Am J Pathol 1981;76:197–200.

139. Millard PR, Yeryet AR. An immunohistochemical study of factor VIII-related antigen and Kaposi's sarcoma using polyclonal and monoclonal antibodies. J Pathol 1985; 146:31–38.

140. Volberding P, Conant MA, Striker RB, Lewis B. Chemotherapy in advanced Kaposi's sarcoma. Am J Med 1983;74:652–656.

141. Volberding P, Abrams DI, Conant M, Kaslow K, Vranizan K, Ziesler J. Vinblastine therapy for Kaposi's sarcoma in the acquired immunodeficiency syndrome. Ann Intern Med 1985; 103:335–338.

142. Krown SE. The role of interferon in the therapy of epidemic Kaposi's sarcoma. Semin Oncol 1987;14:27–33.

143. Mali JW, Kuiper JP, Hamera AA. Acroangiodermatitis of the foot. Arch Dermatol 1964; 92:515–518.

144. Bluefarb SM, Adama LA. Arteriovenous malformation with angiodermatitis, stasis dermatitis simulating Kaposi's disease. Arch Dermatol 1967;96:176–181.

145. Marshall ME, Hatfield ST, Hatfield DR. Arteriovenous malformation simulating Kaposi's sarcoma (pseudo-Kaposi's sarcoma). Arch Dermatol 1985;121:99–101.

146. Kofoed ML, Klemp P, Thestrup-Pedersen K. The Klippel-Trenaunay syndrome with acroangiodermatitis (pseudo-Kaposi's sarcoma).

Acta Derm Venereol (Stockh) 1985;65:75–77.
147. Ackerman AB, Trot JL, Rosen LB, Jerasutus S, White CR, King CR. Pseudo-Kaposi's sarcoma (acroangiodermatitis) vs. Kaposi's sarcoma, plaque stage. In: Ackerman AB, ed. Differential diagnosis in dermatopathology. II. Philadelphia: Lea & Febiger, 1988;98–101.

Part B/ **Muscle**

—C. Harris

Tumors of muscle affecting the foot and leg are associated with smooth and skeletal muscles, exclusively. However, in order to appreciate the differences in evolution and structure of benign and malignant muscle tumors, it is necessary to understand the development and structure of normal muscle tissue.

Normal muscle primarily derives its origin from cells produced in primitive mesenchyme. The cells differentiate along two lines: (a) loosely arranged cells, called fibroblasts, produce collagen, and (b) oval-shaped cells, called myoblasts, with centrally placed nuclei and granular eosinophilic cytoplasm, can form a leiomyoblast or rhabdomyoblast that subsequently gives rise to smooth and striated muscles, respectively (1).

Smooth, or involuntary, muscle is under the control of the autonomic nervous system and usually forms layers of fibers in the walls of tubular structures, such as blood vessels, the uterus, or the trachea. In addition, it forms the pilar arrector muscles of the skin and muscles associated with some glands, e.g., the sweat, lacrimal, and salivary glands. Moreover, smooth muscle consists of individual cells that have a tapered shape and possess centrally located cylindrical nuclei. Thus, a fusiform or tapered muscle cell is usually termed a fiber. Muscle tissue is composed of both muscle and connective tissue fibers. Surrounding the muscle fiber is a connective tissue sheath called the sarcolemma. Muscle fibers, with the capacity to contract and relax, are considered living cells, whereas connective tissue cells are non-living. The size of a muscle cell varies depending upon its location. The ones that encircle very small blood vessels measure approximately 20 μm. Smooth muscle that encompasses the walls of the uterus is reported to be the longest, approximately 0.5 m. The average length, however, of a smooth muscle cell is 2.0 mm. The chief role of smooth muscle is maintenance of muscle tone in blood vessels and the initiation of slow rhythmic contractions in tubular systems, such as the uterus or gastrointestinal tract.

Striated, or skeletal, muscle is appropriately named because of its inherent cross-striations visible under the microscope and its attachment to various components of the human skeleton. In contrast to smooth muscle, striated muscle cells are multinucleated, with peripherally located nuclei. The fibers are much larger and cylindrical. Striated muscle fibers are enclosed in a cell membrane, the sarcolemma that becomes electrically charged when stimulated and initiates muscle contraction. The contractile components contained within each muscle fiber are the myofibrils, which are found in a nutrient-rich environment, called the sarcoplasm, that is analogous to the cytoplasm in other cells. Each myofibril contains two types of smaller filaments termed myofilaments. These ultrastructural filaments are of various lengths and thicknesses, and are called actin and myosin filaments, the former being represented by lightly shaded bands and the latter by thick, darkly shaded bands. The bands associated with striated muscle interdigitate during muscle contraction and thereby initiate voluntary movement of skeletal components, e.g., extension of the upper arm or flexion of the foot on the leg.

Gross movements initiated by skeletal muscle are essential for growth and development during the entire postnatal growing period of each and every muscle fiber. In addition, muscles enlarge in width and length during the postnatal growth period. The mechanisms responsible for this development are an increase of myofilaments synthesized by ribosomes in the sarcoplasm and the production of new sarcomeres that are added to new myofibrils at the muscle-tendon junction, ultimately lengthening the muscle.

As stated above, muscle tissue consists of muscle cells and connective tissue. The outermost, or external, covering of connective tissue of a muscle is referred to as the epimysium. The next type divides a muscle into separate bundles and constitutes the perimysium because it surrounds bundles of fibers. The last and innermost covering of connective tissue envelopes individual myofibrils and is termed endomysium (2).

Now, attention may be directed toward the pathologic aspect of muscle tissue, specifically muscle neoplasms. Neoplasms of muscle originate from both smooth and striated muscles. In addition, they can be subdivided into benign and malignant types.

The group of tumors comprised of striated muscle can be subdivided into two general categories depending on its site of origin. Those arising directly from a constituent element of muscle are primary, whereas those arising by way of metastases or by direct extension from an adjacent neoplasm are secondary (3).

Neoplasms of smooth muscle origin include leiomyomas (multiple cutaneous), leiomyoma (solitary cutaneous or localized to deep soft tissue), angioleiomyoma (vascular), and leiomyosarcoma (cutaneous, subcutaneous, vascular, or osseous). Neoplasms derived from striated muscle include rhabdomyoma, rhabdomyosarcoma (embryonal), rhabdomyosarcoma (botryoid), rhabdomyosarcoma (alveolar), and rhabdomyosarcoma (pleomorphic). In addition, several neoplasms merit discussion because of their similar histologic picture (myoblastoma or granular cell tumor) or because they are classified as tumor-like disorders of muscle (myositis ossificans) (4).

Leiomyomas are benign, neoplastic lesions derived from smooth muscle with a diameter that varies in size from a few millimeters to several centimeters. They are most often found in the uterus and are referred to as "fibroids." When they are localized in other areas of the body, i.e., the foot or leg, the site of origin derives from the arrector pilorum muscles of hair follicles, sweat glands, or cutaneous and subcutaneous blood vessels (5, 6).

Clinically, leiomyomas are firm nodules with a color that ranges from white to pearly gray. Superficial cutaneous leiomyomas tend to be nonencapsulated and attached to the overlying skin. In contrast, subcutaneous leiomyomas tend to be encapsulated and freely movable under the skin. On examination, the most striking clinical feature pertaining to solitary and subcutaneous leiomyomas is nonradiating pain originating from the neoplasm itself. The sudden onset of pain may be precipitated by weather changes, trauma, the menstrual cycle, exercise, and even fatigue. Having attained its maximum size, the proliferative activity of the tumor ceases, but the paroxysmal symptoms of pain continue (7, 8). Moreover, pain and tenderness appear to be associated with lesions of sufficient size that penetrate to the level of the subcutaneous fat (9).

On macroscopic examination, the lesions appear as sharply demarcated circumscribed nodules. Microscopically, leiomyomas are composed of hypocellular masses of interlacing bundles of smooth muscle cells without cytologic atypia (7).

Although once thought to be extremely uncommon in the lower extremity, the literature now states that leiomyomas are not exceptionally rare. They do occur in the foot and leg, associated with hair follicles on the skin as well as small and large blood vessels. Leiomyomas do develop in the walls of large veins and, less frequently, in large arteries (10, 11).

LEIOMYOMA (MULTIPLE CUTANEOUS)

The most common tumor of smooth muscle origin found in the skin, multiple cutaneous leiomyoma, originates from the arrector pilorum muscles. Although of unknown etiology, the neoplasm shows a familial predisposition possibly inherited as an autosomal dominant trait. It is associated with dermatitis herpetiformis and the surface antigen HLA-8. According to the literature, this cutaneous lesion makes its appearance during adolescence, early adult life, or, occasionally appears at birth or during infancy. Multiple cutaneous leiomyomas affect females predominantly.

Typically, the lesion develops as a small discrete papule which may be perceptible upon palpation during the early course of its development, although difficult to distinguish with the unaided eye. It eventually progresses to nodules that may coalesce into a linear pattern following a dermatome distribution (1). Characteristically, the lesions are red but demonstrate considerable variation in color, ranging from shades of brown and yellow to translucency and white (9). The extensor surfaces of limbs are involved frequently with documentation of nearly 50% of reported cases (8). Usually, the tumor grows slowly over the years, thus explaining why patients may not seek medical attention until many years later (1). The presenting feature of pain induced by palpation is associated with most lesions.

Measuring several millimeters in diameter, multiple leiomyomas are located in dermal connective tissue and blend in an irregular pattern with the surrounding dermal collagen and adjacent arrector pilorum muscles.

Microscopically, the lesion shows an absence of connective tissue, with bundles of smooth muscle fibers present. The intersection of the muscle fibers creates the impression of arrector pilorum muscle hyperplasia.

Differential Diagnosis

The differential diagnosis should include multiple glomus tumors that are more vascular in nature and blanch on palpation. Glomus tumors, when found in the adult, tend to affect males predominantly. Skin lesions associated with sarcoidosis can be ruled out because of the absence of symptoms such as pain and the presence of scar formation that may develop residually. Multiple nodular-like lesions of the skin, i.e., xanthoma tuberosum, should also be considered, but they tend to present with a characteristic yellow color and may be associated with early severe atherosclerosis (5, 12–14).

LEIOMYOMA (SOLITARY CUTANEOUS)

Solitary leiomyomas of the skin, once thought to be rare, originate from arrector pilorum muscles of sweat glands and hair follicles. Trauma and certain hereditary factors are implicated in their etiology. They can appear at any age, but the majority seem to appear later in life. Stout (8) reported an equal sex distribution of the lesions between males and females. Documentation shows that the lesions occur on the foot more frequently than previous investigators had thought. Other sites of involvement include the back, chest, and forearms (8, 10).

Upon examination, they appear as freely movable, rounded nodules measuring several millimeters in diameter and fixed to the overlying skin. Solitary leiomyomas occasionally increase in size, approximating the dimensions of a child's head. The lesions tend not to discolor the skin. The most striking clinical feature or symptom associated with this solitary neoplasm is nonradiating pain. Occasionally, paroxysmal symptoms of pain and tenderness may precede the tumor or coincide with its appearance.

Microscopically, solitary leiomyomas are composed primarily of smooth muscle cells arranged in interlacing bands with the presence of fibrous tissue and scant blood vessels that are nutritional in nature. Furthermore, they do not show encapsulation (8, 9).

Differential Diagnosis

Solitary glomus tumors, although painful, can be distinguished from solitary leiomyomas by their characteristic bluish-purple color, encapsulation, and common sites of predilection, such as subungually. These tumors are known to cause erosive changes in bone if found in close association with it. Other benign lesions that should be considered when trying to establish a differential diagnosis include cutaneous fibrosis histiocytoma (dermatofibroma), lipoma, and ganglion (1, 10, 12).

LEIOMYOMA (DEEP)

Located deep in the soft tissues, these leiomyomas are rare. They occur in the deep muscles of the extremities and the abdominal cavity and tend to be much larger than solitary or multiple cutaneous lesions. Age and sex distribution are variable; lesions appear at any age and affect both sexes equally. Calcification is a prominent feature of these deep-seated lesions. Macroscopically, they appear as well-circumscribed gray-white lesions; some have an appearance similar to gelatin.

Microscopically, deep-seated leiomyomas resemble their cutaneous counterparts, but possess the capacity to undergo degenerative changes, especially when present for a long time. In addition, some of the lesions may accumulate large amounts of myxoid ground substance between the cells and lose the fascicular pattern characteristic of muscle fibers.

Differential Diagnosis

The differential diagnosis for deep-seated leiomyomas would include clear cell carcinoma, balloon cell melanoma, and adnexal tumor (1).

ANGIOLEIOMYOMA (VASCULAR LEIOMYOMA)

Angioleiomyomas are benign soft-tissue tumors which originate from the muscular layer of blood vessels, i.e., arterioles and veins of various sizes. Predominantly localized in the dermis and subcutaneous tissues, these lesions can also be found in the fascia layer or intermuscular septa of the extremities. Their etiology has not been firmly established, but infection, trauma, and hormonal influence have been implicated. Mature fat cells have been found in some angioleiomyomas, causing some individuals to suggest that the lesions are of hamartomatous origin. This type of neoplasm accounts for approximately 5% of all benign soft-tissue tumors. Unlike cutaneous leiomyomas, these lesions develop in later life, between the third and sixth decade, as solitary tumors. The female-to-male ratio of tumor involvement is 2:1. The lower extremity is the predominant site where most angioleiomyomas develop, with lesions appearing on the foot, ankle, and lower leg (1, 15–19).

Clinically, they appear as solitary, encapsulated, nodules; however, some lesions found in the skin may not show encapsulation (17, 20). On palpation, they are found to be mobile with uniform size and shape. In addition, angioleiomyomas present as flesh-colored soft-tissue masses which may grow rapidly; others are reported to grow slowly over a longer period of time. The most frequent complaint is a tumor mass with pain and associated tenderness.

Grossly, the lesions appear as circumscribed, glistening white-gray encapsulated nodules. They may also appear red or blue and, at times, flecks of calcium may be visible within the tumor mass (1). The majority of vascular leiomyomas measure between 0.5 and 2.0 cm in diameter, although much larger lesions have been recorded; e.g., one tumor, which was removed from the saphenous vein, measured 12.0 × 6.0 cm in diameter (11).

Microscopically, most tumors possess a fibrous capsule in addition to numerous masses of capillaries and medium-sized blood vessels with thick muscular walls composed of poorly defined smooth muscle fiber proliferation that tends to invade the surrounding collagen. Muscle bundles are also found condensed into tight whorls within the tumor mass. A frequent finding is the presence of dense bundles of muscle that fuse with and become part of the wall of the vessel, producing the appearance of a mass composed of many thick-walled blood vessels. (21) The veins are slit-like in appearance or have large sinusoidal lumina, while a few have a stellate lumen caused by muscle spasm (19).

As mentioned in an article by Freedman and Meland, Hachisuga et al. (22, 23) divide angioleiomyomas into three histologic types: solid, cavernous, and venous. The solid type tumor is composed of smooth muscle bundles that surround, as well as entwine, the vascular channels. The cavernous type tumor is composed of vascular channels that are more dilated; this type has smaller amounts of smooth muscle. Tumors of the venous type are comprised of vascular channels that are primarily venous in nature. The smooth muscle bundles are not as compact as the other types.

Differential Diagnosis

Clinically, it is difficult to differentiate angioleiomyoma from other soft-tissue neoplasia. Glomus tumors may present a similar picture, but angioleiomyomas have not been found under the nails. Both are associated with the subjective symptoms of spontaneous attacks of pain and soreness on pressure or during temperature changes (24).

Fibromas should also be considered; however, paroxysmal symptoms of pain are usually not associated with this lesion. Lipomas and ganglionic cysts tend to transluminate light and usually are not painful unless of sufficient size to cause compression of a superficial nerve branch.

Diagnostic Measures and Follow-up Procedures

Proper evaluation of soft tissue neoplasia, such as leiomyoma or angioleiomyoma, is essential in making a diagnosis. Therefore, appropriate diagnostic measures must follow an orderly logical sequence commencing with soft-tissue radiographs to determine the extent of the tumor and whether or not it is invasive. Additional radiographs should be taken to determine the presence of calcification within the tumor mass and bone erosion (25, 26).

Solitary leiomyomas of sufficient size should be considered for incisional biopsy whereas multiple leiomyomas should be considered for punch biopsy and tissue evaluation on the microscopic level. Appropriate tissue samples can be stained with phosphotungstic acid-hematoxylin (PTAH) and Masson trichrome stain; both are used to demonstrate the presence of myofibrils. Van Gieson's stain is used because of its specificity for collagen (1). A diagnosis established in this manner is highly successful, leading to appropriate treatment.

Treatment and Prognosis

Although benign in nature, multiple cutaneous leiomyomas may be difficult to treat because the large number of lesions make surgical intervention impractical. Recurrence of lesions is common in patients who undergo surgery. Nitroglycerin has been used successfully to shorten severe incapacitating pain attacks, and phenoxybenzamine hydrochloride has been used successfully to decrease pain in general. Complete surgical excision is the treatment of choice for solitary lesions, allowing for relief of symptoms caused by the cutaneous neoplasms. Recurrence is rare. Vascular leiomyomas should be excised by meticulous surgical dissection to avoid recurrence. If successful, the surgery is curative (1).

LEIOMYOSARCOMA (CUTANEOUS AND SUBCUTANEOUS)

These are rare malignant neoplasms of the skin that arise from the arrector pilorum muscles associated with sweat glands and hair follicles. Subcutaneous leiomyosarcomas arise from smooth muscle localized in arterioles and veins. Neoplasms such as these occur with equal frequency in both sexes. They may appear at any age after the neonatal period to well within the eighth to ninth decades; the highest frequency occurs after 60 years of age. The duration of this type of neoplasm is from 2 weeks to as long as 10 years. Thus, some lesions may remain static for long periods with variable growth, and, at a much later stage, show acceleration of growth within the tumor mass. Case documentations have established that the most common location of the tumor is the lower extremity, with the thigh being the predominant site. These tumors are small in diameter, with an average size of 2.0 cm (1, 27).

Clinically, leiomyosarcomas are solitary, unencapsulated nodules that appear on the skin. They tend to proliferate outward in an irregular manner from the central tumor mass (28). The lesions are usually firm and flesh-colored. In relation to the skin, leiomyosarcomas tend to be sessile, although they can be pedunculated and umbilicated. The overlying skin of these tumors is normal, but the surface may be ulcerated, crusted, or scaly in appearance. Multiple nodules may occur, but are extremely rare. When the tumor is localized to the subcutaneous level, the skin is freely movable over the mass. Tenderness on pressure and spontaneous pain, once thought to be nonexistent for these malignant tumors, is a frequent complaint.

Grossly, leiomyosarcomas have an almost white-colored, whorled appearance and adequate circumscription. Lesions in the dermis, however, are not well-circumscribed because of the immersion of tumor fibers with the surrounding collagen and arrector pilorum muscles.

Microscopically, these malignant neoplasms occur in two distinct locations. Lesions of the skin occur in the dermal portion as poorly defined tumor masses that consist of abnormal bundles of smooth muscle that interlace. The periphery of the tumors often display irregular strands of muscle cells that grow between and separate collagen stroma and fat cells. In contrast, leiomyosarcomas of the subcutaneous tissues are not firmly attached but compress the surrounding soft tissue to form a pseudocapsule. Tumors of this type are located at the junction of the lower part of the dermis and subcutaneous layer. They exhibit bizarre-shaped smooth muscle cells with random distribution (27). Because of the smaller size, cutaneous and subcutaneous leiomyosarcomas rarely exhibit hemorrhage, necrosis, hyalinization, or myxoid characteristics. Mitotic figures are easily and readily identified on microscopic examination within the tumors (1).

Differential Diagnosis

Since most leiomyosarcomas of the skin appear as cutaneous nodules that lack significant clinical characteristics, a definitive diagnosis is usually made by studying a biopsy specimen. Those disease entities whose skin manifestations are similar to the above should be included in the differential diagnosis. Such skin or subcutaneous nodules associated with tuberculosis, parasitic infestations, deep fungal infections, and various tumors are a few examples (27).

LEIOMYOSARCOMAS (VASCULAR ORIGIN)

Leiomyosarcomas of vascular origin are extremely rare malignant tumors. In Stout's review (cited by Allison (29) leiomyosarcomas were the third most frequent sarcoma recognized, with the majority found in the uterus. Furthermore, a series of 2095 malignant tumors of soft tissue reported by him included 105 leiomyosarcomas, of which 61 were found located in the retroperitoneal region. Of the entire group, only two originated from large veins: one from the vena azygos and the other from the femoral vein, localized in the thigh (30). The reported incidence of lesions associated with venous involvement is 5 times more frequent than lesions of arterial involvement. In order of decreasing frequency, the vena cava is the most common site, followed by other large central veins, and then the long saphenous vein (31). Statistically, leiomyosarcomas of arterial origin occur in the pulmonary artery and, less frequently, in the large systemic arteries (32). It has been demonstrated that females have a higher incidence of malignant neoplasms involving the inferior vena cava than do males. Because of the high frequency rates of leiomyosarcomas associated with the inferior vena cava found in females and of leiomyomas associated with the uterus, a loose comparison has been suggested to explain the high incidence, but no satisfactory answer has thus far been offered (33).

Aside from vena cava lesions, leiomyosarcomas of the veins affect the sexes equally and most often are in the veins of the lower extremity, i.e., the saphenous, iliac, and femoral veins. Such neoplasms present as large masses that occasionally produce lower leg edema. In addition, they tend to have a variable duration. Pressure on the nerves in proximity to the affected vessel produces additional symptoms of numbness. Angiograms tend to document highly vascular tumors that may create compression of the accompanying artery. Furthermore, compression appears to be the result of entrapment of an artery that resides within the same preformed fibrous sheath as the vein.

Grossly, leiomyosarcomas of vascular origin are described as polypoid or nodular masses, the color of which ranges from gray-white to glistening-like. Neoplasms of this type are firmly attached at some point along a vessel's length and spread to a variable extent on the surface of the vessel.

Microscopically, these tumors are similar to those in the retroperitoneum region, but do not show extensive hemorrhage or necrosis. Also noted is the presence of spindle-shaped cells with blunt-ended nuclei.

Differential Diagnosis

Leiomyosarcomas are sometimes difficult to differentiate from other spindle-cell sarcomas. Thus, fibrosarcoma and malignant schwannoma should be considered. Viewed under a low-power microscope, the appearance of all three lesions are similar, but there is a tendency to see the close proximity of longitudinal and transverse-cut fascicles in leiomyosarcomas. Histopathologically, cells of fibrosarcoma tend to be tapered, whereas those of malignant schwannoma appear buckled, wavy, and characteristically asymmetrical. Usually malignant schwannoma and fibrosarcoma do not

contain glycogen and neither has longitudinal striations (1).

LEIOMYOSARCOMA OF BONE (OSSEOUS LEIOMYOSARCOMA)

Leiomyosarcomas are uncommon tumors, even when they arise primarily from bone. They are known to originate at sites of previous trauma. Clinically, the lesions may present as a mass that may be accompanied by a dull ache or pain.

Grossly, a firm light-colored mass originating from osseous tissue is recognized. Microscopic examination usually reveals spindle-shaped cells and areas of focal necrosis. The nuclei tend to be fusiform, pleomorphic, and hyperchromatic.

Differential Diagnosis

Because of similar characteristics and difficulty in diagnosing this lesion under the light microscope, neoplasms such as nonossifying fibroma, malignant fibroma histiocytoma, and malignant spindle-cell sarcoma should be included in the differential diagnosis (34).

Diagnostic Measures and Follow-up Procedures

The best approach in attempting to establish a diagnosis of a given tumor type, e.g., leiomyosarcoma, is to use all available information on hand, i.e., clinical symptoms, size, location, presence or absence of infiltration, and mitotic counts (35).

Tumor size and location should be determined by initial routine radiographic evaluation; bone scans should be used to detect metastasis to other osseous sites. Computerized tomographic scans and nuclear magnetic resonance imaging are used to demonstrate the size, shape, and extent of tumor involvement. Having localized the tumor mass, a biopsy specimen is of prime importance (36). Incisional biopsy may give rise to seeding; therefore, this technique should be avoided if one suspects a soft-tissue sarcoma. In selected cases, a needle biopsy may be performed instead. Otherwise, wide local excision of the neoplasm is recommended (1, 37).

Sections of formaldehyde-fixed paraffin-embedded tissue samples can be prepared for immunohistochemistry. This technique screens for certain intermediate filament proteins that serve as markers for various soft-tissue neoplasms. The recent development of an antibody (HHF-35) directed against muscle-specific actin may prove useful in the diagnosis of leiomyosarcoma. Smooth muscle actin, desmin, and myosin may also be detected in other types of muscle tumors. Antibodies against desmin are useful in establishing a differential diagnosis of soft tissue. Thus, leiomyosarcomas can be distinguished from malignant fibrous histiocytoma and nerve sheath tumors.

The electron microscope appears to be the definitive diagnostic tool which is most helpful. With good tissue samples and adequate preparation, including Masson trichrome stain, visualization of the number of mitotic cells per high power field can be noted (1).

The importance of the number of mitotic cells cannot be overemphasized, since mitotic activity appears to be the key to predict metastases. Uterine lesions having between 5 and 10 mitoses per 10 high power fields are considered borderline. This level of mitotic activity in soft-tissue lesions always indicates neoplastic lesions capable of metastasis. Thus, even when stringent criteria are applied it is very difficult to be absolutely certain, in all cases, which smooth muscle neoplasms are totally benign, even though histologic features suggest they are (1, 38).

Treatment and Prognosis

When a diagnosis is firmly established for leiomyosarcoma, the treatment of choice is usually wide local excision, provided the patient is free of metastatic disease. On the other hand, if metastatic disease is present, adjuvant therapy should be instituted. In such cases, wide local excision and chemotherapeutic agents and radiation therapy should be attempted (39, 40). Unfortunately, there are situations that make it almost impossible to achieve success with wide local excision. When deep peripheral veins, e.g., the femoral vein, is the origin of the neoplasm, complete extirpation via surgery may be difficult to achieve. In order to totally eradicate a lesion of this nature, amputation of the involved extremity may have to be performed (10).

Tumors of major vessels, although grossly alarming, have a relatively low potential of metastasizing because their slow growth makes surgical palliation or cure feasible.

According to reports, surgical resection of leiomyosarcoma is possible in more than 50%

of the cases, with recurrences occurring in approximately 36%. Lesions that do recur have a greater tendency to increase in size and then to migrate to deeper structures (41). This should not discourage reexcision of the tumor since chemotherapy and radiation therapy are not very effective in such cases. A study of 36 cases by Hare and Cerney (cited by Bernardone and Scarlet (38)) reported the incidence of metastases to be 52.8%. Nineteen patients had metastases to the lung and four to the regional lymph nodes. A study by Ferrell and Frable (cited by Bernardone and Scarlet (38) showed that the mortality rate of leiomyosarcoma was exceeded only by the mortality of rhabdomyosarcoma.

Thus, soft-tissue and subcutaneous leiomyosarcomas have favorable prognoses, similar to those of other forms of sarcomas localized to the soft tissue (e.g., fibrous xanthoma or superficial malignant fibrous histiocytoma). Furthermore, leiomyosarcomas of vascular origin other than vena cava lesions are controversial; one series of tumors studied suggests that small intravascular neoplasms might have a relatively good prognosis, but six case reviews reported by Berlin et al. (cited by Enzinger and Weiss (1)) indicate metastases in all cases, even those with evidence of low mitoses (1). Finally, no definitive prognostic trends could be determined concerning osseous leiomyosarcomas. In an extensive review of 13 patients by Von Hochtetter et al. (cited by Eady et al. (34)) and three case studies by Eady et al. (34) it was found that two patients had been lost to follow-up and seven were deceased. Three other patients were alive with metastases 3–6 years later, and four patients were free of metastatic disease 5–11 years later. The osseous lesions comprised both intracompartmental and extracompartmental neoplasms (34).

RHABDOMYOMA

Benign soft tissue neoplasms frequently outnumber malignant neoplasms by a wide margin. This is not true of striated muscle tumors, however. Benign tumors of striated muscle are commonly called rhabdomyomas. They are exceedingly rare and have a predilection for the head and neck region as well as the genitourinary system in females. Despite their prevalence in other locations, there are no recorded cases of rhabdomyomas originating from muscles of the lower extremities. Both rhabdomyomas and rhabdomyosarcomas are derived from striated muscle and have similar morphologies. Thus, discussion of such benign lesions is included in this chapter.

Morphologically and clinically, rhabdomyomas are categorized as one of three types. The adult type is limited to the head and neck region and commonly affects older persons. The fetal type occurs primarily in children under age four and also has a predilection for the head and neck region. The genital type of rhabdomyoma, mostly localized to the vulva and vagina, occurs in middle-aged females.

Clinically, the lesions tend to be solitary or polypoid masses located in the neck region. They are usually nonpainful but may cause symptoms such as hoarseness, dysphagia, or difficulty in breathing. Tumors have been recorded that range in size from 0.5–6.0 cm in diameter and can either be well-defined, coarsely lobulated, or rounded (1). Rhabdomyomas may be encapsulated; otherwise, they are sharply demarcated from adjacent tissue (42).

Microscopically, these neoplasms are characterized by the presence of cross-striations with small nuclei located on the periphery of the cells. Glycogen and glycoprotein are found contained within cytoplasmic vacuoles. In addition, visible mitotic figures and invasiveness of other tissues by the tumor are practically nonexistent (43).

Differential Diagnosis

In earlier scientific literature, rhabdomyomas were often confused with granular cell myoblastomas. Cells of the latter type lack vacuolation caused by the removal of intracellular glycogen during processing. In addition, there are no cross-striations of muscle filaments found in granular cell myoblastoma. Reticulohistiocytoma must be considered in the differential diagnosis also, but such a tumor lacks glycogen in its various cellular components (i.e., acidophilic histiocytes, fibroblasts, multinucleated giant cells, and xanthoma cells). Clinically, rhabdomyosarcomas are more common and do occur in the lower extremities. In addition to being invasive, these malignant neoplasms are not as well-defined and are composed of poorly differentiated round or spindle-shaped cells in association with varying numbers of rhabdomyoblasts. Mitotic figures, although exceptionally rare in rhabdomyomas, are common in this type tumor (1).

Diagnostic Measures and Follow-up Procedures

Sections of formalin-fixed paraffin-embedded tissue viewed under an electron microscope are used to determine whether the cellular components and diagnostic features are consistent with rhabdomyoma. Histologic studies are used to exclude other tumors and to establish the definitive diagnosis. These benign neoplasms seldom recur, provided all of the tumor is removed. Sometimes, the patient is left with altered vocal sounds following removal of a neoplasm from the larynx or vocal cords (43, 44).

Treatment and Prognosis

Rhabdomyomas are effectively treated by local excision and periodic follow-up to determine recurrence. Examples of recurrence at a much later date have been reported by Czerobilsky et al. (cited by Enzinger and Weiss (1) 5 years after excision. Others, such as Scrivner and Meyer and Andersen et al. (both cited by Enzinger and Weiss (1)) report recurrence after 10 years and 35 years, respectively. It is noteworthy that malignant transformation of this benign tumor has never been observed (1).

RHABDOMYOSARCOMA

Rhabdomyosarcomas are malignant neoplastic lesions derived from striated muscle. Originally, in the early nineteenth century, they were described as having a close resemblance to developing normal tissue. Subsequently, it was determined that many of the tumors described as rhabdomyosarcomas in the 1930s and 1940s, which primarily involved the extremities of patients 50–70 years of age, were sarcomas of other types, e.g., malignant fibrous histiocytoma (1). Between 5 and 15% of all malignant soft-tissue tumors in children under 15 years old have been documented as rhabdomyosarcomas. It is the most common soft-tissue neoplasm in children under 15 years of age, as well as in adolescents and young adults (45). Previously, several national studies, (e.g., the Intergroup Rhabdomyosarcoma Study and the Wilms' Tumor Study) established that rhabdomyosarcoma occurs with approximately the same frequency as Wilms' tumor.

The peak incidence of this neoplastic disease occurs between 2 and 5 years of age, with 70% of documented cases presenting before the age of 10. It has been established that rhabdomyosarcomas occur more often in males than females. Malignant lesions such as these prefer, in order of frequency: the head and neck region (36%), the extremities (24%), the genitourinary tract (18%), the retroperitoneum (7%), the gastrointestinal tract (3%), the thoracic region (2%), and the anal orifice (2%).

Before 1960, the prognosis for 2-year survival of treated patients was 20%. The 2-year survival rate is now extended to above 70% because of the change of treatment from surgery and/or radiation to a multidisciplinary approach, including surgery, radiation therapy, and chemotherapy.

Clinically, the most frequent abnormality noted upon presentation is a swelling or mass (45, 46). The neoplasm grows very rapidly and usually attains considerable size by the time the patient seeks medical attention. Such tumors characteristically have a diameter of approximately 20–25 cm. The tumors, on gross evaluation, may present as gray-red tissue consistent with the feel of "fish flesh." Because of rapid growth, rhabdomyosarcomas simultaneously invade and destroy normal tissue and then undergo hemorrhage and necrosis (4). Subsequently, metastases may result from lymphatic and hematogenous spread. Common sites of metastases include the lung, bone, bone marrow, lymph nodes, brain, and heart.

Having arisen from embryonic mesenchyme, rhabdomyosarcomas tend to differentiate into various subtypes. The four recognized subtypes are: embryonal, alveolar, botryoid, and pleomorphic. They may be found in a "pure" form or as a mixture of subtypes (45).

RHABDOMYOSARCOMA (EMBRYONAL)

Primarily a tumor of the very young, embryonal rhabdomyosarcoma accounts for approximately 75% of all malignant striated muscle neoplasms. It closely resembles normal muscle tissue at different stages of development; however, rhabdomyosarcoma has its origin in undifferentiated mesoderm instead of skeletal muscle myotome. Such tumors commonly originate in the head and neck region, specifically the orbit of the eye and the genitourinary system. Embryonal rhabdomyosarcomas are usually found in areas of the body without striated muscle, e.g., the vagina, urinary bladder, or bile duct. The existence of striated muscle tissue in such areas can be understood when one considers the ubiquitous presence of mesecto-

dermal remnants throughout the body (41, 45). Infrequently, embryonal rhabdomyosarcomas are found localized in the extremities (1). The literature indicates that 4–8% of all malignant neoplastic lesions in children under the age of 15 are embryonal rhabdomyosarcomas. Stout and others (cited by Hadju (41)) grouped botryoid, alveolar, and embryonal types of this tumor into one group and classified it as juvenile rhabdomyosarcoma. However, since some adults and elderly people have been diagnosed with embryonal rhabdomyosarcomas, such a broad grouping may not be appropriate (41).

Grossly, embryonal rhabdomyosarcomas and other forms of the tumor fit the description of other soft-tissue sarcomas: soft or gelatinous-like, fairly well-circumscribed, nonbulky, and gray or pinkish-gray in color. Most of the tumors are highly vascular and it is common to see accellular fibrous bands separating the blood vessels and tumor cells (41, 47).

Microscopically, most embryonal rhabdomyosarcomas exist in several different patterns, i.e., solid, myxoid, trabecular, and alveolar. The cell most commonly seen, however, is a long tapered embryonal rhabdomyoblast with bipolar cytoplasmic processes and a small nucleus that is eccentric in location. There is usually a small amount of eosinophilic cytoplasm as well as fine granular material localized in the cytoplasm adjacent to the nucleus (47).

RHABDOMYOSARCOMA (BOTRYOID)

Considered a variant of embryonal rhabdomyosarcomas, these neoplasms differ from them only in location and configuration. Botryoid rhabdomyosarcomas account for approximately 7% of all rhabdomyosarcomas and are most often found in hollow visceral organs lined with mucosal tissue, e.g., the vagina or urinary bladder. Occasionally, the tumor is also found in the head and neck region (1, 45).

The neoplasms are characterized by distinctive grapelike configurations that are usually soft and semifluid-like in consistency. They possess a relatively smooth surface because of the mucous membrane-covering characteristic of that particular organ system.

Microscopically, a botryoid tumor is identified by a layer of small, rounded cells at its periphery in addition to several layers or zones of cells of myxoid stroma and round, spindle-shaped cells located in the deeper layer. The cells in the compact zone are easily recognized as rhabdomyoblasts because of their cytoplasmic cross-striations (1, 45, 47).

RHABDOMYOSARCOMA (ALVEOLAR)

Alveolar rhabdomyosarcomas account for approximately 18% of all rhabdomyosarcomas. Although the sites of origin are similar to those of embryonal types of striated muscle tumors, these neoplasms are also found in the upper and lower extremities. Forty-five percent of such tumors are localized to the deep tissues of the trunk and 35% are localized to the extremities (1, 45).

Almost half of the tumors tend to have a histologic picture similar to that of embryonal rhabdomyosarcomas. Lesions of this type are characterized by a solid area of small, rounded tumor cells or elongated spindle cells with or without an abundance of eosinophilic cytoplasm (47). The typical microscopic appearance of alveolar rhabdomyosarcomas is important, despite the overlap with the embryonal type, because recognition of the histologic pattern quite possibly enables the pathologist to make a positive diagnosis even without rhabdomyoblasts (1). The typical histologic picture associated with alveolar rhabdomyosarcoma is a tumor composed of moderately large and rounded anaplastic cells arranged in clusters or elongated cleats (45). These cellular masses, which tend to be separated from one another by a collagenous trabeculation, are highly suggestive of normal alveoli separated from one another by fibrous trabeculae (47).

RHABDOMYOSARCOMA (PLEOMORPHIC)

Described as the classic type of rhabdomyosarcoma, pleomorphic rhabdomyosarcomas are reported to be the least common of the four types. Although they can occur at any age, pleomorphic rhabdomyosarcomas are reputed to have a peak incidence in individuals over 45. Males and females tend to be affected in almost equal proportions (1). Having a predilection for patients of middle age, these tumors are thus referred to as the "adult" form of rhabdomyosarcoma. These neoplasms account for approximately 2% of malignant striated muscle tumors (45). Most lesions originate in the lower extremities, specifically the thigh region, but they also occur in the shoulder and upper arm. Inciting factors such as trauma or preexisting intramuscular benign lesions (e.g., rhabdomy-

oma, myositis ossificans) have been proposed as the cause of pleomorphic rhabdomyosarcomas. Compared to liposarcomas, pleomorphic-type tumors tend to be less bulky, although their size may be considerably larger prior to diagnosis. These neoplasms are freely movable and moderately firm. The location of one may be confirmed by a change in its shape when the muscle is relaxed and contracted. Pleomorphic rhabdomyosarcomas are deeply seated within muscle tissue (41, 48).

On gross examination, many tumors appear encapsulated and circumscribed. However, upon careful inspection, this may be an illusion, since the tumors normally exceed the area of circumscription (41).

Microscopically, pleomorphic rhabdomyosarcomas are composed of rounded rhabdomyoblasts and strap-shaped rhabdomyocytes (41). They are distinguished by the presence of large pleomorphic tumor cells that can have many configurations. There is considerable variation due to the size of the cells. Characteristically, cells found in pleomorphic rhabdomyosarcomas may resemble myoblastoma or ganglionic cysts, even when malignant rhabdomyoblasts are the predominant cell type. This occasionally leads to an incorrect diagnosis of malignant granular cell myoblastoma or ganglioneuroblastoma, respectively. Conspicuous amounts of acidophilic cytoplasm with large anaplastic nuclei within giant tumor cells is also a common finding (41, 45). These tumors present with a high degree of cellularity and pleomorphism but generally have a low collagen content (47). As a rule, mitoses in pleomorphic rhabdomyosarcomas are present but scant. Because the histologic picture is similar to that of other soft-tissue sarcomas and lacks striated muscle fibers and cross-striations, the diagnosis may be difficult to establish. However, when other elements, e.g., rhabdomyoblasts, malignant myoblasts, racquet-shaped cells, and constituents of embryonal rhabdomyoblasts, are found, cross-striations are not necessary to make the diagnosis (41).

Differential Diagnosis

Muscle tumors found in children and young adults, i.e., embryonal, alveolar, and botryoid, share histologic similarities with other types of sarcomas when there is poor differentiation of spindle cells and round cells. Because of this confusion, striated muscle tumors may be misdiagnosed as neuroblastoma, Ewing's sarcoma, malignant lymphoma, undifferentiated round cell sarcoma, neuroepithelioma, synovial sarcoma, malignant melanoma, or granulocytic sarcoma. Small cell carcinoma should also be a part of the differential diagnosis when found in patients above the age of 40 (1). Soft-tissue sarcomas, e.g., pleomorphic fibrosarcomas, leiomyosarcomas, and pleomorphic fibrous histiocytomas, derived from undifferentiated mesenchymal cells during embryonic development, may also be confused with rhabdomyosarcomas. Histologically, pleomorphic fibrosarcomas demonstrate a herringbone pattern, as well as trichrome-positive collagenous fibers, but show only occasional pleomorphism. This contrasts with rhabdomyosarcomas, which are characterized by pleomorphism (pleomorphic type) and traces of trichrome-positive collagenous fibers and herringbone patterns. Embryonal or mature rhabdomyoblasts, target cells, and cross-striated myofibrils are characteristic of rhabdomyosarcomas but are notably absent in leiomyosarcomas. Specific stromal patterns, foam cells, and Touton giant cells are histologically consistent with pleomorphic fibrous histiocytoma, but rare in rhabdomyosarcomas (41).

Diagnostic Measures and Follow-up Procedures

When a malignant soft tissue neoplasm, such as rhabdomyosarcoma, is suspected, a complete history, physical examination, and systematic work-up of the patient should be performed. A diagnostic evaluation, commencing with chemistry, hematology, and urine testing, and including plain radiographs of the chest and affected lower extremity, is also warranted (45). Proper diagnosis and effective determination of the tumor extent frequently requires more elaborate testing, i.e., a muscle biopsy, use of immunohistochemical markers, radionuclide imaging (bone scans), computerized tomographic scans, magnetic resonance imaging, or peripheral angiography.

Prior to surgical removal as a curative procedure, various biopsy techniques may be used to help establish the diagnosis for the soft-tissue tumor mass, including incisional, excisional, and semi-open biopsy methods. With the incisional technique, part of the tumor is removed by direct incision through the capsule. The disadvantages are future contamination of fascial planes caused by seeding of tumor cells present within the hematoma and localization of residual amounts of the tumor after surgery. An excisional biopsy is accomplished by removal of the tumor and surrounding pseudocapsule. A frequent sequelae is microscopic tumor cells left in all fascia planes contaminated by the hematoma (49). The semi-open biopsy technique, using an alligator forceps to obtain an adequate amount of muscle tissue, combines the advantages of the open-surgical biopsy method and the needle method. The disadvantages are that the muscle biopsy cannot easily be taken from several muscles or done in a repetitive fashion during the course of the disease and that it is time-consuming (37).

Immunohistochemical markers have also emerged as a diagnostic technique for evaluating soft-tissue tumors, such as rhabdomyosarcomas that, under some circumstances, show poor differentiation. These markers include desmin, creatine kinase (isoenzymes MM and BB), myoglobin, actin, myosin, titin, and vimentin. Sections of formaldehyde and fixed paraffin-embedded tissue are used mostly to detect antigens in suspected tumors. Markers that are specific for cross-striated muscle cell differentiation in tumors include myoglobin, skeletal muscle myosin, and skeletal muscle actin. Of the myosin isoenzymes, only fast myosin has been found to be of value. Antibodies against fast myosin and skeletal muscle actin are preferred to antibodies against myoglobin. The latter are present only in cytoplasm-rich, well-differentiated, tumor cells and, thus, are of little value in the diagnosis of poorly differentiated rhabdomyosarcomas. Creatine kinase M and desmin are not specific markers for the detection of cross-striated muscle differentiation in tumors, but they are useful in the objective evaluation of poorly differentiated rhabdomyosarcomas from other round cell tumors in childhood. Titin is specific for striated muscle tumor but only reacts with a small segment of the cell population. Vimentin, on the other hand, has been identified in most rhabdomyosarcomas, but tumor prominence tends to occur more frequently in undifferentiated neoplasms than in well-differentiated tumors (1, 50).

Radionuclide imaging (bone scans) using technetium-99m diphosphate or pyrophosphate helps to establish the relationship of

soft-tissue sarcomas to adjacent osseous structures (49). In the initial phase of the technique,
the uptake of the isotope is visualized within
the circulation (angiographic). This is followed
by the blood-pool or tissue phase, which demonstrates the radioisotope within the soft
tissues of the extremities. Approximately 3
hours following the initial injection of the ra-
diotracer, bone activity is demonstrated by the
scan (51).

Computerized tomographic (CT) scans appear to be on the increase for use in evaluating
the primary tumor site and chest region (52).
Thus, computed tomography has been considered the standard diagnostic test utilized in the
evaluation and staging of soft-tissue tumors
such as rhabdomyosarcomas. Because of the
difficulty in accurately delineating malignant
striated muscle tumors from adjacent normal
tissue, malignant neoplasms, as well as other
soft-tissue sarcomas, pose a fundamental
problem during evaluation by CT scans. Computerized tomography has the advantage over
plain radiography, however, in being able to
accurately display radiodensities pertaining to
osseous and nonosseous tissues (e.g., fat, muscle, and tendon).

Within the last decade, magnetic resonance
imaging (MRI), a new imaging technique, was
conceived and found to be advantageous in the
evaluation of soft tissue. MRI does not require
radiation, but produces images based on the
magnetic properties inherent in tissues rather
than based on their radiodensities. Thus, MRI
has several advantages over CT scans as a diagnostic tool. MRI does not require ionizing
radiation or contrast dye material to obtain images. It is able to project information anatomi-
cally in a frontal, sagittal, or transverse plane.
Furthermore, the contrast between neoplasm,
vessels, normal tissue, and other structures is
superior to that obtained with CT scans. The
major disadvantages, however, include relatively high cost, increased imaging time, and
difficult detection of small lesions (53).

When necessary, such as during preoperative local staging of malignant tumors of the
extremities, peripheral angiography can be
performed with the use of a vasodilator and
large quantities of contrast media. Angiograms
provide useful information beginning with the
early phase, which demonstrates the location
of the major arterial blood supply and its relationship to the neoplasm. The intermediate or
midphase outlines the extent of the tumor.

Subsequently, the late phase, or the venous
phase, clearly depicts venous drainage from
the tumor mass (49).

Treatment and Prognosis

In general, initiation of treatment of rhabdomyosarcoma occurs only after a biopsy and
resection of lesion has been performed by the
surgeon, followed by careful assessment of the
tumor stage, using radiographs, CT scans,
MRI, and, when necessary, angiograms. Careful staging of the neoplasm is extremely
important prior to planning a treatment regimen and in order to determine the prognosis.
Bone marrow aspiration also should be a part
of the staging process, since rhabdomyosarcomas tend to metastasize to the bone marrow
(1, 45).

Four stages or groups have been recognized
by the Intergroup Rhabdomyosarcoma Study
(IRS). Group I is comprised of tumors that are
completely localized and can be resected entirely. Group II is comprised of tumors grossly
resected but with "microscopic residual" found
at the tumor margins. However, lymph node involvement tends to be absent. Group III is
comprised of incomplete resection of a lesion or
biopsy with gross residual disease. Group IV
demonstrates metastatic disease at the time of
diagnosis (10).

Because of the success of combined chemotherapy and radiation therapy, resulting in
improvement in survival, the surgical approach to rhabdomyosarcomas tends to be an
area of utmost concern, as well as controversy.
For example, with small pelvic tumors, there is
evidence, based on relatively small groups of
patients, that limited surgical excision with
preservation of the organ may be all that is required. The type of surgical procedure depends
on the location of the primary tumor and the
site(s) of metastases. When possible, it has
been shown that wide local resection of the primary tumor, with wide excision of an "envelope" of normal tissue, leads to the best results
and avoids recurrence and metastases. This
approach appears to be more favorable in lesions of the extremities and trunk rather than
those of the head and neck regions. If wide local
excision or radical excision of the neoplasm
cannot be satisfactorily achieved, then amputation appears to be the procedure of choice,
preferable to simple biopsy followed by chemotherapy and radiation. At times, microscopic
examination of the margins of the tumor previ-

ously excised shows residual tumor still present. A second resection may not be required if chemotherapy and radiation are subsequently instituted.

Recent evidence from the Intergroup Rhabdomyosarcoma Study (45) indicates that regional lymph node involvement occurs frequently enough to justify a lymph node biopsy if resection of the nodes along with the primary tumor is not contemplated. Unless one considers using CT scans for follow-up evaluation, metal clips should be placed in areas of lymph node removal that might prove to be positive (45).

When radiation therapy is indicated, a dose of 5000 or 6000 rads in 5 and 6 weeks respectively, is recommended for the primary tumor. Conversely, patients with gross microscopic residual disease treated with doses of less than 4000 rads have been found to develop recurrences, even when chemotherapy was given (45). Indications for postoperative radiation vary in different institutions, but radiation is felt to be unnecessary in group I tumors (1).

Chemotherapy has a significant place in the current treatment of rhabdomyosarcomas, as group II patients should receive various chemotherapeutic drugs. There has been a changing role of adjuvant therapy in the use of these drugs. Chemotherapy is usually given for a period of 1–2 years; its purpose is to arrest occult metastatic disease and further the primary tumor regression. The first-line drugs active against rhabdomyosarcomas are dactinomycin, vincristine, cyclophosphamide, and adriamycin. Because of life-threatening and sometimes fatal toxicities, a thorough knowledge of these drugs is essential. Complications associated with dactinomycin include myelosuppression, abdominal pain, nausea, vomiting, and alopecia. Vincristine may cause constipation, alopecia, and neurologic abnormalities such as parathesias and loss of deep tendon reflexes. Cyclophosphamide may cause bladder toxicity, myelosuppression, and gastrointestinal disturbances. Adriamycin also tends to be associated with alopecia, myelosuppression, and, when given excessively, cardiac toxicity (45).

The prognosis is considered excellent for group I and group II tumors with overall 5-year survival rates of 83 and 70%, respectively. Unfortunately, the overall 5-year survival rate for group III tumors is approximately 52% and group IV tumors have a poor prognosis of about 20% survival. In addition, those with local recurrence of distant metastatic disease at the time of diagnosis rarely survive. As with other soft-tissue sarcomas, a favorable prognosis depends upon early detection and the adequacy of early precise therapy (1).

MYOBLASTOMA (GRANULAR CELL TUMOR)

Myoblastomas are soft-tissue tumors whose origin was previously thought to be striated muscle, but recently that has changed and nerve tissue is now suggested as the true etiology. Suspected of having a myogenic origin because of a morphology similar to that of altered skeletal muscle cells, granular cell tumors were noted by FIsher and Wechsler in 1962 (cited by Berlin et al. (54)) to have similarities to Schwann cells of damaged nerve tissue. Using light and electron microscopes these two investigators established a dissimilarity, both morphologically and enzymatically, between the tumor cells and damaged striated muscle tissue. Hence, a new name, granular cell schwannoma, was proposed because of this tumor's apparent origin in neural tissue. Other synonyms that relate this tumor to one of neural origin include granular cell neuroma and granular cell neurofibroma.

The lesions appear in males and females but have a predilection for females. Myoblastomas occur at any age; however, most have been shown to occur during the fourth, fifth, and sixth decades. Children are rarely affected, if at all. The lesions are found to be present more frequently in Black than in White patients. Malignancy has been reported in approximately 3% of all tumors. Benign tumors average about 2.0 cm in diameter, whereas malignant lesions average 3.0–9.0 cm in diameter. Myoblastomas can occur anywhere on the body, and approximately one-third have been known to occur on the tongue. Other sites of occurrence include the head and neck regions and the skin, subcutaneous tissue, lungs, heart, and gastrointestinal tract.

Clinically, the lesions appear as painless, solitary nodules or tumors which are pedunculated or sessile but rarely ulcerative. They tend to be slow-growing and nonencapsulated and, when found on the foot, especially on weight-bearing areas, are usually covered by a veneer of hyperkeratotic tissue (54).

Microscopically, granular cell tumors are poorly circumscribed, with small centrally placed vesicular nuclei and granular eosino-philic cytoplasm contained within large round-ed-type cells of uniform character. They have a variable growth pattern, and the cells tend to be arranged in sheets or ribbons, with lack of distinctive cellular arrangement. Some tumors may exhibit considerable desmoplasia with age. Granular cells of myoblastomas are devoid of glycogen, unlike cells of both benign and malignant striated muscle tumors. Another frequent histopathologic feature is the replacement or envelopment of small peripheral nerves by granular cells and, to a lesser extent, the replacement of muscle tissue by these cells (55).

Differential Diagnosis

Needless to say, a neoplastic lesion that was originally thought to be derived from muscle can be confused on gross inspection with a variety of other soft-tissue and cutaneous lesions, e.g., malignant granular cell tumor, rhabdomyoma, neurofibroma, fibrosarcoma, papilloma, and squamous cell carcinoma. Macroscopic and microscopic evaluation will help the physician to diagnose and selectively determine the type of lesion present, based on cellular characteristics, clinical features, and tumor behavior (54).

Diagnostic Measures and Follow-up

A variety of methods, such as immunohistochemical analysis, microscopic evaluations, and examination of clinical features have been resorted to in establishing a diagnosis of granular cell tumor. Rarely, however, is this tumor diagnosed prior to examination of the biopsy specimen. Moreover, if the tumor has been adequately resected, recurrence is the exception; adequate follow-up is advocated nonetheless. When malignancy is suspected, the patient should be worked up for possible metastatic disease (54).

Treatment and Prognosis

Wide local excision is the procedure of choice for these neoplasms. Chemotherapeutic agents, as well as radiation therapy, are usually not considered of value in the eradication of the tumor (54). Frequently, adipose and muscle tissue are removed along with the resected tumor because of the tumor's poor circumscription. Since recurrence is extremely rare, surgery should be curative in nearly every case (55).

MYOSITIS OSSIFICANS (HETEROTROPHIC OSSIFICANS)

The term myositis ossificans refers to a benign extraosseous formation of bone, cartilage, and fibrous tissue usually found in association with muscle. Skeletal muscle may not be involved, and inflammation is rarely evident (56). Even supporting structures of the musculoskeletal system, i.e., ligaments, tendons, and subcutaneous tissue, have been linked with myositis ossificans (57).

Various types of calcification, which present as radiodense extraosseous lesions, may appear in the lower extremity and elsewhere as a reflection of dystrophic calcification that is localized and metastatic calcification that is systemic in nature. Both conditions are common findings in the foot under the correct circumstances.

Dystrophic calcification occurs as a result of decreased blood supply and tissue degeneration (56). In connective tissue disorders in which chondroitin sulfate is damaged, the deposition of calcium may be released into the skin and subcutaneous tissue. Normally, the intact chondroitin sulfate of connective tissue inhibits calcification by binding calcium and limiting diffusion (58).

Metastatic calcification occurs as a result of systemic pathology that includes metabolic disorders, renal insufficiency, secondary hyperparathyroidism, and hypervitaminosis D. When the concentration of circulating calcium in milligrams percent, multiplied by the concentration of circulating phosphate in milligrams percent, is in excess of 75 milligrams percent, saturation of the serum takes place and such a phenomenon evolves (58).

Many authorities state that heterotrophic ossification, rather than myositis ossificans, is the correct term for this lesion. Four variants have been recognized. Myositis ossificans progressiva is actually a misnomer, since there is lack of calcification within the muscles themselves; instead, calcification takes place in connective tissue in the musculature. This form is rare and progressively fatal (59). The disease presents usually shortly after birth, with progressive involvement of skeletal muscles in addition to microdactyly of the hallux and anomalies of the metatarsals and phalanges (56, 57). Barr (cited by Pack and Branund (60) believes that this variant of heterotrophic ossification results from a metaplasia of connective tissue to bone. The second variant, myositis ossificans circumscripta, secondary to trauma, is the most common form and results from local trauma of an acute or chronic nature. The third variant is recognized in absence of trauma and, thus, appropriately named myositis ossificans circumscripta, without history of trauma. This lesion occurs in association with chronic infections, burns, neuromuscular disorders, and other diseases. The classification by Jeffreys and Stiles (cited by Mandracchia et al. (56)) sought to label the fourth variant "pseudomalignant osseous tumor of soft tissue." Such ossification occurs locally in normal healthy individuals without a history of trauma (56).

The etiology of heterotrophic ossification is unclear, but several theories have been proposed, including implantation of periosteum in muscle, escape of osteogenic cells from periosteum, metaplasia of connective tissue cells, and ossification of hematomas. However, relating factors (e.g. local tissue reaction, growth relating factors) are probably involved (61).

Clinically, the localized variant of heterotrophic ossificans (myositis ossificans circumscripta) usually presents as localized masses in or near muscle. Symptoms of pain, swelling, and an increase in temperature over the area are characteristic. Antecedent to the development of the lesion, acute trauma or chronic repetitive trauma occurs, resulting in tissue necrosis and hemorrhage (57). Myositis ossificans following a complication of tetanus has been reported in the literature. The causative factor of the trauma appears to be severe muscle spasm from aggressive treatment by physiotherapists in the obtunded individual causing partial rupture of the muscle, which results in hematoma formation in and around muscles that tend to show calcification and ossification (62).

The laboratory findings associated with myositis ossificans include normal serum calcium and phosphorus levels, with a possible elevation of the erythrocyte sedimentation rate and white blood cell count. Macroscopically, heterotrophic ossificans appears as a well-circumscribed mass with a gelatinous consistency in the center surrounded by a periphery of bone (57).

Ackerman's histologic evaluation of the lesion (cited by Kern (63)) is significant because of the pseudosarcomatous growth pattern that can lead to erroneous microscopic diagnoses of bone sarcoma resulting in inappropriate and unnecessary radical surgery. Heterotrophic ossificans demonstrates a zone pattern, the center of which has been described as loosely woven fibroblastic tissue similar to granulation tissue in appearance. The intermediate zone consists of a trabecular pattern of fibroblasts, osteoblasts, and osteoid tissue that may not be readily defined. A third layer, visibly recognized as the outer layer, shows osteoid that has undergone calcification into mature lamellar bone (57, 63, 64). Incidentally, zone phenomenon are not present in soft-tissue sarcomata, although there is pseudoencapsulation (65).

Differential Diagnosis

The histologic picture of myositis ossificans is of utmost importance, since osteogenic sarcoma and extraosseous, or periosteal, osteogenic sarcoma may be mistaken for the lesion. An area of radioluceny between the lesion and bone helps to distinguish myositis ossificans circumscripta from osteogenic sarcoma (61).

Diagnostic Measures and Follow-up Procedures

The diagnosis of myositis ossificans is usually facilitated by a thorough history as it relates to trauma, plain radiology, and zone phenomenon seen on microscopic examination. Ultrasound and CT scans have also been employed as diagnostic tools, especially in preoperative planning (57, 61). In addition, adequate follow-up should be a part of the regimen to establish that the lesion is totally benign, as well as to evaluate symptoms consistent with incomplete excision of the lesion.

Treatment and Prognosis

Myositis ossificans responds well to conservative surgical management; lesions tend not to recur. The prognosis is exceptionally good, with total resolution of symptoms and return of normal function that may have been restricted because of the location of the extraosseous mass (63).

REFERENCES

1. Enzinger FM, Weiss SW. Soft tissue tumors. St. Louis: Mosby, 1988;383–483.
2. Ham AW. Muscle tissue histology. 6th ed. Philadelphia: Lippincott, 1969;546–566.
3. Kakulas BA, Adams RD. Disease of muscle. 4th ed. Philadelphia: Harper & Row, 1985.
4. Robbins SL. Pathology. 3rd ed. Philadelphia: Saunders, 1967.

5. Berlin JS, Binder DM, Emiley TJ, Hatch KL, Mann AL, Milack GP, Palestrant M, Rubinlichl J. Leiomyoma of the foot—a review of the literature and report of cases. J Am Podiatr Assoc 1976;66:450.

6. Spinosa FA. Leiomyoma of the foot. J Foot Surg 1985;24:68.

7. Galinski AW, Aune CJ. Benign leiomyoma of the foot—a case report. Clin Podiatr Med Surg 1988; 5:359.

8. Stout AP. Solitary cutaneous and subcutaneous leiomyoma. Am J Cancer 1937;29:435.

9. Montgomery H, Winkelmann RK. Smooth-muscle tumors of the skin. Arch Dermatol 1959; 79:32.

10. Berlin ST and members of the Maryland Podiatry Residency Research Committee: Soft somatic tumors of the foot—diagnosis and surgical management. Mt. Kisco Futura Publishing Co., 1976.

11. Wilder JR, Lotfi MW. Leiomyoma of the saphenous vein. Postgrad Med 1971;50:154.

12. Galinski AW, Valahos M. Glomus tumor or glomangioma in podiatric medicine. J Am Podiatr Assoc 1975;65:167.

13. Brenner MA, Kalish SR. Glomus tumors with special reference in children's feet. J Am Podiatr Assoc 1978;68:715.

14. Phillsbury DM, Shelley WB, Kligman AM. Dermatology. Philadelphia: Saunders, 1956; 1171–1173.

15. Christopherson WM. Solitary cutaneous and subcutaneous leiomyoma. Arch Surg 1950; 60:779.

16. Templeton AC. Subcutaneous leiomyoma: a neglected tumor. East Afr Med J 1972;49:521.

17. Hosey TC, Jacob T, Kallet HA. Vascular leiomyoma—a case report and review of the literature. J Am Podiatr Assoc 1984;74:93.

18. Genakos JJ, Wallace JA, Napoli AE, Pontarelli A, Terris A. Angioleiomyoma—case report and literature review. J Am Podiatr Med Assoc 1987; 77:101.

19. Tozzi MA, Bodman MA. Angioleiomyoma—a case report. J Am Podiatr Assoc 1978;68:823.

20. Dockery GL, Wendel RE. Benign vascular leiomyoma—angioma of the digit—case report. J Am Podiatr Assoc 1979;69:438.

21. Duhig JT, Payer J. Vascular leiomyoma: a study of 61 cases. AMA Arch Pathol 1959;68:424.

22. Freedman AM, Meland NB. Angioleiomyomas of the extremities: report of a case and review of the Mayo Clinic experience. Plast Reconstruct Surg 1989;83:328.

23. Hachisuga T, Hashimoto H, Enjoji M. Angioleiomyoma: a clinicopathologic reappraisal of 562 cases. Cancer 1984;54:126.

24. Ekeström S. A comparison between glomus tumor and angioleiomyoma. Acta Pathol Microbiol Scand 1950;27:86.

25. Ledesma-Medina J, Kook Sang Oh, Girdany BR. Calcification in childhood leiomyoma. Radiology 1980;135:339.

26. Bulmer JH. Smooth muscle tumours of the limbs. J Bone Joint Surg (Br) 1967;49:52.

27. Jegasothy BV, Gilgor RS, Hull DM. Leiomyosarcoma of the skin and subcutaneous tissue. Arch Dermatol 1981;117:478.

28. White IR, Macdonald DM. Cutaneous leiomyosarcomas with coexistent superficial angioleiomyoma. Clin Exp Dermatol 1981;6:333.

29. Allison MF. Leiomyosarcoma of the femoral vein—report of a case in a child. Clin Pediatr 1965;4:28.

30. Dorfman HD, Fisher ER. Leiomyosarcoma of greater saphenous vein: report of a case and review of literature. Am J Clin Pathol 1963;39:73.

31. Stringer BD. Leiomyosarcoma of artery and vein. Am J Surg 1977;134:90.

32. Kevorkian J, Cento DP. Leiomyosarcoma of large arteries and veins. Surgery 1973;73:390.

33. Humphrey M, Neff J, Lin F, Krishnav L. Leiomyosarcoma of the saphenous vein—a case report and review of the literature. J Bone Joint Surg (Am) 1987;69:282.

34. Eady JL, McKinney JD, McDonald EC. Primary leiomyosarcoma of bone—a case report and review of the literature. J Bone Joint Surg (Am) 1987;69:282.

35. Appelman HD, Halgig EB. Gastric epithelioid leiomyoma and leiomyosarcoma (leiomyoblastoma). Cancer 1976;38:708.

36. Wu KK. Leiomyosarcoma of the foot. J Foot Surg 1988;27:362.

37. Henriksson KG. Semi-open muscle biopsy technique. Acta Neurol Scand 1979;59:317.

38. Bernardone JJ, Scarlet JJ. Leiomyosarcoma—a case report and literature review. J Am Podiatr Med Assoc 1988;78:183.

39. Phelan JT, Sherer W, Perez M. Malignant smooth—muscle tumors (leiomyosarcomas of soft-tissue origin.) New Engl J Med 1962; 266:1027.

40. Wile AG, Evans HL, Romsdahl MM. Leiomyosarcoma of soft tissue: a clinicopathologic study. Cancer 1981;48:1022.

41. Hajdu SI. Pathology of soft tissue tumors. Philadelphia: Lea & Febiger, 1979.

42. Goldman RL. Multicentric benign rhabdomyoma of skeletal muscle. Cancer 1963;16:1609.

43. Parsons HG, Puro HE. Rhabdomyoma of skeletal muscle: report of a case. Am J Surg 1955; 89:1187.

44. Dehner LP, Enzinger FM, Font RL. Fetal rhabdomyoma—an analysis of nine cases. Cancer 1972;30:160.

45. Maurer H. Rhabdomyosarcoma. Pediatr Ann 1979;8:17.

46. Hurley JV. Rhabdomyosarcoma of skeletal muscle. Aust N Z J Surg 1954;24:45.

47. Horn RC, Patton RB. Rhabdomyosarcoma. Clin Orthop 1961;19:99.

48. Charache H. Traumatic rhabdomyosarcoma of thigh. Am J Surg 1936;32:530.

49. Simon MA, Enneking WF. The management of soft-tissue sarcoma of the extremities. J Bone Joint Surg (Am) 1976;58:317.

50. Roholl PJM, Dejong ASH, Ramackers PCS. Application of markers in the diagnosis of soft tissue tumors. Histopathology 1985;9:1019.

51. Fornage BD. Ultrasonography of muscles and tendons: examination technique and atlas of normal anatomy of the extremities. New York: Springer-Verlag, 1989;45–50.

52. Lawrence W, Donegan W, Natarajan N, Mettlin

C, Beart R, Winchester D. Adult soft sarcomas. Ann Surg 1987;205:349.

53. Chang AE, Matory YL, Dwyer AJ, Hill SC, Girton ME, Steinberg SM, Knop RH, Frank JA, Hyams D, Doppman JL, Rosenberg SA. Magnetic resonance imaging versus computed tomography in the evaluation of soft tissue tumors of the extremities. Ann Surg 1987;205:340.

54. Berlin JS, Kovalczyk W, Samuels DB. Granular cell myoblastoma of the foot—a report of four cases. J Am Podiatr Assoc 1984;74:368.

55. Murphy GH, Dockerty MB, Broders AC. Myoblastoma. Am J Pathol 1949;25:1157.

56. Mandracchia V, Mahan KT, Pruzansky J, Uricchio JN. Myositis ossificans—a report of a case in the foot. J Am Podiatr Assoc 1983;73:31.

57. Fuselier CO, Tlapek TA, Sowell RD. Heterotrophic ossification (myositis ossificans) in the foot—a case report. J Am Podiatr Med Assoc 1986;76:524.

58. Siegelmen SS, Jacobson GH. The foot in acquired systemic diseases. Semin Roentgenol 1970;5:436.

59. Riley HD, Christie A. Myositis ossificans progressiva. Pediatrics 1951;8:153.

60. Pack GT, Branund RR. The development of sarcoma in myositis ossificans—report of three cases. J Am Med Assoc 1942;119:776.

61. Flynn JE, Graham JH. Myositis ossificans. Surg Gynecol Obstet 1964;118:100.

62. Mitra M, Sen AK, Deb HK. Myositis ossificans traumatica; a complication of tetanus. J Bone Joint Surg (Am) 1986;58:885.

63. Kern WH. Proliferative myositis: a pseudosarcomatous reaction to injury. Arch Pathol 1960;69:209.

64. Harris DJ, Fornasier VL. Pseudomalignant myositis ossificans (a clinicopathological characterisation of twenty-five cases and review of world literature). J Bone Joint Surg (Br) 1979; 61:246.

65. Ackerman LV. Extra-osseous localized nonneoplastic bone and cartilage formation (so-called myositis ossificans). J Bone Joint Surg (Am) 1958;40:279.

Part C/ **Tenosynovial Neoplasia**

—Thomas M. DeLauro

This chapter part assumes a patient's diagnosis has been confirmed. It does not guide us from the point of initial presentation to that of biopsy. It is of no help to the clinician first confronted with an articular or juxtaarticular soft-tissue mass. Armed with only a nonspecific and interchangeable list of possibilities, we often rush to the point of excision and await a pathologic diagnosis. At times, we take great pride in making the correct diagnosis; however, we have known the surprise and confusion of making the wrong one. Although this chapter cannot solve every problem, it provides the reader with an algorithmic approach to the synovial or tendinous soft-tissue mass.

THE CELLS OF TENDON AND SYNOVIAL TISSUE

Articular, juxtaarticular, or tendinous soft-tissue masses potentially may be of tenosynovial origin. Considering that neoplasia of other histologic types may also affect these regions, it becomes necessary to weigh the relative frequencies of occurrence. While neoplasms affecting the vicinity of joints and tendons are common, those of tenosynovial origin are rare. Neoplasms arising near joints, tendons, and bursae are not always comprised of synovial tissue; nevertheless, it is wise to present some of the latest concepts concerning tendon and synovial cells.

The cells that comprise tendons are known to be of two types, consistent with the surface and innermost portions of the tendon. Tendon collagen is arranged in primary, secondary, tertiary, and even quaternary bundles. The cells that make up the internal portion of the tendon are believed to be of fibroblastic origin, responsible for maintaining this collagen network. Surface tendon cells, on the other hand, are synovial in origin and capable of serving a lubricating and/or gliding function (1).

Synovial lining cells (SLC), as their name implies, exist in the inner layer of the synovial lining. The synovial lining, itself, is the inner, glistening surface of joint capsules and tendon sheaths. The lining does not extend over cartilage but does cover intraarticular ligaments and tendons. It is thought to arise from embryonic mesenchyme.

The synovial lining consists of a SLC layer (known as the synovial intima or intimal layer) and the remainder of the lining (known as the subsynovial tissue or subintima). The subintima contains the neurovasculature of the synovial lining and merges with the joint capsule. Areolar, fibrous, and adipose subintima exist, each type apparently corresponding to a different function. It is the subintima that seems to determine the number and type of SLCs in the synovial intima.

Synovial lining cells form a broken layer between the joint space and the subintima. Synovial lining cells can be of the A type (few in number, with a vacuolar cytoplasm), or of the B type (more numerous, with few vacuoles). The existence of a third or intermediate type, referred to as either C or AB, has been questioned. Each type is capable of division, but does so at a relatively slow rate. Each type appears capable of phagocytic, secretive, and absorptive functions (2).

SPECIFIC DIAGNOSTIC MEASURES AND PROCEDURES

Except for the tenosynovial neoplasias that grow quite rapidly and cause extensive destruction, a history and clinical examination may not be particularly helpful. This may appear to contradict the basic tenets of medical practice but is meant only to reinforce the notion that vague complaints of pain, swelling, or limitation of joint motion do little to identify the neoplastic nature and cellular origin of the mass. Yet these are the very symptoms and signs that patients with tenosynovial neoplasias exhibit because of the location of the tumors. Clinicians have searched, therefore, for alternate ways of imaging as discussed in the following section.

Xeroradiography

When first described, xeroradiography assumed a panaceal status in soft tissue diagnosis. Image resolution was considered superior to anything available through plain film radiography and the medical literature was inundated with articles detailing its use. As newer imaging modalities, capable of differentiating soft tissues from one another, were discovered, the use of xeroradiography declined. It now is difficult to even locate a center that still maintains xeroradiographic equipment; such studies remain somewhat popular only in Europe. There, the superiority of xeroradiography over plain film radiography continues to be expounded for the examination of tumors, tumorous conditions, and Achilles peritendinopathies, not detected by clinical examination alone (3, 4).

Ultrasonography

Ultrasound examinations are most useful because they can differentiate solid from cystic (fluid-filled) lesions, especially when a soft-tissue neoplasm is suspected in the absence of bony findings on plain film radiology. Ultrasonography can disclose even nonpalpable lesions, but it cannot determine the histologic type of a soft-tissue mass or be used to visualize a synovial sheath (5–7).

Ultrasound examinations utilize a tissue's "echogenicity," or ability to emit a signal. Cystic or fluid-filled lesions provide poor signals and are, therefore, said to be hypoechoic. Lesions of similar echogenicity are termed isoechoic, whereas those of greater signal intensity are hyperechoic. Echogenicity is influenced not only by the tissue under study, but also by that tissue's position in relation to the transducer head. This has been demonstrated clearly in ultrasound examinations involving tendons, wherein tendons were hyperechoic (compared to muscle) when the tendons are held perpendicular to the transducer. An angle of only 2–7° away from the perpendicular renders the tendon isoechoic; at greater angles, the tendon becomes hypoechoic (8) (Fig. 5.10, **A** and **B**).

Practitioners will agree quickly that not all tendon enlargements are neoplastic. Ultrasonographic patterns have been described, therefore, to distinguish tenalgia, peritendinitis, tendinitis, and enthesopathy. Tenalgia is the term applied to a painful tendon without other demonstrable change. Peritendinitis results when the highly vascularized paratenon becomes inflamed and exhibits an enlarged anteroposterior tendon diameter with a hyperechoic Kager's triangle. Tendinitis can exist with or without peritendinitis and represents significant pathology of the tendon. Such areas are poorly vascularized, which can lead to rupture. These sites present as thickenings with degenerative hypoechoic nodules within the tendon itself. Enthesopathy occurs at the point of a tendon's attachment into bone and is considered one hallmark of the seronegative spondyloarthropathies. Sonographically, these exhibit a thickening of the distal tendon, microcalcification, and an hypoechoic area behind the tendinous insertion. While plain film radiography and xeroradiography provide similar information concerning a tendon's thickness, ultrasonography is superior to these modalities because of its ability to display the internal structure of a tendon (9) (Figs. 5.3–5.9).

Ultrasonography may also be useful in distinguishing benign lesions from malignant ones, as well as in recognizing sarcomas, since most sarcomas are hypoechoic. Characteristics suggesting a benign lesion include regular margins, homoechogenicity and a spreading or displacement of muscle fibers. The converse appearance suggests malignancy: varying ech-

To the *right* of each *photograph* there is a corresponding *diagram*. In the *photographs*, the "×" and "+" are the markings at which measurements were taken.

In the *diagrams*:
BU, bursa: *CA*, calcaneus: *FHL, flexor hallucis longus:* K, Kager's triangle: *TE*, Archilles tendon: TI, tibia.

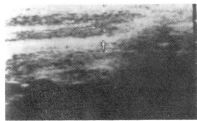

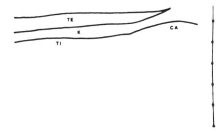

Figure 5.3. Ultrasound image of a normal Achilles tendon. The *two bigger arrows* are placed in the two regular echogenic bands delineating the hypoechogenic structure of the tendon. The *smaller arrows,* in the substance of the tendon, show the waveform structure of the tendon itself. (From Maffulli N, Regine R, Angelillo M, Capasso G, Filice S. Ultrasound diagnosis of Achilles tendon pathology in runners. Br J Sports Med 1987;21:158–162.)

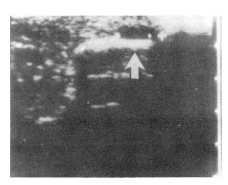

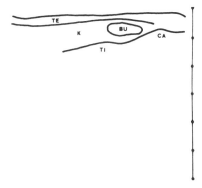

Figure 5.4. Ultrasound appearance of a normal pretendinous bursa: a hypoechogenic area, in front of the tendon, with well-defined borders. The *arrow* points to the posterior wall of the tendon. (From Maffulli N, Regine R, Angelillo M, Capasso G, Filice S. Ultrasound diagnosis of Achilles tendon pathology in runners. Br J Sports Med 1987;21:158–162.)

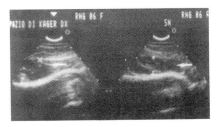

Figure 5.5. Kager's triangle: a homogenous triangle, with a high number of echoes. The *photograph* shows a normal Kager's triangle on both right and left side in a patient suffering from right tenalgia. The "×" (*left side*) and the "+" (*right side*) are the measuring points of the width of the triangle. (From Maffulli N, Regine R, Angelillo M, Capasso G, Filice S. Ultrasound diagnosis of Achilles tendon pathology in runners. Br J Sports Med 1987;21:158–162.)

ogenicity within the mass, irregular margins, and a rupture of muscle fibers (6).

Arteriography

Although it is an invasive procedure associated with some risk, arteriography is useful in assessing a tumor's size, location, extension, and vascularity. Arteriography also provides information concerning the best site for biopsy or amputation in a highly vascular lesion. Arteriography, however, cannot identify the histologic nature of a given soft-tissue mass on

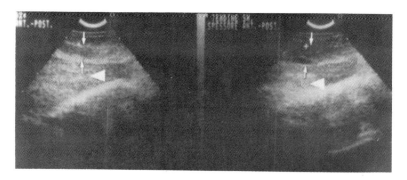

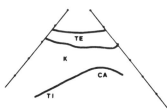
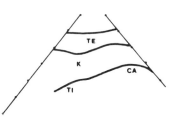

Figure 5.6.   Paratendonitis (*on the right side*): when compared to the normal contralateral tendon (*on the left*), there is an enlargement of the anteroposterior diameter (*arrows*), with some thickening of the anterior border of the tendon. The *arrows* show the anterior and posterior borders of the tendon. The "+" on the right side points to the posterior border of the tendon. The Kager's triangle is not involved in the disease. (From Maffulli N, Regine R, Angelillo M, Capasso G, Filice S. Ultrasound diagnosis of Achilles tendon pathology in runners. Br J Sports Med 1987; 21:158–162.)

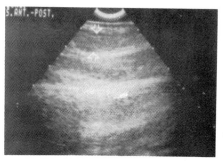
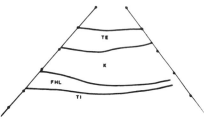

Figure 5.7.   Tendonitis: the tendon is widened, either for its entire length or partially. The *arrows* show the point of discrete changes of echogenic pattern. (From Maffulli N, Regine R, Angelillo M, Capasso G, Filice S. Ultrasound diagnosis of Achilles tendon pathology in runners. Br J Sports Med 1987; 21:158–162.)

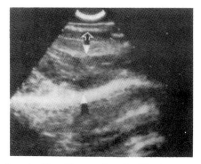
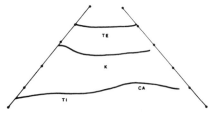

Figure 5.8.   Tendonitis with paratendonitis: increase in the echogenicity of Kager's triangle (delineated by *two triangles*) and of the posterior border of the tendon (*empty arrows*). The *small arrow* points to a definite intratendinous area of dishomogeneity. (From Maffulli N, Regine R, Angelillo M, Capasso G, Filice S. Ultrasound diagnosis of Achilles tendon pathology in runners. Br J Sports Med 1987; 21:158–162.)

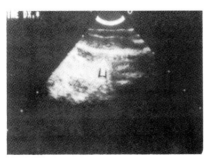
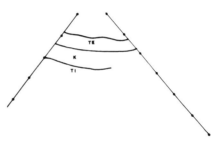

Figure 5.9. Enthesopathy: enlargement of the distal part of the tendon, with alterations of the normal pattern of echogenicity. The *arrow* points to the anterior border of the tendon. (From Maffulli N, Regine R, Angelillo M, Capasso G, Filice S. Ultrasound diagnosis of Achilles tendon pathology in runners. Br J Sports Med 1987;21:158–162.)

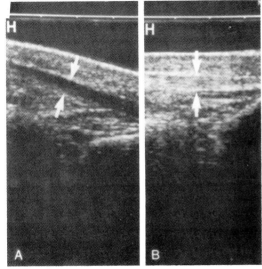

Figure 5.10. Pitfall of tendon sonography. Longitudinal scans of normal patellar tendon. **A,** The tendon is oblique in relation to the ultrasound beam and appears falsely hypoechoic (*arrows*). **B,** Placing the tendon strictly parallel to the probe results in the demonstration of the normal echogenicity of the tendon (*arrows*). **H,** toward subject's head. (From Fornage BD. The hypoechoic tendon: a pitfall. J Ultrasound Med 1987;6:19–22.)

the basis of distinctive vascular patterns. In one study involving synovial sarcoma, the degree of vascularity was found to be dependent upon the histologic type but was determined not to be useful for establishing the primary diagnosis (10).

Contrast Arthrography

The injection of radiopaque material into joints, tendon sheaths, and bursae can aid in visualizing the gross morphology of a mass. Its application appears limited due to the tech-nique's invasiveness and nonspecificity. Although villous and nonvillous lesions may be distinguished, definite conclusions concerning histologic type cannot be drawn.

Computerized Tomography (CT)

The advent of CT scanning represents a significant advance in medical imaging. Its widespread use, availability, and application are well-documented (11, 12). Although it exposes patients to higher radiation dosages than those used for plain film radiography, computerized tomography uses only one-tenth of the dosage of standard x-ray tomography (12). Although CT scanning is excellent for differentiating soft tissue from bone, soft-tissue lesions involving bone, and soft-tissue lesions of varying density, it is limited in its ability to distinguish histologic type or to define soft-tissue masses of the same density as the surrounding tissues.

Magnetic Resonance Imaging (MRI)

Magnetic resonance is the newest imaging modality and the most expensive. However, it is often the least available. Magnetic resonance is similar to computerized tomography in that it is of limited specificity in predicting the histologic nature of a mass. It cannot distinguish a lesion of synovial origin from other origins or distinguish one type of synovial lesion from another. It cannot demonstrate calcification as well as CT scanning can, but is superior to computerized tomography for identifying the borders and relationship of a soft-tissue mass to the underlying bone (13).

A distinct advantage of MRI over CT scanning is its ability to "weight" or manipulate magnetic images to enhance certain pathologic conditions (14). Vascular structures are visible without arteriography, and the sharp borders

Table 5.1. Relative Intensities of Musculoskeletal Tissue[a]

T1-weighted	T2-weighted
High intensity	
Subcutaneous fat	Stationary blood
Bone marrow	Tumor
Stationary blood	Urine
Hyaline cartilage	Subcutaneous fat
Tumor	Bone marrow
Muscle	Hyaline cartilage
Urine	Muscle
Ligaments/tendon	Ligaments/tendon
Compact bone	Compact bone
Air	Air
Low intensity	

[a]From Jacobs AM, O'Leary RJ, Totty WE, Hardy DC. Magnetic resonance imaging of the foot and ankle. Clin Podiatr Med Surg 1987;4:903–924.

of a benign mass and the indistinct borders of a malignancy are more easily visualized.

Except for adipose tissue, most soft-tissue masses have the same signal intensity as muscle on "T1-weighted" examinations, whereas "T2" images will enhance their appearance. In contrast, fatty tumors or masses with a signal intensity similar to that of fat are made more visible on T1-weighted examinations. (14) (Table 5.1).

Fine-needle Aspiration Cytology (FNAC)

Although fine-needle aspiration cytology has been used for almost a century, it is only recently that Swedish investigators have made it a popular procedure. The procedure itself is defined as the gathering and studying of cellular samples that are obtained through a narrow-gauge needle (most frequently 22, 23, or 25 gauge) under vacuum. If a lesion cannot be palpated or visualized by special imaging techniques, such as CT scanning, ultrasonography, or MRI, then fine-needle aspiration cytology should be considered (15). FNAC is helpful in recognizing certain benign lesions, in obtaining cultures for a specific infectious agent, and in the diagnosing, separating, and staging of malignant tumors, both primary and metastatic. The only contraindication to this procedure appears to be a lack of hemostasis when biopsying vascular lesions (e.g., aneurysms) that have been confirmed by angiography. The procedure always should be performed as a sterile one and the skin prepared appropriately (16). The decreased need for general anesthesia and hospitalization, the avoidance of surgery, and the fact that this technique can be performed on an outpatient basis makes percutaneous biopsy a very cost-effective measure, especially in terms of diagnosis-related groups reimbursements (17).

Whereas the efficacy of fine-needle aspiration cytology is well understood and accepted, some disagreement exists as to who should obtain the biopsy and what method or methods should be used. Two basic aspects of the procedure are: (a) the actual collection of the specimen and (b) the preparation and transport of the smear. A high index of suspicion, manual dexterity in needle placement and handling, a good knowledge of anatomy, and experience are reasonable prerequisites for the individual who is planning to obtain the specimen. Any trained practitioner is eligible and capable of collecting the specimen, although many American and European colleagues strongly contend that the pathologist should be the aspirator (18–20). For tumors in highly inaccessible areas where advanced imaging techniques are required to determine needle placement, a radiologist may be the best individual to collect the specimen (18). Since aspiration of simple ganglionic cysts is a common procedure for those who deal with lower extremity pathology, these clinicians should be highly capable of obtaining the specimen.

In terms of specimen collection, the mass in question should be pinched with the thumb and index finger of one hand to fix its position. The other hand should be used to insert the needle vertically. While a continuous vacuum on the plunger of the syringe is maintained, the needle should be moved in both vertical and oblique planes in order to collect an adequate specimen. The visualization of cellular contents in the needle hub indicates that an adequate amount has been collected. At this point, the plunger should be released, allowing the vacuum within the syringe to equalize before the needle is withdrawn. Next, pressure should be applied to the puncture site to promote hemostasis. The needle should never be withdrawn while there is still vacuum in the syringe. Sections of the mass that are fibrotic, previously aspirated, cystic, necrotic, or hemorrhagic may not provide an adequate specimen. Areas that are cystic, necrotic, or hemorrhagic can often be recognized by their soft consistency (16).

A method of collection without aspiration has recently been described (Figs. 5.11–5.16).

As mentioned above, preparation and trans-

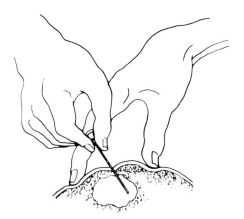

Figure 5.11. The tumor is immobilized with one hand. The fine needle is introduced into the tumor with the other hand. (From Zajdela A, Zillhart P, Voillemot N. Cytological diagnosis by fine needle sampling without aspiration. Cancer. 1987;59: 1201–1205.)

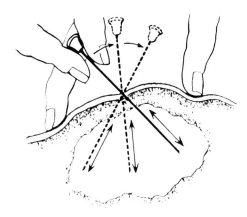

Figure 5.12. The needle is moved back and forth very slightly as it is angled in different depths of the tumor before it is withdrawn. (From Zajdela A, Zillhart P, Voillemot N. Cytological diagnosis by fine needle sampling without aspiration. Cancer. 1987;59: 1201–1205.)

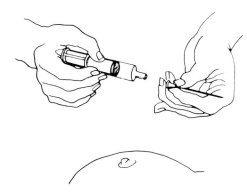

Figure 5.13. The needle is removed and connected to a syringe filled with air. (From Zajdela A, Zillhart P, Voillemot N. Cytological diagnosis by fine needle sampling without aspiration. Cancer. 1987;59: 1201–1205.)

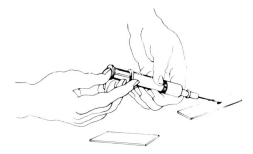

Figure 5.14. The cellular material is expelled onto a glass slide. (From Zajdela A, Zillhart P, Voillemot N. Cytological diagnosis by fine needle sampling without aspiration. Cancer. 1987; 59:1201–1205.)

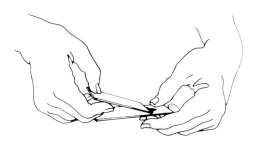

Figure 5.15. The smear is spread gently with a glass slide inclined at an angle of 10°. (From Zajdela A, Zillhart P, Voillemot N. Cytological diagnosis by fine needle sampling without aspiration. Cancer. 1987;59: 1201–1205.)

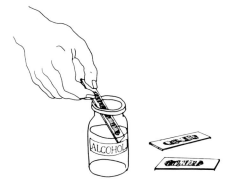

Figure 5.16. The smear is fixed in ethyl alcohol. Other smears are air-dried. (From Zajdela A, Zillhart P, Voillemot N. Cytological diagnosis by fine needle sampling without aspiration. Cancer. 1987;59: 1201–1205.)

port of the specimen pose additional problems. For clinicians unfamiliar with the nuances of these variables, it is highly recommended that they consult their cytology laboratory for the preferred means of transport and leave smear preparation to those best trained to perform it (18, 21, 22).

Fine-needle aspiration cytology has demonstrated its value in the initial diagnosis and confirmation of high-grade malignancies and metastases, and in the exclusion of suspected treatment failures. While not replacing formal open biopsy, FNAC has reduced the need to repeat open biopsies (23).

Fine-needle aspiration cytology, however, is not a panacea. Several authors have reported difficulty in defining the histologic type of sarcoma based upon these aspirations and in separating low-grade malignancies from other conditions such as defibromatosis. Concern over the transplantation of neoplastic cells along the needle tract has been expressed but has rarely been reported when needles of 21 or thinner gauge are used and may be somewhat obviated by needle placement within an area of surgery should that option subsequently become necessary (16, 23). In summary, one may conclude that a routine history and physical examination, in conjunction with numerous imaging modalities, are only of limited value in identifying the tenosynovial nature of a soft-tissue mass and in differentiating one such lesion from another. Despite technological advances, none has supplanted histologic diagnosis at this time. Once a soft-tissue mass is suspected or diagnosed, clinicians should consider using fine-needle aspiration cytology more often. Various imaging methods may be used to better visualize a mass before or during aspiration, or after the histologic diagnosis has been confirmed, in order to plan the best surgical or nonsurgical therapeutic approach.

DIFFERENTIAL DIAGNOSIS

Soft-tissue masses that are within or near joints, tendons, and bursae suggest a tenosynovial origin. Given the large number of such regions in the foot and leg, virtually any soft-tissue mass could be suspicious. While some masses involving or arising from the tenosynovium are truly malignant, most are either nonneoplastic or of a benign neoplastic nature. Hadju's classification (24) therefore is used to separate the tenosynovial neoplasias from nonneoplastic lesions.

Nonneoplastic Lesions (24)

TENOSYNOVIAL CYST (GANGLION)

Those involved in treating lower extremity disorders are most familiar with the tenosynovial cyst or ganglion. These thin-walled, mucin-filled cystic lesions often are found in association with joint capsules, bursae, or tendon sheaths. Although their precise etiology is unknown, three theories of formation have been proposed: herniation, ectopic placement of synovial tissue, and de novo formation secondary to inflammatory or traumatic changes in multipotential cells. Middle-aged patients usually are affected, with a slight female predominance of 2:1. Approximately 35% of patients with this condition admit a history of prior trauma and may also relate that the mass undergoes periods of enlargement and shrinkage. The explanation for this latter phenomenon seems to be a valvular mechanism that regulates the transfer of fluid between the cyst and its associated tendon sheath, joint, or bursae (25, 26).

On plain film radiography, large ganglia may be recognized by adjacent bony pressure effects leading to slight erosion. Computerized tomography, ultrasonography, or radiopaque dye injection may be helpful in visualizing the cyst. Disadvantages of ultrasonography, however, are its inability to recognize small cysts and the difficulty with which it can be used to differentiate debris-laden cysts from solid lesions. Arteriography, although usually unnecessary, can demonstrate the avascular nature of the ganglion (25–27).

TENOSYNOVITIS (TENDINITIS)

As discussed in the section on ultrasonography, tendinitis can range from a simple pain without pathologic change to peritendinitis and degenerative changes within the tendon substance. Chronically inflamed tendons are often the result of overuse in individuals active in sports and can be distinguished from other causes of tendon thickening by the presence of calcification, osseous spurring at the point of tendinous attachment, and occasional cystic changes in the associated bone (28).

Nodular or diffuse Achilles tendon thickening in adults (or in adolescents) at the calcaneal insertion may be secondary to seronegative spondyloarthropathy. Often, these cases are HLA-B27 positive and demonstrate calcaneal erosions on plain film radiography. Recently, however, such tendon thickening was observed in an adult HLA-B27 patient for many years without evidence of spinal disease (29).

SYNOVIAL CHONDROMATOSIS (OSTEOCHONDRITIS DISSECANS)

Although these disorders are grouped pathologically, most practitioners will recognize them as separate clinical disorders. Synovial chondromatosis is thought to be the result of metaplastic changes in subsynovial connective tissue, leading to the development of cartilaginous foci in the synovium. The disorder has been reported to involve the ankle, although rarely. It is usually monarticular but can involve two or more joints. Synovial chondromatosis more frequently is observed in men than women, with a varying history of trauma.

Symptoms are as nonspecific as pain, swelling, and limitation of motion, sometimes to the point of joint locking. Some patients, however, are totally asymptomatic, with a diagnosis being made on x-ray alone. Plain film radiography often will demonstrate intraarticular radiopaque loose bodies and stippling of the synovium. The stippling is the result of cartilaginous foci having become calcified. The loose bodies in this condition generally are considered to be smaller than those seen in osteochondritis dissecans. Computerized tomography may be helpful in identifying the calcified bodies. In the absence of such findings, a synovial biopsy may be required to demonstrate cartilaginous foci within the synovium.

By comparison, pigmented villonodular synovitis also demonstrates nodular masses, but calcification is noticeably absent. While synovial chondromatosis is usually intraarticular and free of bony involvement, synovial sarcoma often is extraarticular, with adjacent bone destruction. Since synovial chondromatosis and synovial sarcoma exhibit calcification on x-ray, this finding is not particularly helpful (30).

In contrast to synovial chondromatosis, osteochondritis dissecans more often represents a posttraumatic event at any age or a traction apophysitis in children. In younger age groups, these are considered overuse syndromes secondary to repetitive microtrauma or a single episode of macrotrauma at the apophysis during growth spurt periods. The hypothesis that muscle tendon units may not elongate as rapidly as their accompanying osseous segments,

therefore leading to enhanced tension, has been advanced to explain the development of these disorders. Classic lower extremity sites include the tibial tubercle (Osgood-Schlatter disease), the inferior pole of the patella (Sinding-Larsen-Johansson syndrome), the calcaneal apophysis (Sever's disease), and the accessory navicular (os tibiale externum syndrome) (31). All produce localized swellings capable of being erroneously diagnosed as neoplasia.

When associated with a finite history of trauma, plain film radiography, triphasic technetium bone scans, and magnetic resonance imaging have been helpful in determining the mechanical stability of the osteochondritic fragment and in assessing whether conservative or surgical therapy is warranted. On plain film radiography, the larger the involved area and more intense the sclerotic rim, the greater the chance of loosening. The presence or absence of an ossification center has no bearing. The presence of focal hyperemia is a strong sign of loosening, with MRI permitting direct visualization of fragment-loosening or displacement (32).

XANTHOMA

Xanthomas are discrete lipid collections usually seen in the hyperlipoproteinemias and in patients with diabetes mellitus or obstructive liver disease. As solitary or multiple peritendinous masses, they can easily be confused with true neoplasia. (33, 34).

Paradoxically, xanthomas also have been observed in normocholesterolemic and normolipemic patients. One will recall that cholesterol is carried in the bloodstream by low-density lipoproteins (LDL), very low-density lipoproteins (VLDL), and high-density lipoproteins (HDL). HDL seem to exert a protective effect by transporting intracellular cholesterol to the liver for degradation; decreases in this fraction, therefore, will interfere with the removal of intracellular cholesterol. As a result, three types of normocholesterolemic xanthomatosis now are known: (a) altered lipoprotein content or structure, as in cerebrotendinous xanthomatosis, in which the lipid component is abnormal, and situations wherein the protein portion of the lipoprotein is abnormal, (b) association with underlying lymphoproliferative disease, such as cryoglobulinemia, multiple myeloma, etc., and (c) situations in which the elements of (a) and (b) above are absent, with abnormalities primarily due to local tissue alteration such as inflammation or trauma (35, 36).

Granulomatous Synovitis. Reported most commonly in the knee and ankle, these usually are tuberculous joints which can mimic a tumor with an occasional draining sinus through the skin. On plain film radiography, one notes early swelling of soft tissue followed by periarticular demineralization and marginal erosions in nonstress areas. In time, the process results in destruction of articular cartilage. The healing process usually results in ankylosis with soft-tissue calcification. Arteriography demonstrates the hypervascular nature of the lesion (27).

Benign Neoplastic Lesions
SYNOVIAL HEMANGIOMA

Primarily affecting the knee and synovial tendon sheaths, these rare lesions usually are associated with angiomas of skin and deeper tissues. Adolescent or young adult women are chiefly affected. In its localized form, the synovial hemangioma frequently leads to joint locking as a result of its often pedunculated shape. In contrast, diffuse forms of synovial hemangioma present with hemarthrosis as well as associated skin and visceral hemangiomas. Ipsilateral increases in limb length may be observed in some arteriovenous shunts, as well as in cases of diffuse synovial hemangioma because of the hypervascular effect these lesions have on an immature epiphysis. Both the localized and diffuse forms can be visualized with contrast arthrography (seen as multiple filling defects with a villous configuration) on computerized tomography. The hypervascular nature of these lesions can be demonstrated by arteriography (27).

PERITENDINOUS FIBROMAS AND LIPOMAS

Covered in greater detail in other portions of this text, these are included in the present discussion for the sake of completeness. One must guard against mistaking the firm nature of a desmoplastic or fibrotic malignancy from that of a benign fibroma.

PIGMENTED VILLONODULAR SYNOVITIS

Histologically, this lesion consists of a fibrous stroma, hemosiderin deposits, a histiocytic infiltrate, and giant cells in the affected synovial tissues (37). Its multicellularity has led to a vast array of well-documented synonyms, as well as an equal number of theories concerning its pathogenesis. Young adult males and females are affected equally, with lesions developing within joint linings, tendon sheaths, fascial planes, or ligaments. It is usually a monarticular disorder most commonly affecting the knee, followed by the ankle. Again, presenting complaints are as nonspecific as pain, swelling, and in some cases, a palpable mass. The finding of a palpable mass is observed more frequently in the ankle than in the knee (38).

Localized and diffuse forms exist, each appearing as a synovial lesion with hyperplastic and villous projections on gross examination. In the diffuse form, extensive pigmentation is found, often leading to the discovery of blood on joint aspiration. On plain film radiography, extensive hemosiderin deposition may appear more radiodense; however, no more than marginal erosion or cystic change is noted (Figs. 5.17–5.18). Calcification is usually noticeably absent. Arthrography will demonstrate clearly the villous configuration of both the localized and diffuse forms. Arteriography will reveal this lesion's early hypervascular nature and will demonstrate a more avascular pattern in chronic lesions or lesions with a great deal of fibrosis. CT scanning demonstrates intense signals in areas of hemosiderin deposition. MRI, by virtue of its inverse image, demonstrates hypointense signals in areas of hemosiderin deposition, and hyperintense signals where the synovium has been inflamed and congested (27, 38–41) (Figs. 5.19–5.20).

GIANT CELL TUMOR OF THE TENDON SHEATH (GCTTS)

This condition is considered by most authors as a variant of pigmented villonodular synovitis that affects the tendon sheath and is considered second only to the ganglion (tenosynovial cyst) in terms of its frequency of occurrence in the foot and leg (42–45). In one study of the antigenic and enzymatic properties of GCTTS cells, it is concluded that they are true histiocytes that most closely resemble osteoclasts (46). One case is reported in association with hypophosphatemic osteomalacia. Only 50 such cases are documented and recognized by the concomitant findings of osteomalacia, normocalcemia and hypophosphatemia. In addition to tumors, other causes of this presentation include Fanconi's Syndrome, X-linked hypophosphatemic rickets, and adult sporadic osteomalacia (47).

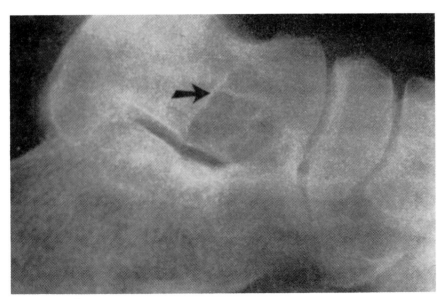

Figure 5.17. Lateral view of the talocalcaneal joint with thin-walled cysts (*arrow*). (From Mrose HE, DeLuca SA. Pigmented villonodular synovitis. Am Fam Physician 1988;37:195–196.)

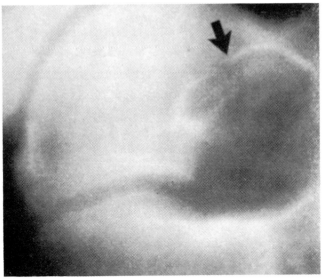

Figure 5.18. Computed tomographic scan of talocalcaneal joint, showing thin-walled cystic changes in the bone (*arrow*). (From Mrose HE, DeLuca SA. Pigmented villonodular synovitis. Am Fam Physician 1988;37:195–196.)

One series makes a distinction between giant cell tumor of the tendon sheath and pigmented villonodular synovitis on histologic grounds (the presence of villous projections in pigmented villonodular synovitis and their absence in GCTTS). Giant cell tumors of the tendon sheath were subdivided into a large-joint type involving ankles and knees, and a digital-type involving fingers and toes. The digital-type often presents as painless subcutaneous masses, most frequently involving the first and second toes in females. The large-joint type, on the other hand, presents more often as a large intraarticular mass with nonspecific

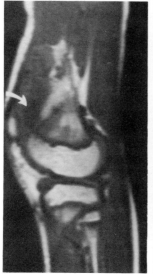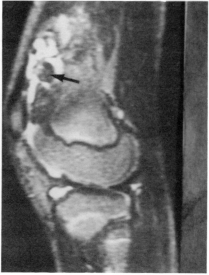

Figure 5.19–5.20. *Left,* Sagittal 600/25 ms image of the knee. Proliferating synovium is expanding the suprapatellar bursa and appears intermediate in signal (*arrow*). *Right,* 2500/80 ms image showing hemosiderin-laden synovium as areas of low signal (*arrow*) surrounded by high signal areas of fluid and congested synovium. (From Spritzer CE, Dalinka MK, Kressel HY. Magnetic resonance imaging of pigmented villonodular synovitis: a report of two cases. Skeletal Radiol 1987;16:316–319.)

symptoms. Since the large-joint type is able to grow with fewer anatomic restrictions, it can approach a histologic picture similar to that of pigmented villonodular synovitis, except for the latter disease's villous projections. The digital-type tumor has too many anatomic restrictions and, therefore, retains its appearance. The painful nature of tendon sheath fibromas, as well as their male predominance, help to distinguish them from the digital type of GCTTS (48) (Table 5.2).

Malignant Neoplastic Lesions
MALIGNANT GIANT CELL TUMORS

Although usually benign, the potential for malignant transformation for these lesions does exist (45).

TENOSYNOVIAL SARCOMAS (SYNOVIAL SARCOMAS)

Six different neoplasias comprise the tenosynovial sarcomas: biphasic sarcoma, monophasic spindle cell sarcoma, monophasic pseu-

Table 5.2. Clinicopathologic Differences between Digit and Large Joint Tumors of Giant Cell Tumor of the Tendon Sheath[a]

	Digit Tumors	Large Joint Tumors
Anatomic site	Synovial tissue of tendon sheath or small joints of a digit	Intraarticular synovial tissue of a large joint
Size and no. of nodules	Small (average, 1.1 cm), usually multiple	Relatively large (average, 2 cm), usually single
Covering of the nodule	Surrounded by a thin fibrous capsule	Covered by one or more layers of synovial cells
Synovial-lined spaces	Small numbers of cleft-like spaces	Large or numerous pseudoglandular spaces sometimes filled with foam cells
Fibrous elements within the nodule	Thick bundles of collagenous tissue, sometimes hyalinized	Loose-meshed appearance
Inflammatory cells	Rare or sparse	Mild or moderate

[a]From Ushijima M, Hashimoto H, Tsuneyoshi M, Enjoli M. Giant cell tumor of the tendon sheath (nodular tenosynovitis). A study of 207 cases to compare the large joint group with the common digit group. Cancer 1986;57:875–884.

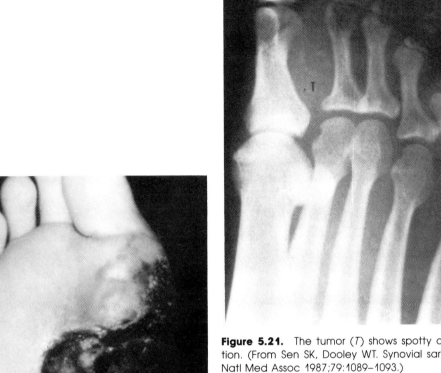

Figure 5.21. The tumor (*T*) shows spotty calcification. (From Sen SK, Dooley WT. Synovial sarcoma. J Natl Med Assoc 1987;79:1089–1093.)

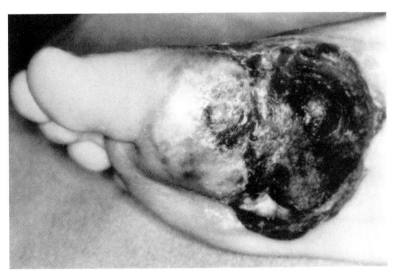

Figures 5.22–5.23. Preoperative pictures of a foot with a recurrent synovial sarcoma show that the tumor has produced extensive necrosis of the soft tissue on the medial and medioplantar aspect of the forefoot. (From Wu KK. Synovial sarcoma of the foot. J Foot Surg 1987;26(4):359–364, © by American College of Foot Surgeons, Inc.)

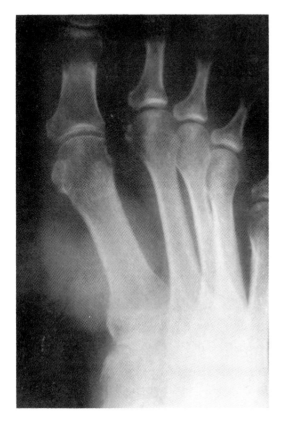

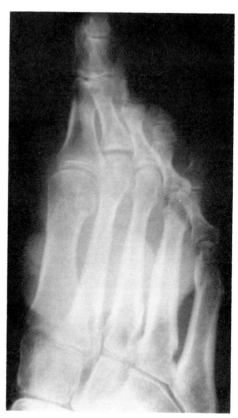

Figures 5.24–5.26. Anteroposterior, lateral, and oblique x-rays of the same foot show the presence of a slightly radiopaque and lobulated tumor on the medioplantar aspect of the foot. (From Wu KK. Synovial sarcoma of the foot. J Foot Surg 1987;26(4):359–364, © by American College of Foot Surgeons, Inc.)

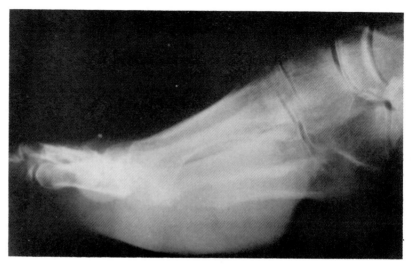

doglandular sarcoma, epithelioid sarcoma, cordoid sarcoma, and clear cell sarcoma (24). Variations within the fibrous stromal component or the epithelial component differentiate these lesions. As a group, they represent less than 10 percent of all soft-tissue malignancies and tend to predilect for males in their second through fourth decades. Tenosynovial sarcomas tend to arise near, but not necessarily from, joints, tendon sheaths, and bursae, presenting most frequently in the lower extremities as a slow-growing, painless mass. A history of trauma often can be elicited, but is not felt to be a predisposing factor. Plain film radiography usually demonstrates a soft-tissue mass with smooth or indistinct margins. Calcifications within the mass are noted in approximately one-third of affected patients (Fig. 5.21). Adjacent bony erosion, secondary to a pressure effect, can sometimes be observed. Computerized tomography often aids in visualization, and angiography generally exhibits a hypervascular pattern (27, 49–51) (Figs. 5.22–5.30).

TREATMENT AND PROGNOSIS

Nonneoplastic tenosynovial lesions most often are treated conservatively, using rest, immobilization, and antiinflammatory medications. Lesions, such as the tenosynovial cyst

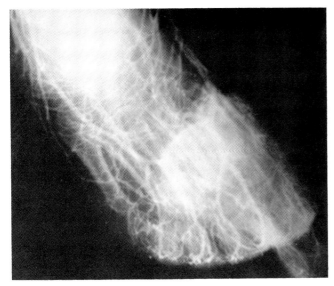

Figures 5.27–5.28. Arteriograms of the same foot show a marked increase in vascularity in the metatarsal region. (From Wu KK. Synovial sarcoma of the foot. J Foot Surg 1987;26(4):359–364, © by American College of Foot Surgeons, Inc.)

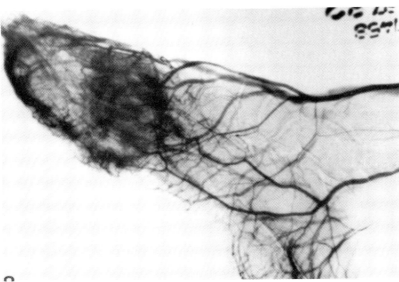

Figure 5.29. Nuclear magnetic resonance imaging of the foot shows that the tumor is basically confined to the region which indicates that a Syme's amputation or a below-knee amputation is the treatment of choice. (From Wu KK. Synovial sarcoma of the foot. J Foot Surg 1987;26(4):359–364, © by American College of Foot Surgeons, Inc.)

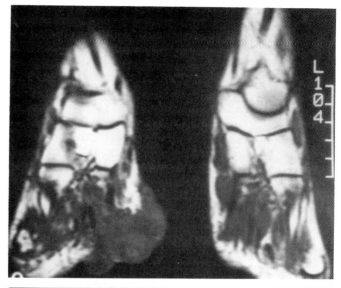

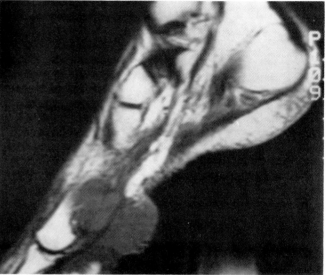

(ganglion), may be aspirated with the subsequent installation of a corticosteroid (52). Persistent symptoms or recurrence may necessitate surgical excision of the offending lesion. In the case of nonneoplastic masses that result from metabolic defects, such as xanthomas, consultation or referral to manage the underlying problem is paramount.

In patients with a truly benign neoplasm, conservative measures may be undertaken, but often only delay the eventual need for surgical excision prompted by interference by the neoplasm with pain-free ambulation or footgear use.

The greatest therapeutic concern centers around malignant tenosynovial lesions, wherein treatment can vary from wide excision (with chemotherapy and/or radiation) to amputation. The following features have been associated with a better prognosis: calcification, occurrence in children or females, distal location on the extremity, a strong glandular or epithelial tumor component, and tumor diameter of less than 5 cm (49, 53–56). Of these variables, a tumor diameter of less than 5 cm seems to be the most favorable prognostic indicator (24, 53, 54). One author has recommended a Syme's amputation if the lesion involves

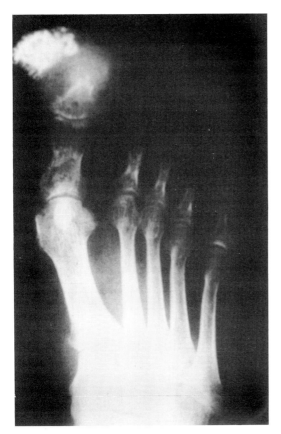

Figure 5.30. Anteroposterior foot x-ray shows a very large synovial sarcoma with extensive intralesional calcification in the distal portion of the great toe. (From Wu KK. *Surgery of the Foot*, Lea & Febiger, Philadelphia, 1986.)

the forefoot, sparing the heel and anterior ankle. A below-knee amputation is usually recommended if the rear of the foot is involved (57). Metastasis most often occurs to the lungs, although it has been reported to the skin as well and can occur months to years after the initial diagnosis (49, 53). Local recurrence is common and has been associated with a poor prognosis (27).

CONCLUSIONS

The location of the soft-tissue mass near a joint, tendon, tendon sheath, or bursae should make one consider a tenosynovial neoplasia. Malignant tumors of these tissues are rare but must be seriously considered at the time of initial presentation. Available forms of imaging may help to recognize benign from malignant lesions and to differentiate one synovial disor-

der from another. Absolutely nothing available today, however, can replace pathologic diagnosis available through fine-needle aspiration cytology (a nonaspiration method has recently been described (58)), or formal open biopsy. Earlier and greater reliance on these procedures is, therefore, strongly recommended. True malignancies require a seriously undertaken team approach during the periods of diagnosis, treatment, and follow-up.

REFERENCES

1. Banes AJ, Donlon K, Link GW, et al. Cell populations of tendon: a simplified method for isolation of synovial cells and internal fibroblasts: confirmation of origin and biologic properties. J Orthop Res 1988;6:83–94.
2. Henderson B, Pettipher ER. The synovial lining cell: biology and pathobiology. Semin Arthritis Rheum 1985;15:1–32.
3. Skotnikov VI, Chazov PD. Comparison of film radiography and electroroentgenography (xeroradiography) for the investigation of soft tissue tumors. Radiol Diagn (Berl) 1985;26:389–396.
4. Pignatelli V, Maffei G, Ruiu U, Orsitto E, Savino A. Xeroradiographic study of Achilles tendinopathies and paratendinopathies. Radiol Med (Torino) 1987;73:407–413.
5. Fornage BD, Rifkin MD. Ultrasound examination of tendons. Radiol Clin North Am 1988;26:87–107.
6. Vincent LM. Ultrasound of soft tissue abnormalities of the extremities. Radiol Clin North Am 1988;26:131–144.
7. Fornage BD, Rifkin MD. Ultrasound examination of the hand and foot. Radiol Clin North Am 1988;26:109–129.
8. Crass JR, van de Vegte GL, Harkavy LA. Tendon echogenicity: ex vivo study. Radiology 1988; 167:499–501.
9. Maffulli N, Regine R, Angelillo M, Capasso G, Filice S. Ultrasound diagnosis of Achilles tendon pathology in runners. Br J Sports Med 1987;21:158–162.
10. Lois JF, Fischer HJ, Mirra JM, Gomes AS. Angiography of histopathologic variants of synovial sarcoma. Acta Radiol [Diagn] (Stockh) 1986;27:449–454.
11. Sartoris DJ, Resnick D. Pictorial review: cross-sectional imaging of the foot and ankle. Foot Ankle 1987;8:59–80.
12. Sartoris DJ, Resnick D. Computed tomography of podiatric disorders: a review. J Foot Surg 1986;25:394–403.
13. Sundaram M, McGuire MH, Fletcher J, Wolverson MK, Heiberg E, Shields JB. Magnetic resonance imaging of lesions of synovial origin. Skeletal Radiol 1986;15:110–116.
14. Jacobs AM, O'Leary RJ, Totty WE, Hardy DC. Magnetic resonance imaging of the foot and ankle. Clin Podiatr Med Surg 1987;4:903–924.
15. Hammers LW, McCarthy S, Williams H, et al. Computed tomographic (CT) guided percuta-

neous fine needle aspiration biopsy: the Yale experience. Yale J Biol Med 1986;59:425–434.

16. Phillips JN, Goodman BN. Clinching the diagnosis: fine needle aspiration cytology. Pathology 1987;19:371–376.

17. Paolella LP, Cronan JJ, Dorfman GS, Esparza AR. Dollars and sense of percutaneous biopsy demonstrates the cost effectiveness of the procedure. RI Med J 1987;70:127–132.

18. Young GP. Enabling more physicians to do aspiration biopsy. Diagn Cytopathol 1986;2: 229–230.

19. Champ CS, Mason CH, Coghill SB, Powis SJ. Role of fine needle aspiration cytology (letter). J Clin Pathol 1988;41:234.

20. Kline TS. The hows of aspiration biopsy. Diagn Cytopathol 1986;2:228.

21. Anderson G, Cross HJ. Safe and efficient procedure for fine needle aspiration biopsy (letter). Med Lab Sci 1987;44:298–299.

22. Harris SC, Currie A, Anderson G, Howat AJ. Transport media for fine needle aspiration cytology (letter). J Clin Path 1987;40:1263.

23. Miralles TG, Gosalbez F, Menendez P, Astudillo A, Torre C, Buesa J. Fine needle aspiration cytology of soft-tissue lesions. Acta Cytol (Baltimore) 1986;30:671–678.

24. Hajdu SI. Pathology of Soft Tissue Tumors. Philadelphia: Lea and Febiger, 1986:165–226.

25. Rosenberg A. Dorsal tendosynovial cyst. J Am Podiatr Med Assoc 1986;76:455–457.

26. Wenig JA, McCarthy DJ. Synovial cyst of the hallux. J Am Podiatr Med Assoc 1986;76:7–12.

27. Sartoris DJ, Resnick D. Neoplastic processes of synovial origin. Contemp Diagn Radiol 1988;11:1–5.

28. Hunter SC, Poole RM. The chronically inflamed tendon. Clin Sports Med 1987;6:371–388.

29. Olivieri I, Gemignani G, Gherardi S, Grassi L, Ciompi ML. Isolated HLA-B27 associated Achilles tendinitis. Ann Rheum Dis 1987;46: 626–627.

30. Bauer M, Jonsson K. Synovial chondromatosis of the ankle. ROFO 1987;146:548–550.

31. Micheli LJ. The traction apophysitises. Clin Sports Med 1987;6:389–404.

32. Mesgarzadeh M, Sapega AA, Bonakdarpour A, Revesz G, Moyer RA, Maurer AH, Alburger PO. Osteochondritis dissecans: analysis of mechanical stability with radiography, scintigraphy and MR imaging. Radiology 1987;165:775–780.

33. Nakayama H, Mihara M, Shimao S. Perineural xanthoma. Br J Dermatol 1986;115:715–720.

34. Doyle JR. Tendon xanthoma: a physical manifestation of hyperlipidemia. J Hand Surg (Am) 1988;13:238–241.

35. Caputo R, Monti M, Berti E, Gasparini G. Normolipemic eruptive cutaneous xanthomatosis. Arch Dermatol 1986;122:1294–1297.

36. Parker F. Normocholestolemic xanthomatosis. Arch Dermatol 1986;122:1253–1257.

37. Flandry F, Hughston JC. Pigmented villonodular synovitis. J Bone Joint Surg (Am) 1987; 69:942–949.

38. Ushijima M, Hashimoto H, Tsuneyoshi M, Enjoli M. Pigmented villonodular synovitis. A clinico-pathologic study of 52 cases. Acta Pathol Jpn 1986;36:317–326.

39. Mrose HE, DeLuca SA. Pigmented villonodular synovitis. Am Fam Physician 1988;37: 195–196.

40. Spritzer CE, Dalinka MK, Kressel HY. Magnetic resonance imaging of pigmented villonodular synovitis: a report of two cases. Skeletal Radiol 1987;16:316–319.

41. Kottal RA, Vogler JB III, Matamoros A, Alexander AH, Cookson JL. Pigmented villonodular synovitis: a report of MR imaging in two cases. Radiology 1987;163:551–553.

42. Lisch R, Marczak L. Giant cell tumors of the tendon sheath. J Am Podiatr Med Assoc 1986; 76:218–220.

43. Agostinelli JR, Amendt W, Banerjee M. Giant cell tumor of tendon sheath. A case report. J Am Podiatr Med Assoc 1987;77:510–512.

44. Frankel SL, Chioros PG, Sidlow CJ. Giant cell tumor of the plantar fascia: a case report. J Am Podiatr Med Assoc 1987;77:557–559.

45. Gold AG, Bronfman RA, Clark EA, Comerford JS. Giant cell tumor of the extensor tendon sheath of the foot. A case report. J Am Podiatr Med Assoc 1987;77:561–563.

46. Wood GS, Beckstead JH, Medeiros LJ, Kempson RL, Warnke RA. The cells of giant cell tumor of tendon sheath resemble osteoclasts. Am J Surg Path 1988;12:444–452.

47. Prowse M, Brooks PM. Oncogenic hypophosphatemic osteomalacia associated with a giant cell tumor of a tendon sheath. Aust NZ J Med 1987;17:330–332.

48. Ushijima M, Hashimoto H, Tsuneyoshi M, Enjoli M. Giant cell tumor of the tendon sheath (nodular tenosynovitis). A study of 207 cases to compare the large joint group with the common digit group. Cancer 1986;57:875–884.

49. Reale CD, Sinclair G. Synovial sarcoma of the foot. J Foot Surg 1986;25:124–127.

50. Fuselier CO, Cachia VV, Wong C, et al. Selected soft tissue malignancies of the foot: an in-depth study with case reports. J Foot Surg 1985; 24:162–204.

51. Sen SK, Dooley WT. Synovial sarcoma. J Nat Med Assoc 1987;79:1089–1093.

52. Estebon JM, Oertel YC, Mendoza M, Knoll SM. Fine needle aspiration in the treatment of ganglionic cysts. South Med J 1986;79:691–693.

53. Fletcher CD, McKee PH. Sarcomas—a clinicopathological guide with particular reference to cutaneous manifestation III. Angiosarcoma, malignant haemangiopericytoma, fibrosarcoma and synovial sarcoma. Clin Exp Dermatol 1985;10:332–349.

54. Soule EH. Synovial sarcoma. Am J Surg Path 1986;10(Suppl 1):78–82.

55. Southerland CC Jr, Spinner SM. Synovial sarcoma presenting as tarsal tunnel syndrome. J Am Podiatr Med Assoc 1987;77:70–72.

56. Majeste RM, Beckman EN. Synovial sarcoma with an overwhelming epithelial component. Cancer 1988;61:2527–2531.

57. Wu KK. Synovial sarcoma of the foot. J Foot Surg 1987;26:359–364.

58. Zajdela A, Zillhart P, Voillemot N. Cytological diagnosis by fine needle sampling without aspiration. Cancer 1987;59:1201–1205.

Part D/ **Neural Neoplasms of the Lower Extremity**

—Gerald A. Weber

Mary Ann Cardile

Neural neoplasms of the lower extremity are entities which are often undetected, misdiagnosed, or improperly managed. Through a basic yet thorough overview of the lesions' pathogenesis, clinical manifestations, differential diagnosis, histopathologic patterns, and classification, such a dilemma may be avoided. This chapter includes methods of diagnosis, treatment regimens, and prognostic indicators which are outlined according to each tumor subtype, thereby serving as a guide to providing optimal patient care to those individuals afflicted with a neoplasm of the lower extremity.

Peripheral neural neoplasms of the lower extremity pose a diagnostic challenge because of their complexity and relative rarity. Although extensive clinical and histopathologic studies have been performed, definitive criteria have not been established. Often, benign and malignant growths are unrecognized or misdiagnosed, lending credence to their reported infrequency in the foot and leg.

This chapter presents the salient features of these nerve lesions through a basic yet thorough overview of their classification, histopathologic patterns, pathogenesis, and clinical manifestations. Therapeutic regimens and prognostic indicators have been outlined according to the various tumor subtypes as a guide in providing optimal patient management of these neural processes. Pertinent observations in the literature to date of considerable interest to neuro-oncology have been summarized. It is the authors' intent to familiarize the readers with these poorly understood tumors. Additional emphasis is placed upon a comprehensive, as well as deductive, methodical approach in establishing a differential diagnosis, with its subsequent delineation toward the prompt and concise detection and treatment of neural neoplasms of the lower extremity.

INCIDENCE

The incidence of neoplasms of the nervous system varies according to each specific type. Influencing factors may include a positive family history, developmental defects, and other individual features.

For instance, the incidence rate of neurofibromatosis is one in 3000 births, and 50% of cases have a strong family history (1). According to Holt and Wright (2), 5.5% of neurofibromas will undergo malignant transformation to a neurofibrosarcoma, fibrosarcoma, or spindle-cell sarcoma. Associated soft-tissue tumors have been estimated to be 5–16.4% (3, 4). In summary, benign neurofibromas constitute approximately 75% of all the peripheral nerve neoplasms (5).

Conversely, malignant schwannomas possess a very small incidence rate. Based on the data by Ducatman's group (6), the incidence of malignant peripheral nerve sheath tumors during the period of 1950 to 1952 was 0.001%. Yet, its frequency sharply escalates with the coexistence of von Recklinghausen's disease. These researchers estimate that the risk of developing malignant schwannomas is 4600 times greater in patients with neurofibromatosis than in the general population at the Mayo Clinic. From 1912 to 1983, of 120 cases reviewed, 52% had concurrent neurofibromatosis and an additional 23% had a positive family history. Unlike the pattern of neurofibromas, malignant schwannomas are rarely multifocal in occurrence.

Benign schwannomas are also uncommon tumors of the peripheral nervous system. Cellular schwannomas constitute 9.8% of all benign peripheral nerve sheath tumors and 2.83% of 635 reviewed neoplasms of the peripheral nervous system (7).

Thus, when a patient presents with manifestations which are suspect of a neural tumor, the incidence rate of each lesion subtype becomes one delineating determinant.

AGE

The propensity for neoplasms of neural derivation to affect certain age groups assists in the differential diagnosis. The likelihood that a specific tumor will involve a young child may be remote, but may be much higher in adults. Such a characteristic helps the practitioner to confirm clinical and laboratory suspicions, and to arrive at a more probable diagnosis.

Neuroblastoma is basically a lesion occurring in young children, and rarely in adolescents and adults. In the study by Phillips (8), only 40 of 623 reported cases (1933–1952) were in adults.

Based on 65 cases of neuromas, the average age was 57, with a range of 25–83 years (9).

Peripheral nerve sheath tumors, both malignant and benign, correlate with aging. They are generally found in patients over 60 years of age. However, this percentage decreases in patients older than 70 years (10).

The average age may be younger with various tumors. In the study by Fletcher et al. (7), 18 cases of cellular schwannoma had an average age of 40.9 years, with a range of 15–73 years. The mean age of diagnosis of malignant schwannomas with associated neurofibromatosis was 32 years, based on 46 cases (11).

The discrepancy in average ages in these neoplasms may be due to a lack of timely detection or by the presence of coexistent disorders. Neurofibromatosis decreased the mean age of diagnosis of malignant schwannomas from 34 to 28.7 years in 120 cases at the Mayo Clinic from 1912 to 1983 (6).

In a review of 678 patients with von Recklinghausen's disease at the Mayo Clinic, D'Agostino et al. (12) reports a median age of 28 years, with a range of 12–57. Neurofibromatosis may occur in patients from birth to the 70s or 80s. However, the initial appearance of manifestations is usually at puberty (with bouts of exacerbations during this period), pregnancy, menopause, or times of emotional stress (2).

SEX

Certain nerve tumors predominantly affect one sex. Diagnosis cannot be based on this sole finding, but, rather, on the entire clinical presentation.

Invariably, females are more often afflicted by Morton's neuroma. In the study by Gaynor's group (9) of 65 cases, 90% were female. Influencing factors may include constrictive footgear, occupational demands of excessive or prolonged walking and/or standing, and a marked degree of forefoot varus.

Neurothekeoma is a neoplasm of neural derivation which invariably involves female patients. In a series of 53 such cases by Gallagher and Helwig (13) during a 22-year period, this tumor appears in women 4 times more often than in men.

Other tumors with a strong predilection for females include nonrecurring neurofibromas and schwannomas. Yet, in percentage distribution, males were affected to a greater degree (10).

Malignant schwannomas occur more frequently in females (14). The presence of von Recklinghausen's disease is noncontributory; in the study by Ducatman et al. (6) on cases of malignant schwannoma with and without neurofibromatosis, both groups demonstrate a female preponderance. The coexisting disorder serves to enforce female predominance. In a review of 165 cases of malignant schwannoma by Sordillo et al. (15), the male:female ratio with concomitant neurofibromatosis was 26:39. However, regarding the malignant evolution of neurogenic sarcoma in patients with a prolonged duration of neurofibromatosis, males tend to be affected to a greater degree (16). Neuroblastomas also involve males predominantly (17).

SITE

Neoplasms of the nervous system have a tendency to originate in particular anatomic locations. This trait often guides the diagnostician toward the feasible pathologies.

Neuromas in the foot tend to develop at the common digital nerve formed by the union of the medial and lateral plantar nerves. Such lesions have been named "Morton's neuromas," in honor of the physician who presented 12 cases of neuralgia in this site (18).

Dermal nerve sheath myxomas have a predilection for the hands and feet. Angervall et al. (19) relate a case of a patient presenting with an asymptomatic superficial nodule about the proximal phalanx of a digit following a traumatic incident. Therefore, this type of tumor should be included in the differential diagnosis of nonulcerated and painless masses of the foot.

The sites where neuroblastomas evolve differ according to the patient's age group. With the classic presentation in the child, primary locations include the retroperitoneum, pelvis, extremity, and neck. Sites of metastasis involve mainly the skeletal system, followed by, in decreasing order of frequency, the lungs, pleura, liver, lymph nodes, breast, diaphragm, meninges, pancreas, testes, blood vessels, intestine, prostate, skin, spleen, thyroid; and, least likely, the appendix, bladder, heart, ovary, pericardium, pituitary, spinal cord, and stomach. In rarer instances, when a neuro-blastoma involves adolescents and adults, the most common primary site is the mediastinum, as well as the adrenal, retroperitoneum, and pelvis. Metastatic lesions are also found in the skeletal system. However, the lung is one site of metastasis which frequently occurs in older patients, but not children (17).

Schwannomas generally originate along the peripheral nerves and major nerve plexuses, but not in small cutaneous nerves. They may also occur on dorsal nerve roots of the spinal cord, forming dumbbell-shaped masses with growths on both sides of the intervertebral foramina. The presence of von Reckling-hausen's disease alters the anatomic locations of these neoplasms. Only in this syndrome will schwannomas of the brain occur. Additionally, bilateral acoustic schwannomas almost exclusively belong in the realm of neurofibromatosis. Multiple lesions are usual with this coexisting disorder, yet solitary schwannomas of peripheral nerves are infrequently associated with von Recklinghausen's disease (20).

Melanotic schwannomas have been reported in peripheral nerves, spinal nerves, cranial nerves, and sympathetic ganglia (21).

According to Fletcher et al. (7), common anatomic locations of cellular schwannomas include the mediastinum, retroperitoneum, pelvis, and lower extremity. Thus, lesions in the proximal aspect of the leg may present with manifestations in the foot.

Malignant peripheral nerve sheath tumors most commonly involve the sciatic nerve (14). In decreasing order of frequency, other sites are the brachial plexus, spinal nerve roots, vagus and femoral nerves, median sacral plexus, and popliteal, obturator, posterior tibial, and ulnar nerves (6). The lesions tend to occur near the central axis of the body (e.g., the pelvic girdle) more often than in the limbs proper (e.g., thigh and leg) (11). As mentioned previously, impingement on vital structures by these proximal neoplasms may produce symptomatology distally. Thus, pain, weakness, and paresthesias of the foot may be secondary to suprastructural causes such as these.

Plexiform neurofibromas reportedly occur in large nerves, particularly in the legs and neck, and in major nerve plexuses (i.e., the lumbosacral and brachial) (20). Basically, all lesions are a constituent of von Recklinghausen's disease. Local gigantism of the affected area, e.g., leg or arm, may ensue.

Various lesions of neurofibromatosis are localized in the trunk region of the body. However, several studies state that they occur in the lower extremities as well. Of particular interest is that sparing of the palmar and plantar aspects have been noted. Gazivoda et al. (22) discuss a rare case of a plantar, von Recklinghausen's neurofibroma of 5-years duration (see Fig. 5.31).

The incidence of malignant transformation of both schwannomas and neurofibromas is greater in the extremities than the trunk (10). In a review of 20 neurofibrosarcomas, Storm et al. (23) state anatomic locations (e.g., proximal arm and leg, distal leg, chest wall, and, less frequently, the distal arm, pelvis, and retroperitoneum). These findings support the view that malignant neurogenic tumors arise more commonly in the extremities.

Metastatic sites of malignant schwannomas include the lung, and, with decreasing frequency, soft tissue, bone, liver, intraabdominal cavity, adrenal glands, diaphragm, mediastinum, brain, ovaries, kidneys, and retroperitoneum. The presence of von Recklinghausen's disease increases the propensity for metastasis (6).

CLASSIFICATION

Neurogenic tumors are derived from the neural crest. They may be melanocytic, as are nevi and malignant melanomas, or may be nerve sheath lesions (e.g., neurofibromas or schwannomas (24)). Some neoplasms contain features of both types: the pigmented schwannoma or neurofibroma, cellular blue nevus, neurotrophic melanoma, and "melanocytoma" of the meninges (25).

Peripheral nerve neoplasms may be benign or malignant, aggressive or slowly growing, or metastatic. The following is an outline of these tumors (26).

Classification of peripheral nerve neoplasms
  I. Benign primary nerve sheath cell tumors
     A. Schwannomas (Variants: ancient, cystic, and plexiform)
     B. Neurofibroma, cutaneous
     C. Neurofibroma of a peripheral nerve
  II. Locally aggressive primary nerve sheath cell tumors that undergo malignant transformation (plexiform neurofibroma)
  III. Malignant primary nerve sheath tumors
     A. Malignant schwannoma

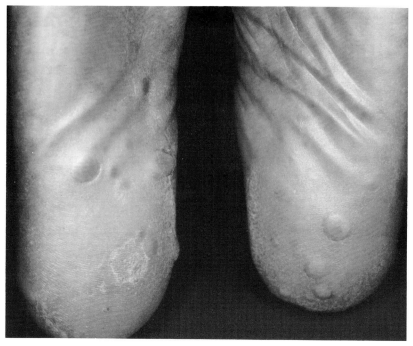

Figure 5.31. Plantar cutaneous markers in von Recklinghausen's disease are rare occurrences which should nonetheless be considered in the differential diagnosis of dermal lesions of the sole. (Courtesy of Dr. Harvey Lamont.)

B. Nerve sheath cell sarcoma (neurogenic sarcoma)
IV. Neuroectodermal tumors of primitive type and tumors with nerve cell differentiation
A. Neuroblastoma
B. Ganglioneuroma
C. Pheochromocytoma
V. Tumors metastatic to peripheral nerves.

Some lesions of the peripheral nervous system are not neoplastic. They include neuromas of the amputation, Morton's, and traumatic forms, hypertrophic neuropathies, and degenerative abnormalities, such as axonal, Wallerian, and segmental demyelination (27).

Several examples of nerve sheath tumors exist. There are benign forms, which are characteristically encapsulated, yet not in all instances. Malignant schwannomas are typically aggressive, and often metastasize to other anatomic sites of the body. Other nerve sheath variants include the classic (Verocay) schwannoma, cellular schwannomas, granular cell schwannomas, cranial nerve schwannomas, plexiform neurofibromas, nerve sheath myxo-

mas, "ancient" schwannomas, and epithelioid schwannomas (28).

It has been proposed that the benign peripheral nerve sheath lesions be classified according to their sources; i.e., schwannoma, perineurinoma, and neurofibroma, since they are derived from Schwann cells, perineural cells, and fibroblasts, respectively (29).

Malignant peripheral nerve sheath tumors may be grouped on a histologic basis. They may be considered epithelioid, homologous, or heterologous (metaplastic) (24). Schwannomas may be divided by the histologic classification of Harkin and Reed (1969): (a) malignant, (b) malignant epithelioid, (c) malignant melanocytic, (d) nerve sheath fibrosarcoma, and (e) malignant nerve sheath mesenchymoma (30).

Neurofibromatosis may be demonstrated by a multitude of clinical presentations. Four types have been reported: (a) schwannomas, central gliomas, meningiomas, and neurofibromas of the central nervous system, (b) visceral neurofibromas and schwannomas of the autonomic nervous system, (c) schwannomas and neurofibromas of the peripheral nervous system (exclusively), and (d) forme fruste, an incomplete expression of manifestations (1). Specific clinicopathologic types of neurofibromas exist: common, plexiform, Pacinian, storiform, pigmented, epithelioid, granular cell, and perineurioma (24).

With this brief overview of the vast assortment of neural neoplasms, it immediately becomes obvious why their diagnosis is difficult to ascertain without a biopsy.

PATHOGENESIS

Several theories exist that propose the etiology of neoplasms of the peripheral nervous system.

Heredity is considered to influence the incidence of these tumors to a certain degree. Certain neurocutaneous entities are associated with congenital angiomas that are further related to pathologic growths of the nervous system. They may consist of Bourneville's syndrome with tuberous sclerosis, or von Recklinghausen's disease and angiomas of the skin.

Neurofibromatosis may be a major etiologic determinant, since it often occurs concomitantly with other nervous system tumors (31).

The following section reviews the histopathogenesis of peripheral nervous system neoplasms, with an emphasis on those lesions with a higher propensity of growth in the lower extremity.

The common ancestry of Schwann cells and melanocytes is generally accepted (25). The neuroectoderm is the originating site of the melanin-producing cells of the human body. Due to the ultrastructural description of pigmented schwannomas, the melanocytic potential of Schwann cells has been recognized (21).

Schwann cells usually exist in conjunction with axons or nerve cells. Their long, slim cell processes contain interdigitations. Electron microscopic studies have demonstrated that these processes enfold around axons, forming mesaxons. Though entrapped by a continuous basement membrane, Schwann cells possess intercellular junctions.

In comparison, melanocytes do not possess distinct cell junctions and are not ensheathed within the basal lamina. Normally, they occur separately within the dermis or between the basal cells of the epidermis.

Certain neoplasms derived from the neural crest contain histologic aspects of both cell types. Thus, theses tumors are considered transitional lesions. Such growths may include the pigmented schwannoma or neurofibroma, cellular blue nevus, neurotrophic melanoma, and melanocytoma of the meninges (25).

Neurofibromatosis was initially described by Smith (32), and thought to be associated with molluscum fibrosum. It was not until 1882 that von Recklinghausen established its non-acquired nature. Preiser and Davenport (33) further demonstrated that neurofibromatosis occurs in both sexes and follows Mendelian laws as a dominant trait.

The pathogenesis of a neurofibroma is not yet known. It has been theorized to be due to a neural crest deficit. The neuroectoderm is a transient embryonic mass the cells of which form neuronal, endocrine, pigmentary, and other structures in the body. Thus, it becomes apparent that neurofibromatosis may affect structures of ectodermal, mesodermal, and endodermal origin. This disorder involves all nerve sheaths and other enveloping membranes of the nervous system.

Recently, the origin of von Recklinghausen's disease has been associated with a malfunctioning pericentromeric region of chromosome 17 in human DNA. This results in deficits in tyrosine metabolism. This proposal reinforces the close relationship between Schwann cells and melanocytes (34).

The accepted criteria for the diagnosis of peripheral nerve sheath tumors is that they are closely related to von Recklinghausen's disease and stem off the nerve trunk. Originating structures may include the Schwann cell of the endoneurium, the perineural cells located in the perineurium, and fibroblasts situated in the perineurium of large nerve fascicles (24).

Schwann cells are derived from the neural crest. However, perineural cells may originate in mesenchyme. Certain Schwann cells possess perineural histologic features that may be the neoplastic aspect in the tumors and in neurofibromas. Yet, it is also feasible that the neuroectoderm contains cells that demonstrate melanocytic and fibrocytic expressions when they migrate to unanticipated, yet "normal," milieus in the human body.

Laserus and Trombetta (35) propose that benign peripheral nerve sheath tumors be placed in three categories: schwannoma, neurofibroma, and perineurinoma; each type corresponds to its origin from a Schwann cell, a fibroblast, and a perineural cell, respectively.

It is probable that the majority of malignant

nerve sheath tumors arise from Schwann cells since they may be able to synthesize collagen and since they express phagocytic activity. The term "malignant schwannoma" is reserved for those tumors which demonstrate Schwann cell derivation, whereas lesions of possible fibroblastic mesenchymal origin are "neurofibrosarcoma," "fibromyxosarcoma of nerve," "peripheral fibrosarcoma," "neurogenic sarcoma," and "fibrosarcoma of nerve" (36).

The term "neurogenic sarcoma" is now largely avoided. The suffix "sarcoma" was originally affixed to explain the considerable amounts of entangling fibrous tissue. When these neoplasms were believed to arise from nervous tissue, the prefix "neurogenic" was adapted. Today, the terms schwannoma and neurilemoma are preferred.

CLINICAL MANIFESTATIONS

Specific findings, either subjective or objective, do not exist for neoplasms of the peripheral nervous system. Pain may only occasionally be the patient's chief complaint. More commonly, an asymptomatic mass, which was not initially palpable, is reported. Neurologic signs, such as paresthesia or weakness, may then ensue. Often, symptoms which develop are contingent on the adjacent tissues that are affected by the presence and growth of the tumor.

This section presents a brief overview of the clinical symptomatology of the major neural tumors that involve the lower extremity.

DESCRIPTIONS

Benign peripheral nerve sheath tumors (or schwannomas) occur in the average healthy individual, yet are encountered more frequently in patients with von Recklinghausen's disease. When the tumor originates in the extremities, the flexor surface is generally affected (31) (See Fig. 5.32).

These neoplasms are asymptomatic during their early stages. Pain and paresthesia, secondary to nerve impingement, may evolve as the growth enlarges. Arising from posterior spinal roots, the accompanying symptoms are generally sensory in nature. Motor manifestations later develop, with continued pressure of the anterior nerve roots or the spinal cord.

Upon inspection, benign schwannomas are found to be mobile, but with movement in a horizontal direction, not a longitudinal plane.

Common findings of malignant schwannomas include a mass—occasionally palpable, tender, or painful. Previous rapid swelling may be noted prior to diagnosis (see Fig. 5.32). Pain in the lower extremity may be induced by neoplasms situated on the retroperitoneum and the sciatic nerve. Paresthesias and motor weakness may be associated with them.

In the study by Guccion and Enzinger (11) of 46 malignant schwannomas, the duration of time between the onset of manifestations and diagnosis ranged from 1 month to 2 years, with a median of 6 months. Longer histories of objective and subjective findings were recorded in patients with von Recklinghausen's disease. In this analysis, the duration of neurofibromas varies from 3 to 36 years in 16 cases. An addi-

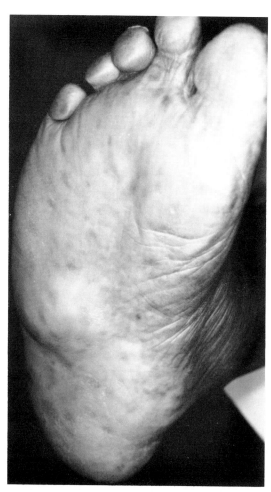

Figure 5.32. The clinical presentation of a peripheral nerve sheath tumor (schwannoma) of unknown duration. (Courtesy of Dr. Harvey Lamont.)

tional five patients state their lesions were present for their entire lives. A family positive history of neurofibromatosis was recounted by nine patients with malignant schwannomas.

CELLULAR SCHWANNOMA

The course of this benign peripheral nerve sheath tumor is extremely variable, ranging from weeks to years. In a review of 18 cases, Fletcher *et al.* (37) note the duration of time before diagnosis, after onset of preceding symptoms, spanned from 2 weeks to 10 years. The most common objective finding is a painless, tediously developing growth. In the aforementioned study, five tumors were detected incidentally during routine radiographic evaluations.

Neuroblastoma

Frequently cited manifestations of this rare neural tumor are an asymptomatic mass or sensations of pain induced by the growth impinging on adjacent tissues. Weight loss, anemia, and bouts of fever may be secondary findings (17). Common complaints include a palpable tumor mass, gastrointestinal disturbance, fever, pallor, and locomotor disturbances (18).

Neurothekeoma

This benign neoplasm of nerve sheath origin usually presents as an asymptomatic and slowly developing nodule. In the case report highlighted by Goette (38), the lesion is described as a cutaneous lesion which is dermal-colored, firm, adherent to the underlying fascia, and situated near the patient's ankle.

In the review of 53 cases of neurothekeoma, Gallagher and Helwig (13) state that this tumor customarily appears as a solitary, slightly erythematous, and seemingly soft mass averaging 10 mm in size, with a range of 4–18 mm in diameter.

Neuroma

The neuroma evolves from the degenerative process of intraneural fibrosis. It should be recognized as a "pseudotumor." The most frequent subjective findings are pain, tingling, numbness, or other parasthesias. The lesion usually affects the third interdigital nerve, a branch formed by the conjoined lateral and medial plantar nerves. Symptoms are generally reported as localized in the third and fourth interspaces, with manifestations radiating to the involved toes.

Symptomatology increases with excessive ambulation and constrictive footgear. Upon clinical examination, a palpable mass is not likely to be noted (see Fig. 5.33). When present for prolonged periods, neuromas may produce splaying between the third and fourth toes. Pain may be elicited by direct palpation of the third interspace, between the third and fourth metatarsal heads, along with lateral compression of the foot. On radiographic evaluation, a widened area between the third and fourth metatarsal heads may be noted.

Neurofibromatosis

Von Recklinghausen's disease is autosomal dominant, and expressed by a myriad of diverse symptoms. An incomplete development of manifestations, or forme fruste, is the most frequent presenting pattern. For this reason, neurofibromatosis may be undetected and misdiagnosed for years.

Characteristic findings of neurofibromatosis include hamartomatous lesions and irregular cell growths. Examples of such include local gigantism, scoliosis, café-au-lait dermal lesions (produced by excessive melanin in the basal layer of the epidermis), neurofibromas of varying dimensions, schwannomas, and associated malignancies.

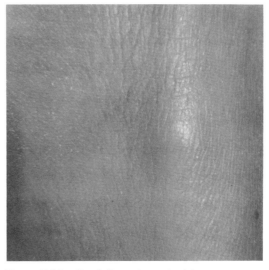

Figure 5.33. Depiction of a palpable mass, representing an underlying Morton's neuroma of prolonged duration, and constituting a rare finding in this entity. (Courtesy of Dr. Harvey Lamont.)

Pain, potentially accompanied by a palpable mass, may be the initial chief complaint. Paralysis due to impingement on vital structures may be a later finding. A familial history may support the suspicion of neurofibromatosis. In the review of 678 patients with von Recklinghausen's disease at the Mayo Clinic, D'Agostino et al. (12), estimated the duration of symptoms prior to diagnosis ranges from several weeks to 18 years.

The presence of cutaneous neurofibromas may cause a slight prominence of the skin. The texture may be rubbery and not necessarily painful. Neurofibromas are superficially situated in the dermis and subcutaneous tissue. In general, they do not undergo malignant transformation (see Fig. 5.34).

Whereas the appearance of a dermal neurofibroma does not confirm the diagnosis of von Recklinghausen's disease, extensively enlarged lesions are almost always associated with this syndrome (20).

Café-au-lait spots are characteristic of von Recklinghausen's disease and are present in over 99% of patients. A criterion for neurofibromatosis includes the presence of six or more lesions 1.5 cm (or larger) in diameter.

Café-au-lait spots may be present at birth or may gradually develop within 12 months. Sparing of the face is noted. With time, the amount and size of the spots may increase. Additionally, exacerbation of the lesions and other manifestations may occur with puberty, pregnancy, menopause, or physiologic stresses (31).

Lisch nodules, or pigmented iris hamartomas, may also be present.

Molluscum fibrosum, or skin tumors which are soft and pedunculated, is another dermal manifestation of von Recklinghausen's disease.

Elephantiasis neuromatosa is a clinical presentation of diffuse peripheral nerve lesions, osseous hypertrophy, and periosteal generation, leading to local gigantism.

The central nervous system is also affected in neurofibromatosis. Related pathologies include meningiomas, astrocytomas, spongioblastomas, gliomas, and intracranial tumors. Acoustic neuromas are frequently associated with this syndrome. In a study of five family generations with bilateral deafness (39), acoustic neoplasms were accompanied by neurofibromatosis in 84% of the cases.

Brooks and Lehman (40) classified the osseous changes secondary to von Recklinghausen's disease. Three categories were reported: scoliosis, subperiosteal cyst, and abnormal bone growth. Congenital anomalies, bowing and pseudarthrosis of the leg, and intraosseous cysts also were reported. These researchers surmised that skeletal irregularities were caused by neurofibromatous matter in the periosteal nerves. With growth, pressure

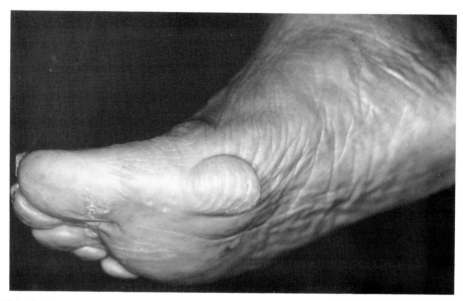

Figure 5.34. Delineation of a neurofibroma is appreciable along the plantar medial aspect of this patient's first metatarsal-phalangeal joint. (Courtesy of Dr. Harvey Lamont.)

is exerted against the adjacent bony cortex, creating erosive defects. Brooks and Lehman (40) also proposed that hyperplastic changes in the lymphatic system result in increased bone porosity and weakening. Due to this osteoporosis, spontaneous fractures and pseudarthroses ensue.

Scoliosis is a common objective finding in von Recklinghausen's disease. Several etiologic factors are feasible: osteoporosis, neurofibromata in the spinal nerves, developmental abnormalities, and limb length discrepancies.

Erosive defects ("pit" or "cave" defects) are characteristic in the extremities (2). These deformities may be induced by the enlargement of contiguous neurofibromas.

Regarding osseous growth disorders in neurofibromatosis, overgrowth of one or more bones is most often reported (2). In clinical presentations of local gigantism, adjacent soft tissue became elephantiasic when infiltrated by plexiform or cirsoid neurofibroma. Serial radiographic examinations may reveal gradual, yet progressive, periosteal hypertrophy, leading to an increased bone diameter. Increased vasculature secondary to lymphatic stasis may be a cause of longitudinal overgrowth.

These researchers also presented less overt manifestations of von Recklinghausen's disease. In their review of 127 cases, two patients demonstrated bones which elongated with concurrent diameter diminution. Surprisingly, these atrophied bones contained normal calcium concentrations. In one of the two patients, the metatarsals of the left foot were similarly elongated and thinned. Interestingly, osteoporosis was not present.

Congenital tibial bowing, with subsequent pseudarthrosis has been considered a pathognomonic sign of neurofibromatosis (2). The pseudarthrosis may evolve after trauma, due to a nonhealing fracture, may be a complication of a failed surgical procedure, or may be propagated by an intraosseous neurofibroma.

Additional skeletal anomalies related to von Recklinghausen's disease include spina bifida, clubfoot, congenital hip dislocations, vertebral ankylosing, and other congenital defects.

A multitude of associated features in this syndrome include macrocephaly, short stature, headaches, hypertension, seizures, speech disorders (30–40% of patients), congenital heart defects, constipation (10% of cases), intellectual deficits (40% of patients), strokes, and visceral tumors (22).

The stigmata of von Recklinghausen's disease may also contain hirsutism, Sturge-Weber syndrome, von Hippel-Lindau disease, mesodermal tumors (e.g., lipomas, fibromas, etc.), and congenital defects of the fingers and toes (31) (see Fig. 5.35).

Malignant tumors arising from nervous and other tissue are encountered in the clinical presentation of von Recklinghausen's disease. They include malignant schwannomas, neurofibrosarcomas, liposarcomas, rhabdomyosarcomas, and other soft-tissues neoplasms. Malignant transformation of neurofibromas or the de novo appearance of a neurofibrosarcoma should be suspected when there is an insidious onset of pain in a previously asymptomatic mass or when there is development of a palpable lesion.

HISTOPATHOLOGY

The diagnosis of neoplasms of neural origin is based on presenting manifestations and distinct histopathologic features. The tumors comprise a vast spectrum of clinical and microscopic heterogeneity. They include the typically encapsulated benign schwannomas, the clinically aggressive malignant schwannomas with mainly pleomorphic fusiform cells, the

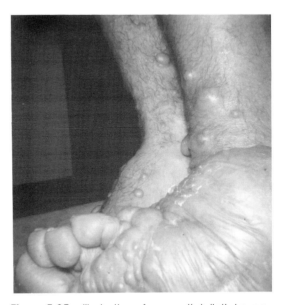

Figure 5.35. Illustration of congenital digital anomalies, rarely manifested in von Recklinghausen's disease, and seen in conjunction with the more prevalent findings of dermal lesions observed diffusely throughout this patient's lower extremity. (Courtesy of Dr. Harvey Lamont.)

characteristically nonencapsulated neurofibromas, and endless variants.

This section is an overview of the microscopic and gross aspects of nerve tumors, particularly those affecting the lower extremity.

Neurofibroma

Neurofibromas are benign growths, generally nonencapsulated, and consist of various cell types (e.g., Schwann cells and excessive collagenous matrix). The lesions may be situated in the dermis or subcutaneous layers.

Compared to nerve sheath tumors, neurofibromas are less cellular (41). It was demonstrated that the principal cell is spindle-shaped, with long and extremely thin bipolar (rarely tripolar) cytoplasmic processes. The cells usually disperse in stroma comprised of random groups of collagen fibrils and fibrillogranular material. Small blood vessels with one to three layers of spindle-shaped pericytes may be seen. Occasional mast cells, lymphocytes, and fibroblasts may be noted. Endothelial cells and pericytes exhibit a thin, continuous basal lamina (see Fig. 5.36).

The origin of cutaneous neurofibromas is rarely identified. On cross-section, the lesion is localized, but not encapsulated. It is often pale gray and glistening. Its cells are fusiform or stellate. This tumor type is mainly composed of extracellular collagen. The overlying epidermis may be flattened.

The neurofibroma of a peripheral nerve may be pale gray, gelatinous, and rubbery. This tumor's origin from a nerve is usually apparent, and it is often sharply demarcated. Histologically, the lesion resembles its dermal counterpart, but possesses a much looser extracellular matrix.

The gross appearance of a plexiform neurofibroma has been likened to a batch of different-sized worms. The tangled nerve fascicles of the gelatinous lesion tend to blend into adjacent soft tissues. Microscopically, the nerve fascicles are seen to be hypocellular, swollen, and made of endoneural cells, Schwann cells, and a minimal amount of axons. Typically hypocellular, and following a long pattern of slow growth, plexiform neurofibromas may increase the tumor's cellularity as it undergoes malignant transformation.

Myxoma of the Nerve Sheath

Observations by light and electron microscopy of this rare neoplasm have been concisely reported by Goldstein and Lifshitz (42). The growths tend to involve the dermis and subcutaneous tissue at different levels. They are typically nonencapsulated, nodular, and well-delineated. Its cells are pleomorphic, being either elongated, stellate, or bipolar. The intercellular matrix is abundant, thus giving a "foamy" appearance. Long cytoplasmic extensions form a net-like pattern.

Neurothekeoma

This tumor is typically nonencapsulated with round to oval well-demarcated lobules. Its cells are generally spindle- and round-shaped, with eosinophilic cytoplasm. Cutaneous and peripheral nerves may be seen blending into the lobules of neurothekeoma. In the article by Goette (38), diffuse fine-granular calcinosis was reported in this recently described neoplasm of nerve sheath derivation.

Ancient Schwannoma

In the study by Gould *et al.* (28), a spectrum of nerve sheath neoplasms were investigated by immunofluorescence microscopy, two-dimensional electrophoresis, and immunoblot analysis. Ancient schwannomas, a benign variant, demonstrates encapsulation and has distinct, yet atypical, hyperchromatic nuclei scattered throughout. It also possesses the Antoni types A and B growth patterns as illustrated in characteristic benign schwannomas.

Cellular Schwannoma

Based on 18 cases, Fletcher *et al.* (7) lend great insight to this recently delineated neural

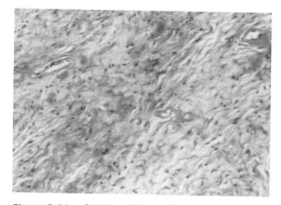

Figure 5.36. Outline of histopathologic features of a neurofibroma, consisting predominantly of spindle-shaped cells located in stroma composed of collagen fibrillogranular matrix. (Courtesy of Dr. Harvey Lamont.)

tumor. They found this benign variant to be well-circumscribed and to usually have a dense fibrous capsule.In cross-section, the mass is described as translucent or pinkish-gray. Foci of yellowish-brown gelatinous tissue are occasionally encountered. Variably sized blood vessels with thick hyalinized walls, microthrombi, and microscopic foci of hemorrhage may be visualized, but necrosis was never evident.

Reproducible histologic features include extremely cellular Antoni type A growth patterns, but neither Verocay bodies nor nuclear palisading. Rather, the spindle-shaped cells are interlacing fascicles arranged in whorls. Understandably, cellular schwannomas may be initially misdiagnosed as smooth muscle tumors or fibrous histiocytomas. Malignant tumors are a differential diagnosis due to the frequent presence of nuclear pleomorphism and mitotic activity in this tumor.

Glandular Schwannoma

This rare, malignant, peripheral nerve sheath tumor contains both malignant spindle and seemingly benign glandular features. Its ultrastructure was initially detailed by Uri *et al.* (43). The tumor is described as possessing amorphous, granular, and multilayered substances, abundant collagen fibers, and complex cytoplasmic processes. Mitotic activity is prominent, with as many as 40 mitoses/10 high power fields (HPF).

The epithelial lining of the glands is nonciliated cuboidal or columnar. Also present are distinct aspects such as microvilli with core rootlets, glycocalyx, and Russell bodies. These latter findings confirm the epithelial nature of glandular schwannoma, whereas the aforementioned principal cells support the hypothesis of Schwann cell origin.

Benign Peripheral Nerve Sheath Tumors

Benign schwannomas (neurilemoma) are generally encapsulated with multicellular components of Schwann cell differentiation: Antoni type A and B growth patterns and Verocay bodies.

Antoni type A tissue consists mainly of compactly arranged entangled Schwann cells with distinct cell membranes, sparse stroma, and scattered collagen fibrils (24). The cell cytoplasm is uniformly pale in this area. Verocay bodies (parallel and long cell processes separated by prominent basement membrane and converging to a central area with thickened external lamina and collagen fibrils) are also present (see Fig. 5.37). A characteristic feature of the cytoplasmic processes of Antoni type A growth pattern is their propensity to entrap extracellular material, defined as pseudomesaxon formation (41).

The more loosely arranged, less cellular Antoni type B tissue invariably contains lipid-laden histiocytes, lymphocytes, and small blood vessels with thick hyalinized walls. Its pleomorphic cells are broadly separated by a pale myxomatous and edematous matrix (see Fig. 5.38). This pattern is theorized to be a degenerative form of Antoni type A tissue (44).

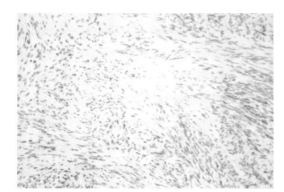

Figure 5.37. Demonstration of Antoni type A tissue pattern in peripheral nerve sheath tumors. Note the compactly arranged Schwann cells in sparse stroma. Verocay bodies are occasionally visualized. (Courtesy of Dr. Harvey Lamont.)

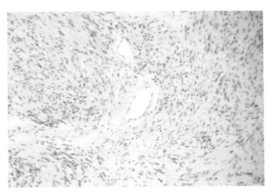

Figure 5.38. Loosely arranged and relatively less cellular Antoni type B tissue pattern seen in schwannomas, containing pleomorphic cells situated in myxomatous matrix. The hyalinization of small blood vessels is also demonstrable in this presentation. (Courtesy of Dr. Harvey Lamont.)

Malignant Peripheral Nerve Sheath Tumors

A myriad of nonspecific histologic patterns exist for malignant peripheral nerve sheath tumors (malignant schwannomas). This neoplasm has been called malignant schwannoma, neurofibrosarcoma, malignant neurilemoma and other terms since, theoretically, it has been thought to originate from either fibroblasts, perineural cells, or most likely, Schwann cells.

On gross examination, malignant peripheral nerve sheath tumors appear reddish-gray and firm. They extend into adjacent soft tissues without a sharp line of demarcation (20). A majority are nonencapsulated and demonstrate an infiltrative growth. On cross-section, areas of necrosis and hemorrhage may be visualized.

Malignant schwannoma are considered to be an extremely cellular neoplasm of randomly arranged fusiform cells. Necrosis appears frequently. Pleomorphism is notable and mitotic rate is high (28). Its spindle ("serpentine") cells appear in fascicles, having a "herringbone" design. Other histologic features include nuclear hyperplasia, cellular density, terminal cytoplasmic processes, and a myxoid stroma.

Another characteristic microscopic finding of malignant schwannoma is its prominent vascular pattern. In the analysis of 40 cases, Guccion and Enzinger (11) noted gaping, thin-walled blood vessels forming a pericytoma-like arrangement. Smaller blood vessels were also seen, with a cuff of proliferated cells.

The diagnosis of malignant schwannoma is based on various factors. Increased cellularity, a high mitotic index, nuclear atypia, and necrosis are considered the most reliable histologic criteria (6). Infiltrating growth with ill-defined borders is another sign of malignancy (36).

With regard to recurrence, the presence of basal lamina around the Schwann cells is a crucial histogenetic criterion (35).

Malignant schwannoma may be differentiated microscopically in patients with or without associated von Recklinghausen's disease. With it, the sarcomas are highly vascular and predominantly collagenous, have mast cells, and infrequently have areas of necrosis and calcification. Without the diagnosis of neurofibromatosis, malignant schwannoma appears to be highly mitotic, with minimal stroma, and poor differentiation (15).

The sarcomas are graded from low to high malignancy according to their cytologic and histologic patterns. Low-grade tumors demonstrate significant nuclear atypia, minimal to moderate hypercellularity, and an only slightly elevated mitotic index (grade 1, 1–2/10 HPF; grade 2, 2–6/10 HPF). High-grade neoplasms present with extreme hypercellularity, advanced mitotic activity (more than 6/10 HPF), and prominent pleomorphism.

Neurofibrosarcoma

Neurofibrosarcoma is a rare neoplasm which may or may not be associated with von Recklinghausen's disease. Its diagnosis and grading is generally based on its histopathologic pattern (23).

Grade One of this type tumor contains abundant collagen formation, minimal to moderate hypercellularity and a mitotic index of less than 5/50 HPF. Grade Two demonstrates an increased mitotic activity (at least 5 and up to 75/HPF). In comparison to Grade One, the amount of collagen is reduced. Lastly, Grade Three is characterized by sparse collagen production, dense cellularity, and a mitotic count of at least 20 and up to 300/50 HPF.

Neuroma

Neuroma in the foot occurs most frequently at the third interdigital nerve, which is formed by the union of the medial and lateral plantar nerves. On gross examination, this pseudotumor appears to be yellowish-white, firm to palpation, generally ovoid, and with substantial dense fibrous connective tissue that ensheathes the nerve portion. According to Tate and Rusin's study on 50 specimens (45), the lesions rarely exceed 1 cm in diameter. Microscopically, abundant fibrosis and collagenous collection is noted, along with swirls of unorganized axons.

The size of the neuroma tends to be a differential in the histologic pattern (46). Relatively large neuromas contain a somewhat normal and uniform intraneural pattern, whereas smaller growths possess an irregular and poor internal organization. Regardless of gross dimensions, axonal degeneration affects larger myelinated axons more often than smaller unmyelinated axons. Also of interest is the finding that the amount of connective tissue coincides with the duration of the neuroma (45).

DIFFERENTIAL DIAGNOSIS

Cutaneous Neurofibroma

The cutaneous lesions of individuals with neurofibromas grossly resemble dermal nevi, lipomas, dermatofibromas, or granular cell tumors (myloblastomas) (see Fig. 5.39). However, these various growths may be differentiated histologically (20).

NEUROFIBROMA OF A PERIPHERAL NERVE

These neoplasms are derived from Schwann cells and often contain a considerable amount of mucoid material. They can be distinguished from a lipoma or lipofibromatous hamartoma of nerve (47). Upon physical examination, the lesions are similar to cysts around joints (20).

PLEXIFORM NEUROFIBROMA

The primary differential diagnosis of plexiform neurofibroma is a malignant nerve sheath tumor. This is of great import since the malignant transformation of the former into the latter has been reported and drastically decreases the prognosis of the patient. A developing traumatic neuroma histologically resembles a plexiform neurofibroma, yet the history and symptomatology usually separates these pathologies.

The plexiform schwannoma is grossly similar to plexiform neurofibroma but is microscopically distinct.

Almost without exception, plexiform neurofibromas are associated with von Recklinghausen's disease. Other presentations of individuals with these lesions may be local gigantism (20).

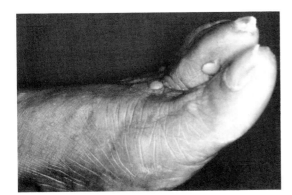

Figure 5.39. The differential diagnosis of the neurofibromas noted on the dorsum of this patient's foot includes fibromas, lipomas, and other cutaneous lesions. (Courtesy of Dr. Harvey Lamont.)

NEUROFIBROMATOSIS

A myriad of disorders comprise the classic stigmata of von Recklinghausen's disease. They may include central nervous system neoplasms such as meningiomas, acoustic neuromas, and optic nerve gliomas. Other entities included in the presentation of this pathology are: Sturge-Weber syndrome, tuberous sclerosis, von Hippel-Lindau disease, mental retardation of unknown etiology, hirsutism, mesodermal tumors (lipomas, fibromas, etc.), abnormal nonneoplastic hypertrophy of the bones and skin, congenital malformations (spina bifida, hypospadias, cerebral meningocele), and congenital defects of the toes and fingers (31).

Whenever a patient manifests one of the aforementioned abnormalities, the diagnosis of von Recklinghausen's disease must be ruled out.

Distinct osseous changes have been reported in neurofibromatosis. While there appears to be a vast range of skeletal abnormalities, the majority are classified as erosive defects, scoliosis, disorders of growth, bowing and pseudoarthrosis of the lower leg, intraosseous cystic lesions, and congenital anomalies (2).

Erosive changes may be secondary to various tumors or aneurysms. However, the presence of smooth erosions, especially of the spine and ribs, raises strong suspicions of von Recklinghausen's disease.

Though scoliosis is prevalent in this pathology, its multifactorial etiology reduces the consideration of neurofibromatosis when present as an isolated finding.

Underdevelopment or atrophy of bones may occur in postparalytic or debilitating disorders. Yet, a crucial differential feature of neurofibromatosis is the absence of osteoporosis, which is noted in osteogenesis imperfecta.

Osseous overdevelopment may be present in chronic osteomyelitis, hemangioma, lymphangioma, and hemihypertrophy. Advanced maturation and hypertrophy of the epiphyses may be due to hemophilia, secondary to recurrent hemarthrosis.

The characteristic finding of anterior tibial bowing in neurofibromatosis is also identified in osteogenesis imperfecta and rickets. It may also result from pseudarthrosis from the malunion or nonunion of fractures which are frequently sustained in these individuals.

Intraosseous cystic lesions may be encountered in reticuloses, hyperparathyroidism, bone cysts, Ollier's disease, and Albright's syndrome, as well as in localized fibrous dysplasia.

Calcifying Neurothekeoma

This recently described tumor of nerve sheath origin must be grossly separated from neurofibroma, dermatofibroma, eccrine peroma, or a foreign body granuloma. Differentiation is made upon histologic inspection (38).

Peripheral Nerve Sheath Tumors

The basis of differentiation of a nerve sheath cell tumor, benign or malignant, from other soft-tissue sarcomas is the presence of a growth extending from a nerve which possesses a histologic pattern consistent with this diagnosis (20).

The differential diagnosis of peripheral nerve sheath tumors, namely malignant, includes fibrosarcoma, leimyosarcoma, monophasic synovial sarcoma, malignant fibrous histiocytoma, and rhabdomyosarcoma.

Leimyosarcoma can be distinguished by blunt, oblong nuclei and abundant cytoplasm containing longitudinal myofibrils.

Synovial sarcoma's markers include focal calcification, a biphasic cellular pattern, and a pericytoma-like vascular pattern (11).

Identification of the origin of a nerve sheath neoplasm may be facilitated when the lesion evolves from a plexiform neurofibroma. Cellularity and mitotic activity separates the two entities.

When the tumor source is difficult to ascertain, Bodian staining for axon visualization may prove beneficial (16).

The concomitant occurrence of von Recklinghausen's disease may aid in diagnosis. However, it is pertinent to note that not all sarcomas in neurofibromatosis are nerve sheath tumors. Rather, they may range from liposarcoma, angiosarcoma, and rhabdomyosarcoma to leukemia (29).

In Table 5.3 from Asbury and Johnson (48), the differential features of schwannomas and neurofibromas, respectively, are outlined.

DIAGNOSTIC METHODS

Once the possibility of a neural neoplasm of the lower extremity arises, a methodic approach to diagnosis must be used. A multidisciplinary team consisting of an oncologist, a pathologist, a podiatrist, a vascular surgeon, and other specialists may be necessary to differentiate the lesion. A battery of radiologic, immunohistochemical, microscopic, and clinical examinations must be performed to promptly identify and treat the potentially lethal tumors.

Table 5.3.   Schwannoma—Neurofibroma Differential Features

	Schwannoma	Neurofibroma
Setting	Usually solitary.	Often multiple. May be solitary especially if cutaneous.
Parent nerve	Frequently identified.	Uncommonly identified in cutaneous tumors. Usually identified in plexiform tumors.
Gross	Usually encapsulated; rarely plexiform.	Nonencapsulated. Occasionally plexiform.
Cut surface	Tan-brown, may be cystic and hemorrhagic.	Homogeneous gray and gelatinous.
Histology	Compact, long spindle cells, sometimes palisaded, forming Verocay bodies (Antoni A tissue) and zones of loose spindle cells (Antoni B tissue)	Roughly parallel spindle cells with small nuclei separated by variably collagen bundle and a loose stroma.
Interstitium	Devoid of acid mucopolysaccharide.	Often containing acid mucopolysaccharide.
Vessels	Dilated, thick-walled, hyalinized.	Inconspicuous and thin-walled.
Ultrastructure	Resemble differentiated Schwann cells.	Spindle cells resembling perineural cells. Myelinated and nonmyelinated nerves sometimes entrapped within tumor.
Relation to von Recklinghausen's disease	May be seen in von Recklinghausen's disease	Predominant type in von Recklinghausen's disease.
Malignant transformation	Almost never.	Occasionally.

Special emphasis should be placed on the particular manifestation of the tumor, the patient's age and sex, the site of occurrence, the tumor's duration, and other clinical features. These factors may support specific disease entities and rule out other disorders. For example, cellular schwannomas notoriously evolve on the flexor aspects of the limbs (49). This characteristic facilitates tumor recognition.

A history of a previous malignancy in another body region may also direct a physician to the possibility of a neural neoplasm in the lower extremity. Carcinomas of the thyroid, breast, and lung classically metastasize to peripheral nerves (20). However, these unsuspected metastatic lesions are generally excised and not thoroughly investigated, since they are assumed to be innocuous ganglions or sites of nodular synovitis. A comprehensive history and physical examination are paramount for all patients.

Light microscopy is usually the basis for the detection and differentiation of neural neoplasms. Ultrastructurally, benign neurofibromas have a looser and less complicated cellular pattern than do schwannomas. A malignant nerve sheath tumor is less distinct by conventional microscopic studies, since marked anaplasia occurs with increased cellularity and the trademarks of nerve origin become less apparent (25).

Typical benign nerve sheath tumors are encapsulated and have characteristic Antoni type A and B growth patterns (28). In contrast, light microscopic criteria for malignant schwannomas include pleomorphism, accelerated mitotic rate, necrosis, or signs of necrosis, invasion, and metastasis (25). It has been estimated that approximately one-fourth of malignant-peripheral nerve sheath tumors can be definitively identified via light and electron microscopic techniques (20).

Neurofibromas may be poorly visualized by light microscopy and appear to encroach upon adjacent nonpathologic structures (28). The probability of neurofibromatosis is accentuated by a positive family history. More than six café-au-lait lesions, measuring over 1.5 cm in diameter, are necessary for its diagnosis. Associated clinical features may be present (see Fig. 5.40). Differential testing such as radiography, computed tomographic scanning, evaluation of the epinephrine and norepinephrine levels, electrocardiography, and psychologic testing should be considered (1). The diagnosis of a ma-

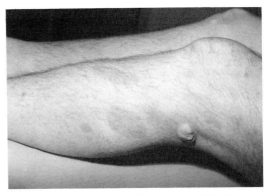

Figure 5.40. Myriad manifestations exist in the presentation of von Recklinghausen's disease, often making the diagnosis of this syndrome a challenge. (Courtesy of Dr. Harvey Lamont.)

lignant schwannoma is the demonstration of its origin from a nerve or its association with a contiguous neurofibroma. Ducatman *et al.* (6) observed that those tumors related to von Recklinghausen's disease fit into a more advanced malignancy grade.

Apart from clinical features, the diagnosis of a neuroblastoma may be based on a positive myelogram, as well as by tumor sections of biopsy (17). The lesion should be excised with a border of normal surrounding tissue for optimal identification.

Computed tomography appears to be an invaluable method of differentiation of neural neoplasms. Lesion classification is made according to attenuation values. Kumar *et al.* (50) found schwannomas, plexiform neurofibromas, and, occasionally, neurofibrosarcomas to be hypodense, yet found neurofibromas to be unpredictable.

Uri *et al.* (43) recommend repeated computed tomographic testings to monitor treatment regimens. Mass shrinkage correlates with a better prognosis. Magnetic resonance imaging and ultrasonography are also useful in the detection, differentiation, and monitoring of neural neoplasms and their management. The realm of immunohistochemical studies has successfully tackled the diagnostic challenges which many nerve tumors of the lower extremity have posed. This method of detection has served as an objective means of identification because of its specificity, a characteristic often lacking in microscopy, radiography, and clinical examination.

Antibodies to nervous system antigens, such as S-100 protein, Leu-7, neuron-specific enolase (NSE), and neurofilament, may be isolated (25). S-100 protein is found in Schwann cells of the peripheral nervous system, melanomas, nevi, granular cell tumors, central nervous system glia, and other cell types. Therefore, it is nonspecific for schwannomas, since it is present in most neural crest derivatives. Leu-7 is an antibody that recognizes myelin-associated glycoprotein (MAG) in the nervous system, thus being an important marker for neural sheath lesions.

In a study of 202 soft-tissue lesions in 1983, Weiss et al. (51) found that neural tumors were consistently positive for S-100 protein, particularly the benign nerve sheath tumors, neurofibromas, and benign granular cell tumors. The benign schwannoma demonstrated the most intensity in response. Unfortunately, this antibody is not always present in malignant schwannomas; therefore, another reliable means of detection is necessary for this tumor, as well as for neuroblastomas.

Cellular schwannomas are invariably positive for S-100 protein due to their predominant composition of Antoni A type tissues (37). Gould et al. (28) also stated that this type of lesion and ancient schwannomas stained readily for this antibody, whereas neurofibromas were only weakly positive. Johnson et al. (52) reported that S-100 immunoreactivity was detected in all traumatic neuromas and in a majority of schwannomas and neurofibromas.

Vimentin is acknowledged as the predominant, if not only, cytoskeletal intermediate filament protein in regenerating Schwann cells. The study by Gould et al. (28) demonstrated that samples representative of the entire spectrum of nerve sheath neoplasms expressed immunoreactivity to vimentin.

The diagnosis of schwannomas may be facilitated by confirming the Leu-7 immunoreactivity in Schwann cells and peripheral nerve sheaths (52). Intense positively was also noted in all traumatic neuromas, as was an extreme reaction to the myelin basic protein (MBP) in this pseudotumor.

Furthermore, these researchers encountered a greater sensitivity using anti-S-100 protein antibody, which marked 90% of schwannomas. In contrast, anti-Leu-7 antigen stained in only 66% of Schwann cell neoplasms. However, Perentes and Rubinstein (53) claim that 68% of 69 nerve sheath tumors, including 80% of the schwannomas, contained anti-Leu-7 positive cells. Despite these per-

centage discrepancies, it is obvious that this determinant is an insightful aid in diagnosis.

In the analysis of malignant schwannomas, Matsunou et al. (36) observed NSE in cells undergoing differentiation, such as neuroblastoma and neuroepithelioma. Unfortunately, this enzyme is also isolated in normal cells, including Langerhans' cells of the skin, and amine precursor uptake and decarboxylation (APUD) cells (54). Although several peripheral nerve tumors (e.g., neuroblastoma and ganglioneuroma) stain positively for NSE, these researchers (and others) conclude that this nonspecific marker is of little value in the differentiation of nervous system neoplasms.

The utilization of electromyography and nerve conduction studies is extremely resourceful in the differentiation of the various types of neural neoplasms. These examinations may provide confirmation of the location and extent of involvement, the level of advancement, and the response to treatment regimens.

When the nerve sheath is affected, the nerve study is consistent with a prolonged latency and a decreased conduction velocity which is directly proportionate to the degree of demyelinization. Electromyographic determinants at this stage may reflect a relative degree of fibrillation potentials at rest, and perhaps, a slight increment of polyphasic potentials of normal duration and amplitude, in view of normal recruitment patterns.

Once axonal changes evolve, relative and proportionate reductions in amplitude will manifest in all involved sensory and motor fibers. In the presence of axonal degeneration, electromyographic findings will be consistent with that of the presence of relative degrees of acute as well as chronic denervation within the distribution of all affected motor nerves.

The presentation of abnormal spontaneous activity at rest will reflect the amount and nature of acute denervation. The degree of polyphasic motor unit potentials at rest, in view of alterations in amplitude and duration, will signify the presence of denervation and reinnervation. Decreasing recruitment patterns will be directly proportionate to the degree of chronic denervation, as well as being indicative of the likelihood of permanent pathogenesis pertaining to the polyphasic motor unit potentials during minimal voluntary contractions.

The development of a neuroma of digital

nerves may best be appreciated upon nerve conduction evaluation. The anticipated nerve conduction parameters will contain a course of initial prolonged latencies that will evolve into subsequent concomitant decreasing amplitudes of all affected nerves in the absence of appropriate therapeutic intervention. Ultimately, a conduction block of all involved nerves may ensue, should appropriate therapeutic measures be deterred. Therefore, it is recommended that, should progressive axonal changes be observed upon serial nerve conduction studies, the treatment regimen be altered in order to prevent irreversible nerve damage (that could otherwise have been averted with suitable management).

It must be emphasized that the manifestation of digital neuroma formation in the presence of an underlying subclinical tarsal tunnel syndrome reflects a major dichotomy from the existence of an isolated occurrence of neuroma formation within a single digital nerve. In such an instance, it is strongly advisable to treat the underlying tarsal tunnel syndrome concurrently, while acknowledging that the therapy for most presentations of tarsal tunnel syndrome at this stage may be managed sufficiently in a conservative manner.

Treatment

The treatment regimen for a neural neoplasm is outlined according to several fundamental principles, i.e., general patient history, type of tumor, site of occurrence, whether the lesion is primary, recurrent, or metastatic, and other salient considerations. Ultimate management relies on organized interaction between the surgeon, oncologist, neurologist, radiotherapist, and other faculties throughout the entire evaluation period.

Of primary importance, the histologic constituents of the mass must be identified in order to rule out the possibility of malignancy. Superficial, small, or clinically benign lesions may be locally incised. However, deeper or expansile tumors may necessitate exploration. Unfortunately, this incisional type of biopsy may be disadvantageous, since further growth may ensue following incidental penetration of the neoplasm's pseudocapsule. Intractable hemorrhage may occur due to this procedure (31). It has been recommended that a formal biopsy, meticulously carried out under general anesthesia, be performed when a malignant le-

sion is suspected. Thus, paraffin sections and the pathologist's impression will guide the planning of therapeutic measures (31).

Anatomic region is paramount in determining the choice and amount of resection. When the tumor involves an isolated muscle, excision of the entire muscle is desirable. Wide excisions of muscle sections recur in approximately 50% of cases (31). Amputation of an extremity is advisable when major nerves or blood vessels are affected. Occasionally, nerves may be sacrificed and vessels excised and grafted. Shortcomings secondary to these methods should be anticipated by the patient. Amputation is again recommended when joint invasion is detected.

A combined protocol of surgical resection, chemotherapy, and radiation treatment is often used in managing a neuroblastoma. The latter two modalities may not always be incorporated when amputation is performed. Better prognosis is correlated with complete or partial removal of the lesion. Chemical agents (which are selected individually for each case) may include mercaptopurine, nitrogen mustard, thiopeta, adriamycin, daunomycin, thioguanine, vincristine sulfate, cyclophosphamide, actinomycin D, methotrexate, and vinblastine sulfate (17).

The sole treatment of von Recklinghausen's disease is generally that of observation for further expansion and unexpected changes. Some exacerbating factors may be prevented (extreme emotional and physical stress); others may not be (puberty, pregnancy, menopause). Sterilization may be considered early on to decrease complications from this disease.

Surgical management may be decided upon when cosmetic deformities develop; infection or hemorrhaging occurs; lesions cause neurovascular impingement, hinder normal activity, or are symptomatic; or malignant transformation appears feasible (31).

Small lesions may be completely excised without concern for increased growth. Extirpation may be necessary for infiltrative and irregular masses such as plexiform neurofibromas. However, major nerves should not be removed in the existence of lesions in this syndrome unless malignancy is highly suspected. Amputation may then become the palliative procedure of choice if the tumor attains dimensions sufficiently enormous to create acute and potentially threatening symptomatology.

Associated malignant neoplasms often complicate the clinical presentation of multiple neurofibromatosis. Based on 678 cases of von Recklinghausen's disease at the Mayo Clinic, D'Agostino *et al.* (12) identified 21 patients with a vast assortment of associated malignant tumors of somatic tissues or peripheral nerves. Nine individuals in this group were managed with wide local excision; seven of these experienced local recurrences and six then died, secondary to the pathology. Due to extensive expansion, eight individuals received no definitive surgical intervention and subsequently died. Four patients were treated by amputation for local recurrences following local excision. Three individuals are deceased due to pulmonary metastasis.

One theory of neurofibromatosis proposes that malignant transformation ensues surgical management of benign growths. However, 12 of the 21 cases in this study had no antecedent history of surgical procedures; this finding lends no credence to the hypothesis. It appears that, regardless of the therapeutic regimens adapted for the management of von Recklinghausen's disease and its associated malignant neoplasms, its prognosis is extremely guarded.

The surgical procedure for a Morton's neuroma is customarily the exploration of the third interspace of the foot, with the excision of the intermetatarsal nerve formed by the conjoined medial and lateral plantar nerves. Today, this surgical technique is still used with a variety of skin incisions, such as dorsal, plantar, or interspacial approaches. To prevent the evolution of a "stump" neuroma, the hypertrophic nerve is exposed and excised as proximally as feasible in the interspace.

Conservative therapy (e.g., injections, wider shoes, a metatarsal crest raise, orthoses, and taping) should be attempted before considering surgical intervention. Comparing both forms of management, the surgical method demonstrates greater success and relief from pain and paresthesia.

Refractory neuroma pain may plague patients despite the most meticulous surgical finesse. Several theories may explain this phenomenon. It has been estimated that in approximately 30% of cases, an accessory nerve trunk, plantar to the metatarsal head, joins the common digital nerve distal to the transverse metatarsal ligament, is undetected and, therefore, not excised (55). Occasionally, the common digital nerve adheres to surrounding tissue, creating fibrosis and traction (55). Symptomatology associated with a "stump" neuroma may actually be due to axonal regeneration of the proximal section of the interdigital nerve.

Management for recalcitrant neuroma pain, subsequent to neuroma excision, may include an accommodative or functional orthoses with a metatarsal pad. Local injection therapy with a steroid solution, local anesthetic, and hyaluronidase is recommended, along with immobilization via a compressive, soft cast over cast padding. Often, this method is poorly tolerated by the patient due to hyperesthesia initiated by decreased threshold as a result of axonal regeneration. In our experience, helium-neon cold laser therapy has provided partial to total symptomatic relief with unseen recurrence.

Electroacupuncture, in the form of transcutaneous electrical nerve stimulation (TENS), induces analgesia by modifying pain perception. A TENS system incorporates a battery-operated stimulator emitting continuous waves of electrical impulses through silicone electrodes which are placed directly on skin that has been coated with conduction gel (56). It has been reported that the TENS modality prevents pain formation through the release of endogenous, morphine-like substances, namely endorphins and enkephalins. These compounds activate a descending pain-inhibition pathway by binding to specific morphine receptors situated in the periaqueductal gray area (57).

Benign schwannomas are generally encapsulated and, therefore, treated with local excision. They are characteristically dissected from the nerve trunk and excised without extreme difficulty. Sacrifice of the nerve section is not indicated in this presentation (see Fig. 5.41).

The initial treatment of malignant schwannomas should consist of a biopsy to ascertain the ultimate diagnosis through histopathologic evaluation. Therefore, a therapeutic regimen may be outlined according to gross and microscopic findings, as well as by clinical presentation. Prompt radical surgery is mandated once a malignant peripheral nerve sheath neoplasm is identified. Aggressive local resection and amputation must be considered. Inadequate excision permits recurrence and metastasis to evolve. Local resection should be performed en bloc (i.e., the lesion and all adjacent and adher-

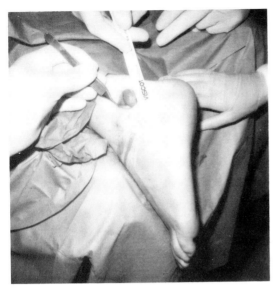

Figure 5.41. Superficial, small, or clinically benign lesions may be locally excised. This figure illustrates the surgical resection of a benign schwannoma present in a 30-year-old Caucasian male. An asymptomatic palpable mass noted on the lateral aspect of his left ankle with no acute changes caused gradual increasing discomfort in footgear. (Courtesy of Dr. Daniel Girardi.)

ent blood vessels, muscles, bone, and nerves should be sufficiently extirpated). If satellite foci are detected, the treatment of choice to prevent recurrence and metastasis is an amputation at the most proximal site. Amputation subsequent to the formation of serial recurrences will not, however, prolong the patient's life (10).

Grade 1 malignant neurofibromas or schwannomas mandate less radical management. The incompletely encapsulated neoplasms must be thoroughly excised, along with their nerve origins.

When the sciatic nerve is affected by a malignant tumor and necessitates sacrifice, partial limb function is restored to the patient with a triple arthrodesis and a custom-made foot and leg brace (31).

Several factors limit total removal of soft-tissue sarcomas. Site becomes a crucial determinant, especially when one is located in the trunk,neck, pelvis, or head. Expansion of the lesion also restricts complete eradication. Size, in particular a diameter over 5 cms, may also limit complete resection and, thus, negatively affect the ultimate prognosis.

In situations which only permit subtotal resection, high-dose radiation and chemotherapy may be incorporated into the management regimen. Their efficacy in reference to malignant neural neoplasms remains nondelineated, and their utility in treating aggressive lesions appears minimal. Based on a review of 120 cases of malignant peripheral nerve sheath tumors, Ducatman *et al.* (6) concluded that the adjuvant therapeutic modalities did not alter the survival rates. Responses to radiation and chemotherapy were consistently poor in malignant schwannomas in both the presence and absence of von Recklinghausen's disease (15).

Neurofibrosarcoma, considered a highly malignant neoplasm, is generally managed with an aggressive wide en bloc resection or amputation. Storm *et al.* (23) advocate adjuvant radiation and chemotherapy to reduce local recurrence. Based on 20 cases, they recommend radiation levels of 3000–6500 rads, with the higher ranges reserved for lesions affecting the extremities. Good response was noted using combined chemotherapeutic agents, namely cyclophosphamide, vincristine, adriamycin, and dimethyltriazene imidazole carboxamide (CY-V-A-DTIC). Additionally, patients received intraarterial adriamycin preoperatively and then high-dose methotrexate and adriamycin postoperatively. Radical surgical measures, along with radiation and chemotherapy, achieved local disease control in 80% of the patients.

PROGNOSIS
Neuroma

Depending on whether palliative care or surgical management is employed, varying levels of symptomatic relief may be achieved. Based on one comparative analysis between the treatment modalities, surgery demonstrates a much greater probability of success.

Gaynor's *et. al.* (9) study of 60 subjects claims positive results following surgery in 76% of the cases. Less encouraging outcomes accompanied conservative regimens (poor results 73%, fair results 70%). Data by other researchers give credence to the percentages. Miller (58) relates an 80% success rate for surgical excision and less than 20% improvement with nonsurgical approaches.

There are no accurate statistics for neuromal

recurrence status-post surgery. Contributing factors may include neural entrapment, secondary to substantial fibrotic formation, lingering intermetatarsal bursitis, inadequate excision, or regeneration of the proximal nerve segment with concomitant inflammation. Another etiologic consideration of recurrence is that initial objective and subjective findings were insufficiently investigated and, therefore, improperly diagnosed.

Often, paresthesias located interdigitally (especially in the third interspace) are hastily labeled neuromas. However, a presentation such as this may actually be a component of a tarsal tunnel syndrome. Such a suspicion should be thoroughly addressed by definite diagnostic modes (e.g., nerve conduction velocity studies) prior to enlisting any therapeutic plan. By utilizing this methodic approach to differentiation, patients will less likely undergo needless procedures for these "recurrent neuromas," and the podiatric practitioner will enjoy a greater success rate in the management of neuromas.

According to the literature, malignant transformation of neuromas appears unlikely.

Neuroblastoma

Prognostic indicators of neuroblastoma include the tumor's stage, extent, and morphology, its primary site, and the location of metastases. Other pertinent factors include age, form of treatment, and follow-up.

The retrospective study by Tang and Hajdu (17) lists the following sites of metastasis, in decreasing frequency: skeletal system; lungs and/or pleura; liver and lymph nodes; breast, diaphragm, meninges, pancreas, and testis; blood vessels, intestine, prostate, skin, spleen, and thyroid; and, least likely, appendix, bladder, heart, ovary, pericardium, pituitary, spinal cord, and stomach.

To demonstrate patient's age as a differentiating variable, metastasis to the lung is common in adults and infrequent in children. The overall 1-year survival rate in adults with neuroblastomas is 67%, far more hopeful than the estimated 18.8% in child counterparts (59).

Furthermore, these researchers demonstrated that complete or partial excision of this tumor coincides with a better prognosis. Patients who undergo radical procedures (such as amputation) for the eradication of neuroblastoma are more likely to survive longer.

Peripheral Nerve Sheath Tumors

Prognostic predictors of peripheral nerve sheath tumors (PNST) may include growth pattern, nuclear polymorphism, mitosis, vascularity, cellularity, and other determinants. In the study by Horak et al. (10), the neoplasms are categorized into four groups: (a) benign tumors without recurrences, (b) recurring benign tumors, (c) recurring tumors that underwent malignant transformation, and (d) primary malignant tumors. Based on a retrospective review of 118 subjects, they report that the variety of tumor cellularity is the most pertinent feature. Histologic examination of these lesions distinguishes three pathomorphologic subtypes: (a) typical, (b) cellular, and (c) sarcomas. This group relates a 10-year survival rate of 94% in their set of "typical" tumors, whereas a 67% 10-year survival rate was found in those individuals with primary "cellular" neoplasms. Approximately 50% of this cellular subtype underwent malignant transformation and the majority recurred. On the other hand, Horak et al. (10) consider the cellular neurogenic growths to be potentially progressive, with the possibility of recurrence and malignant transformation.

The patient's sex proved to be a differentiating factor. The incidence rate was higher in males, and nonrecurring neurofibromas and schwannomas were more common in females.

Neurofibromas and schwannomas were more frequent in patients older than 60 years of age. However, the proportion of schwannomas decreased in patients 70 years and older. These researchers further recount a higher incidence of malignancy in the extremities when compared to the trunk. Sheath tumors associated with von Recklinghausen's disease have a higher incidence of malignant transformation than do other sheath tumors. Therefore, whenever a patient presents with symptomatology in the lower extremity that is neurologically suspect, the podiatric practitioner should thoroughly investigate such cases to rule out neoplasm formation.

Prognostic correlations can be drawn regarding tumor size. In this review by Horak et al. (10) most of the lesions less than 2 cm in diameter were benign and demonstrated no recurrences. Conversely, it was found that the larger primary neoplasms were initially diagnosed as being malignant. Some investigators claimed that infiltrating growth and tumor size correlate with local recurrence.

Das Gupta and Brasfield (61) think that inadequate surgical excision is a factor responsible for recurrence. This point of view may support the option of amputation and other radical procedures as the ultimate treatment of PNST, yet this has not been established.

Malignant Peripheral Nerve Sheath Tumors

A poor prognosis customarily accompanies the diagnosis of malignant peripheral nerve sheath tumors (MPNST). Its clinical course is generally one of multiple local recurrences. Pertinent clinical features which may adversely influence its prognosis include the presence of von Recklinghausen's disease, a tumor size of more than 5 cms, and the extent of resection (6). Other salient clinical aspects that correlate with a guarded outcome is a lesion located near the central axis of the body and an elevated rate of mitotic activity (more than 6 mitotic figures/10 HPF) (11). For this reason, patients with tumors in the extremities fared slightly better than those with lesions in other anatomic regions. Statistically, however, location does not appear to be a major prognostic factor. This may enforce the fact that most extremity neoplasms originate in proximally situated major nerves.

No significant differences were found in survival distributions between sexes, or between patients younger or older than 40 years (15).

The use of adjuvant radiation and chemotherapy did not appear to alter the prognosis. In fact, patient responses to these treatment modalities were consistently poor (6, 15). The study by Ducatman's group (6) demonstrates the high frequency of malignant transformation of neurofibromas to MPNST in patients with von Recklinghausen's disease (81%), as compared with nonaffected individuals (41%). This finding supports the theory that the presence of this disorder greatly enhances the risk of developing MPNST in certain cases. It has not established why the sarcomas associated with neurofibromatosis are more aggressive clinically, and hence, have a reduced patient survival rate and a poorer prognosis.

Tumors present with an extremely guarded survival rate. In a review of 46 malignant schwannomas by Guccion and Enzinger (61), 32 patients died within 2 years. The 5-year survival rate for patients with this neoplasm and neurofibromatosis was estimated to be 15%.

Of great interest is their finding that certain individuals, whose lesions were located in the peripheral extremities, were tumor-free at a 5–15-year follow-up examination. They surmise that the data demonstrate that neural sarcomas in this site tend to be smaller and have a lower rate of mitotic activity.

Pulmonary metastasis from malignant schwannomas is most common. In decreasing order of frequency, the usual sites of metastasis are soft tissue, bone, liver, intraabdominal cavity, adrenal glands, diaphragm, mediastinum, brain, ovaries, kidneys, and retroperitoneum (16).

Patients with neurofibromatosis had a dismal prognosis: 84% in this group with locally recurrent lesions had distant metastasis, as compared to 52% in those individuals without this disorder.

Various pathologies have been associated with malignant peripheral nerve sheath tumors. Several examples of these conditions are listed in Table 5.4, based on a review of 165 cases of malignant schwannomas by Sordillos' group (15).

Table 5.4. Conditions Associated with Malignant Schwannoma[a]

	VRMS[b]	SMS
Retardation	3	0
Seizure disorder	3	0
Cryptorchidism	2	0
Deafness	0	2
Spina bifida	1	0
Scoliosis	1	1
Congenital strabismus	2	0
Associated malignancies (total)	8	18
Breast carcinoma	1	1
Prostate carcinoma	1	2
Carcinoma of cervix	1	2
Carcinoma of uterine corpus	1	0
Malignant melanoma	1	2
Basal cell carcinoma	1	2
Epidermoid carcinoma of skin	0	1
Neuroblastoma	0	1
Acoustic neuroma	1	1
Ganglioneuroma	1	1
Lymphoma	0	5
Hodgkin's disease	0	1
History of brain tumors in immediate family	4	4

[a] VRMS, von Recklinghausen's disease associated with malignant Schwannomas. SMS, subjects with malignant Schwannomas.
[b] Patients in this group were diagnosed as having von Recklinghausen's disease.

Von Recklinghausen's Disease

There appears to be a higher rate of malignant transformation to neurogenic sarcoma in patients with long-term von Recklinghausen's disease, compared to individuals having the condition for a shorter duration, or with solitary peripheral schwannoma or neurofibroma (16). In the series by Holt and Wright (2), malignant changes in neurofibroma have an incidence of 5.5%; varying occurrences have been reported more recently.

Pathologic studies have listed malignant tumors from multiple neurofibromas as being neurofibrosarcoma, fibrosarcoma, or spindle-cell sarcoma. It is claimed that transformation follows the excision of cutaneous lesions, and may evolve into a malignant neoplasm in a remote site elsewhere in the body. However, this view has been refuted. In a review of 21 cases of neurofibromatosis by D'Agostino et al. (12), 12 patients with no antecedent history of surgical treatment were diagnosed as having developed a malignant tumor. Therefore, there is substantial conflicting scientific evidence to discredit the view that surgical intervention of neurofibromatosis predisposes the person to malignant transformation.

In addition to local recurrences, metastasis to the lungs is most common. The incidence of sarcoma of neural and somatic soft tissues arising in association with von Recklinghausen's disease has been estimated as approximately 5–16.4% (12). Glioma of the central nervous system is frequently described.

Symptomatology that may raise suspicion of malignancy include the insidious onset of acute pain, rapid enlargement of a preexisting lesion, or sudden occurrence of new masses. The mortality rate for those with neurofibromatosis that are affected by such lesions has been estimated to be between 80 and 97% (16). Incidentally, the histologic type and the site of the sarcoma did not appear to directly influence the ultimate prognosis.

Neurofibrosarcoma

Prognostic indicators include primary lesion size and its histopathologic grade of malignancy, which is based on mitotic activity and pleomorphism (62). In the review of 20 patients with neurofibrosarcoma by Storm et al. (23), a positive correlation was made between clinical stage and survival rate for the initial 36 months. However, both stages II and III demonstrate equally poor prognosis by 5 years. It was estimated that the 5-yea survival rate for stage II lesions was 40%, and 30% for stage III tumors. Contrary to what is assumed, those individuals with tumors unrelated to neurofibromatosis did not fare better. The frequent occurrence of pulmonary metastasis within the first 2 years highlights the systemic nature of this neoplasm.

CONCLUSION

This chapter has presented the salient features of neural neoplasms affecting the lower extremity. Their pathogenesis and classification have been reviewed in order to categorize various tumor subtypes. Commonly encountered clinical manifestations and characteristic symptomatology of each lesion group have been emphasized, as have frequently used modes of detection. In addition, the comparative analysis of the diverse histopathologic patterns and the comprehensive deductive methodic approach toward differential diagnosis given in this chapter will provide a prompt and concise way to detect the neoplastic processes. Therapeutic regimens and prognostic indicators have been outlined to assist in providing optimal patient management of individuals afflicted with a neural neoplasm of the lower extremity.

REFERENCES

1. Riccardi VM. Von Recklinghausen's neurofibromatosis. N Engl J Med 1981;305:1617.
2. Holt JF, Wright EM. The radiologic features of neurofibromatosis. Radiology 1948;51:647.
3. Stout AP. Tumors of the peripheral nervous system. In: Atlas of tumor pathology, sect 2, fasc 6. Washington DC: Armed Forces Institute of Pathology, 1949.
4. Preston FW, et al. Cutaneous manifestations and incidence of sarcoma in 61 male patients. AMA Arch Surg 1952;64:813.
5. Martuza RL, Eldridge E. Neurofibromatosis. N Engl J Med 1988;318:684.
6. Ducatman B, et al. Malignant peripheral nerve sheath tumors: a clinicopathologic study of 120 cases. Cancer 1986;57:2006.
7. Fletcher CD, et al. Cellular schwannoma: a distinct pseudosarcomatous entity. Histopathology 1987;11:21.
8. Phillips R. Neuroblastoma. Ann R Coll Surg Engl 1953;12:29.
9. Gaynor R, et al. A comparative analysis of conservative versus surgical treatment of Morton's neuroma. J Am Podiatr Med Assoc 1989;79:27.
10. Horak E, et al. Pathologic feature of nerve sheath tumors with respect to prognostic signs. Cancer 1983;51:1159.

11. Guccion JG, and Enzinger FM. Malignant schwannoma associated with von Recklinghausen's neurofibromatosis. Virchows Arch [A] 1979;383:43.

12. D'Agostino AN, et al. Sarcomas of the peripheral nerves and somatic soft tissue associated with multiple neurofibromatosis (von Recklinghausen's disease). Cancer 1963;16:1015.

13. Gallagher RL, Helwig EB. Neurothekeoma: benign cutaneous tumor of nerve origin. Am J Clin Pathol 1980;74:759.

14. Ducatman B, et al. Malignant peripheral nerve sheath tumors with divergent differentiation. Cancer 1984; 54:1049.

15. Sordillo P, et al. Malignant shwannoma—clinical characteristic, survival, and response to therapy. Cancer 1981;47:2503.

16. Enzinger FM, Weiss SW. Soft tissue tumors. 2nd ed. St. Louis: Mosby; 1988;719–815.

17. Tang C-K, Hajdu S. Neuroblastoma in adolescence and adulthood. NY State J Med 1975; 75:1434–1438.

18. Morton TG. A peculiar and painful affection of the fourth metatarsophalangeal articulation. Am J Med Sci 1876;71:37.

19. Angerall, et al. Dermal nerve sheath myxoma. Cancer 1984;53:1752.

20. Harkin J. Differential diagnosis of peripheral nerve tumors. In: Omar G, Samner M, eds. Philadelphia: Saunders, 1980:657–668.

21. Mennmeyer RP, et al. Melanocytic schwannoma: clinical and ultrastructural studies of three cases with evidence of intracellular melanin synthesis. Am J Surg Pathol 1979;3:3.

22. Gazivoda PL, et al. Surgical management of plantar von Recklinghausen's neurofibroma. J Foot Surg 1988;27:52.

23. Storm F, et al. Neurofibrosarcoma. Cancer 1980;45:126.

24. Erlandson R. Peripheral nerve sheath tumors. Ultrastruct Pathol 1985;9:113.

25. Bruner JM. Tumors of Schwann cells and pigmented skin cells. Clin Lab Med 1987; 7:181.

26. Harkin JE, Electron microscope studies of goldfish tumors previously termed neurofibromas and schwannomas. Am Pathol 1969;55:191–202.

27. Hajdu SI. Pathology of soft tissue tumors. Philadelphia: Lea and Febiger, 1979;427.

28. Gould VE, et al. The intermediate filament complement of the spectrum of nerve sheath neoplasms. Lab Invest 1986;55:463.

29. Chitale AR, Dickerson GR. Electron microscopy in the diagnosis of malignant schwannomas. Cancer 1983;51:1448.

30. Daimaru Y; Hashimoto H. Malignant peripheral nerve sheath tumors (malignant schwannomas). An immunohistochemical study of 29 cases. Am J Surg Pathol 1985;434–444.

31. Ariel I. Current concepts in the management of peripheral nerve Tumors. In: Omar G, Spinner, M, eds. Management of peripheral nerve problems. Philadelphia: Saunders, 1980:669–693.

32. Smith, T. Multiple neuromata. Trans Pathol Soc Lond 1860–1;xii:2.

33. Preiser SA, Davenport CB. Multiple neurofibromatosis (von Recklinghausen's disease) and its inheritance; with description of a case. Am J M Sci 1918;156:507.

34. Barker, D, et al. Gene for von Recklinghausen neurofibromatosis is in the pericentromeric region of chromosome 17. Science 1987;236:1100.

35. Laserus SS, Trombetta LD. Ultrastructural identification of a benign perineural cell tumor. Cancer 1978;41:1823.

36. Matsunou H, et al. Histopathologic and immunohistochemical study of malignant tumors of peripheral nerve sheath (malignant schwannoma). Cancer 1985;56:2269.

37. Fletcher et al. Dermal nerve sheath myxoma. Histopathology 1986;10:135–145.

38. Goette DK. Calcifying neurothekeoma. J Dermatol Surg Oncol 1986;12:958.

39. Gardner WJ, Frazier CH. Bilateral acoustic neurofibromas. Arch Neurol Psychiatry 1930; 23:266.

40. Brooks B, Lehman EP. Bone changes in Recklinghausen's neurofibromatosis. Surg Gynecol Obstet 1924; 38:587.

41. Erlandson RA, Woodruff JM. Peripheral nerve sheath tumors: an electron microscopic study of 43 cases. Cancer 1982;49:273.

42. Goldstein S, Lifshitz A. Myxoma of the nerve sheath. Am J Dermatopathol 1985;429:423.

43. Uri A, et al. Electron microscopy of glandular schwannoma. Cancer 1984;53:493.

44. Sian CS, Ryan SF. The ultrastructure of neuroleoma with emphasis on Antoni b tissue. Hum Pathol 1981;12:145.

45. Tate R, Rusin J. Morton's neuroma: its ultrastructural anatomy and biomechanical etiology. J Am Podiatr Med Assoc 1978;68:797.

46. Woodhall B, et al. Neurosurgical implications in peripheral nerve regeneration. [Monograph]. Washington DC: Veterans Administration, 1957:567.

47. Seddon H. Surgical disorders of the peripheral nerves. Baltimore, Williams & Wilkins, 1972.

48. Asbury AK, Johnson PC. Pathology of peripheral nerve, vol 9. Philadelphia: Saunders, 1978; 210.

49. Hennessee MT, et al. Benign schwannoma: clinical and histopathologic findings. J Am Podiatr Med Assoc 1985;75:310.

50. Kumar AJ, et al. Computed tomography of extracranial nerve sheath tumors with pathological correction. J Comput Assist Tomogr 1983; 7:857.

51. Weiss S, et al. Value of S-100 protein in the diagnosis of tissue tumors with particular reference to benign and malignant Schwann cell tumors. Lab Invest 1983;49:299.

52. Johnson MD, et al. Immunohistochemical evaluation of leu-7, myelin basic protein, glial-fibrillary acidic-protein, and LN3 immunoreactivity in nerve sheath tumors and sarcomas. Arch Pathol Lab Med 1988;112:155.

53. Perentes E, and Rubenstein LJ. Immunohistochemical recognition of human nerve sheath tumors by anti-leu7 (hnk-1) monoclonal antibody. Acta Neuropathol (Berl) 1985;68:319.

54. Vinores S, et al. Immunohistochemical demon-

stration of neuron-specific enolase in neoplasms of the CNS and other tissues. Arch Pathol Lab Med 1984;108:536.

55. Mann RA, Reynolds JC. Interdigital neuroma: a critical clinical analysis. Foot Ankle 1983; 3:238.

56. Melzack R, Wall PD. Acupuncture and transcutaneous electrical nerve stimulation. Postgrad Med J 1984;60:893.

57. Chan CS, Chow SP. Electroacupuncture in the treatment of post-traumatic sympathetic dystrophy (Sudek's atrophy). Br J Anaesth 1981; 53:899.

58. Miller SJ. Morton's neuroma. In: McGlamry ED, ed. Comprehensive textbook of foot surgery, vol. I. Baltimore, Williams and Wilkins, 1987.

59. Fortner, J, et al. Neuroblastoma: natural history and results of treating 133 cases. Ann Surg 1968;167:132.

60. Das Gupta TK, Brasfield RD. Solitary malignant schwannoma. Ann Surg 1970;419.

61. Guccion JG, Enzinger FM. Malignant schwannoma associated with von Recklinghausen's neurofibromatosis. Virchows Arch [A] 1979; 383:43–57.

62. Russell WO, et al. A clinical and pathological staging for soft-tissue sarcomas. Cancer 1977;40:1562.

Part E/ **Fibrous Tumors of the Foot and Leg**

—Donnamarie Stewart

Hal F. Abrahamson

The incidence of fibrous tumors of the foot and leg is difficult to assess. Differences in categorization (e.g., benign versus malignant of any histologic origin, or benign versus malignant of the extremities versus trunk versus foot) contribute to the difficulty.

In 1980, Berlin (1) reviewed 2720 lesions of the foot over a 5-year period and determined that tumors of fat and connective tissue origin constituted the fourth largest category (i.e., 274 lesions). Based on a classification system to be discussed later, fibrous lesions accounted for 6.9% of the total. Subsequently, Berlin (2) assessed some 67,000 tumors of the foot, concluding that those of fat and fibrous origin represented the fifth largest group (i.e., 1136 lesions) or 1.7%. As both studies included osseous lesions and classified fibrous tumors with those of adipose origin, the results are biased. Additionally, the two studies analyze lesions of the foot rather than the entire lower extremity.

Differentiating benign neoplasms from malignant ones will also facilitate determination of the incidence of fibrous tumors in the lower extremities.

Benign tumors, generally, resemble normal tissue histologically and clinically, have low potential for local invasion, and demonstrate a low rate of local recurrence following conservative treatment (3). Additionally, benign tumors demonstrate slow growth and tend not to metastasize (4).

Malignant tumors, conversely, exhibit aggressive behavior locally with rapid growth and tend to disseminate throughout the body (3). Grading and staging of malignant tumors are based on histologic and clinical presentations and allow for prediction of local recurrence and metastatic potential and for selection of adequate treatment and prognosis.

In a study conducted on a hospital population, Rydholm and Berg (5) estimated that benign soft-tissue tumors are approximately 100 times more common than malignant ones. However, Enzinger and Weiss (3) indicate the study is not reflective of the general population.

Further studies conclude that malignant soft-tissue lesions are rare. Analysis of soft-tissue sarcomas of the extremities and limb girdles conducted by Rantakko and Ekfors (6) based on 240 lesions concludes that the annual incidence rate is 1.35/100,000 population. The annual incidence rate is age-specific for many types of neoplasms, and the vast majority of clinical studies do not consider the occurrence of these lesions confined to the lower extremity.

The classification of fibrous tumors is highly variable. Lesions such as neurofibromas are included by some authors and omitted by others. Lever (7) identifies the following as fibrous tumors: dermatofibroma, soft fibroma, recurrent infantile digital fibroma, multiple perifollicular fibromas, fibrous papules of the face (nose), tuberous sclerosis, hypertrophic scar and keloid, giant cell tumor of tendon sheath, giant cell epulis, desmoid tumor, congenital generalized fibromatosis, fibrous hamartoma of childhood, juvenile hyalin pilomatosis, nodular pseudosarcomatous fasciitis (cranial fasciitis of childhood), dermatofibrosarcoma protuberans, atypical fibroxanthoma of skin, malignant fibrous histiocytoma, epithelioid sarcoma, fibrosarcoma, focal mucinosis, digital mucous cyst, mucous cyst of oral mucosa, and myxosarcoma.

Samitz (8) considers fibrous skin tumors

of the lower extremity to be in four categories: benign, premalignant, malignant, and pseudomalignant.

The benign tumors are dermal and subcutaneous neurofibromas with or without von Recklinghausen's disease (see Figs. 5.42 and 5.43), periungual fibroma with tuberous sclerosis (see Fig. 5.44), keloid, plantar fibromatosis, nodular subepidermal fibrosis (dermatofibroma, histiocytoma, and sclerosing hemangioma), myxoid cyst, fibroma, fibrolipoma, radiation fibromatosis, and reticulohistiocytoma.

The malignant classification includes malig-nant fibrous histiocytoma, dermatofibrosarcoma protuberans, and sarcoma (fibrosarcoma and neurofibrosarcoma).

As pseudomalignant he classifies nodular pseudosarcomatous fasciitis, atypical fibroxanthoma, and atypical fibrous histiocytoma (8).

Samitz (8) also concludes that certain tumors have a predilection for the lower extremities. These are plantar fibromatosis, nodular subepidermal fibrosis, periungual fibromas occurring in tuberous sclerosis, and fibrosarcoma.

C. J. Campbell (9) categorizes fibrous tumors and tumor-like lesions as follows: fibroma, fibromatosis (cicatricial fibromatosis, keloid,

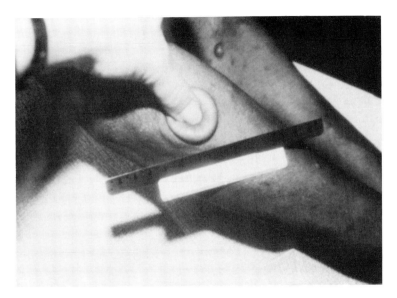

Figure 5.42. A neurofibroma in a 43-year-old patient with von Recklinghausen's disease.

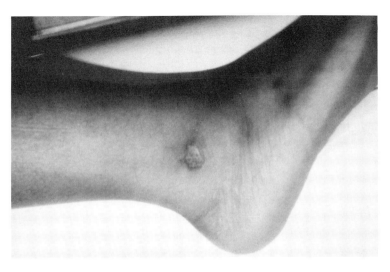

Figure 5.43. Same patient as depicted in Fig. 5.44. Neurofibroma of lateral malleolus.

Figure 5.44. Periungual fibromas in a female patient with tuberous sclerosis. (Courtesy of Dr. M. A. Kosinski.)

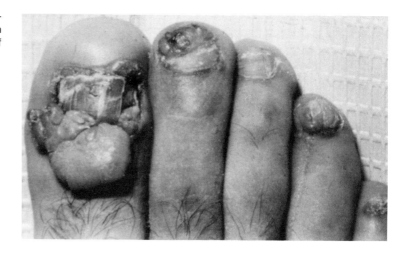

nodular fasciitis, plantar fibromatosis, aggressive fibromatosis, and congenital generalized fibromatosis), dermatofibrosarcoma protuberans, fibrosarcoma, and resembling neoplasms (fibroxanthoma and xanthoma).

Another classification of fibrous tumors, by Hajdu (10), distinguishes nonneoplastic lesions from neoplastic ones, with the latter subdivided into noncollagenous and collagenous tumors.

The designation of nonneoplastic lesions refers to fasciitis, keloid, elastofibroma, and fibromatosis.

Neoplastic-noncollagenous fibrous tumors include (a) fibroblastic fibrous histiocytomas (sclerosing hemangioma, myxoma, and dermatofibrosarcoma protuberans), (b) histiocytic fibrous histiocytomas (histiocytoma, giant cell tumor of tendon sheath, and giant cell tumor of soft parts), and (c) pleomorphic fibrous histiocytomas (xanthoma, atypical fibroxanthoma, and xanthosarcoma).

Neoplastic collagenous fibrous tumors include fibroma, ganglion, fibrolipoma, angiofibroma, neurofibroma, desmoid tumor, fibroblastic fibrosarcoma, and pleomorphic fibrosarcoma.

A detailed histologic categorization of fibrous tumors is presented by Enzinger and Weiss (3). This classification considers both fibrous and fibrohistiocytic varieties. Tumors and tumorlike lesions of fibrous tissue are divided into benign, those occurring in infancy and childhood, fibromatosis, and malignant forms.

Benign tumors include fibroma, nodular fasciitis, proliferative fasciitis, fibroma of tendon sheath, elastofibroma, nuchae fibroma, nasopharangeal fibroma, and keloid.

Fibrous tumors of infancy and childhood are fibrous hamartoma, myofibromatosis (solitary and multicentric), fibromatosis callus, infantile digital fibromatosis, infantile fibromatosis desmoid, giant cell fibroblastoma, gingival fibromatosis, calcifying aponeurotic fibroma, hyaline fibromatosis.

Fibromatosis tumors are either superficial (palmar and plantar fibromatosis, Peyronie's penile fibromatosis, and knuckle pads) or deep (abdominal fibromatosis, extraabdominal fibromatosis, intraabdominal fibromatosis, mesenteric fibromatosis (Gardner's syndrome), postirradiation fibromatosis, and cicatricial fibromatosis).

The malignant tumors are adult fibrosarcoma, congenital and infantile fibrosarcoma, inflammatory fibrosarcoma, postirradiation fibrosarcoma, and cicatricial fibrosarcoma.

Fibrohistiocytic tumors are divided into (a) benign lesions (cutaneous or dermatofibroma fibrous histiocytoma, deep fibrous histiocytoma, atypical fibroxanthoma, juvenile xanthogranuloma, reticulohistiocytoma, and xanthoma), (b) intermediate tumors (dermatofibrosarcoma protuberans and Bednar's tumor), and (c) malignant tumors (malignant fibrous histiocytoma, storiform or pleomorphic tumor, myxofibrosarcoma, giant cell tumor, malignant xanthogranuloma and xanthosarcoma inflammatory tumors, and angiomatoid tumor).

Enzinger and Weiss' classification of fibrous tumors, and those of Lever and Hajdu are based on soft-tissue tumors of the entire body, not those exclusive to the lower extremity. However, the organization and histologic detail of the former, we think, will enhance discussion of fibrous tumors of the foot and leg.

DIAGNOSTIC PROCEDURES

As noted by many researchers, the clinical presentation of a soft-tissue tumor may be highly variable, ranging from a small, painless mass to a large tumor that causes pain and dysfunction (3, 9–12).

In addition to a thorough physical examination noting the consistency, adherence or lack thereof to surrounding structures, and the actual size of the lesion, specific diagnostic tests may facilitate prompt and accurate diagnosis. Certain diagnostic examinations may also assist in the selection of surgical approaches and/or options for adjuvant therapy.

Although there is no pathognomonic finding obtainable by any of the following modalities that enables distinction between benign and malignant lesions, the examinations may be useful in corroboration with clinical findings.

RADIOGRAPHY

Radiography may yield results generally considered nonspecific for differential diagnosis of soft-tissue masses (13). However, it may provide characteristic findings for lipomatous lesions (11, 14–16).

Soft-tissue calcifications that occur in both benign and malignant lesions can be visualized radiographically (17). Such calcifications may be demonstrated in the benign lesions nodular (pseudosarcomatous) fasciitis (18) and myositis ossificans (19, 20).

In addition to indicating size and location, plain radiography may be useful in demonstrating or refuting involvement of adjacent soft tissue, bones, and joints. Margins of the mass may either be sharp or ill-defined, the former exhibited more frequently by benign lesions and the latter by malignant lesions (11).

Soft-tissue masses that occur adjacent to osseous structures may evoke periosteal reactions that can be seen radiographically. Solid periosteal reactions are more typical of benign lesions and interrupted patterns are more suggestive of malignant ones (21). One can also distinguish between soft-tissue mass invasion of bone and osseous invasion of soft tissue.

Plain film radiography at low kilivolt tech-

nique enhances differences in radiographic densities between fat and muscle and may accentuate soft-tissue detail (18, 22–24). In predicting the presence and type of osseous involvement, some authors state plain film radiography is superior to other techniques. (25).

XERORADIOGRAPHY

Xeroradiography offers excellent contrast and delineation of soft-tissue detail (18, 21, 26, 27), however, some shortcomings have been noted.

Heiken et al. (25) states that the differentiation between soft-tissue tumor and adjacent soft tissue, as indicated on a xeroradiogram, is most pronounced with lipoma, and that this modality is less useful in the differentiation of soft-tissue masses with densities similar to that of muscle. Bernadino et al. (21) note the inability of xeroradiograms to detect the clinical aspect of tumors. Other researchers have questioned the use of xeroradiography over conventional x-rays under optimal conditions (11, 28–30).

SCINTIGRAPHY

The use of radionucleotide scanning with phosphate and other radiopharmaceutical agents is useful in the evaluation of soft-tissue masses, as these lesions demonstrate uptake (11, 18, 21, 25, 32, 33–54). Particular usefulness of scintigraphy is for dynamic scanning of vascular soft-tissue lesions (34) and for determining osseous involvement of soft-tissue sarcomas (35).

Its disadvantages are invasiveness of the procedure and occurrence of allergic reactions to contrast media. Additionally, scintigraphy is inconclusive if local extent of the mass is poorly defined (36). This modality lacks spatial resolution as well (37).

ANGIOGRAPHY

Angiography is of value in assessing soft-tissue sarcomas, particularly in determining the vascular supply of the lesion and the effect of the mass on adjacent vascular structures (11, 25, 38–44). It appears most useful in the extremities where adipose tissue is sparse (45–48).

Neovascularity, pooling, and "tumor blush" are some of the features of malignant tumors (44). However, these features are not unequivocal evidence of malignancy as they may also be demonstrated by benign lesions.

Hudson et al. (49) asserts that a great difficulty in the interpretation of the arteriogram is differentiating reactive vascularity from wound healing.

Although arteriography is appreciated as an excellent modality for planning surgical resection (46, 47), some researchers think there is a consistent underestimation of tumor size (11, 49).

Additional difficulties in the interpretation of arteriograms include differentiation of pathologic fracture from neoplasm vascularity, inconclusive results in areas of complex anatomic structure such as the pelvis (49), and failure to demonstrate relationships of structures instead of simple displacement in relatively "avascular" tumors (50).

As with radiography, xeroradiography, and the modalities yet to be discussed, angiography cannot differentiate benign from malignant lesions (48, 51); however, it appears to be somewhat more useful in assessing the malignancies (49).

ULTRASONOGRAPHY

This noninvasive imaging technique provides accurate information as to the size and location of soft-tissue masses in the extremities. Sonography is particularly useful in differentiating cystic from solid masses (52), although little information is revealed regarding adjacent bony and neurovascular structures (11, 49). Lipomatous masses are also difficult to scan (25, 49).

Lange et al. (53) found that greater homogeneity of the internal pattern correlates with general histologic features; therefore, the more homogeneity noted, the greater the cellularity of the mass.

As with other modalities, sonography cannot accurately differentiate malignant from benign lesions.

COMPUTED TOMOGRAPHY

Computed tomography is well-documented as a diagnostic technique in the evaluation and management of soft-tissue tumors (11, 21, 25, 49, 52–58, 102). This modality provides excellent detail of cortical description and demonstrates soft-tissue mass relationships better than magnetic resonance imaging does (59). It

also differentiates lipoma from other soft-tissue masses and, when contrast-enhanced, differentiates vessels (60).

As with other modalities, computed tomography has disadvantages. Visualization of structures in the distal extremities is less than acceptable (61). The use of contrast enhancement renders it more invasive than other modalities and, as with other imaging techniques, there are no specific findings for differentiating benign from malignant lesions.

MAGNETIC RESONANCE IMAGING

The introduction of magnetic resonance imaging (MRI) has revolutionized medicine and is invaluable for detecting and managing soft-tissue masses. Despite high costs of acquisition and operation, many facilities are adding MRI to their armamentaria of diagnostic and treatment techniques.

MRI affords three-dimensional information (49, 52, 62–66), unlike computed tomography and ultrasound. This modality is employed with neither ionizing radiation nor contrast enhancement, which gives it an advantage over computed tomography. Moon et al. (67) assert that MRI can differentiate fibrous from nonfibrous lesions. Additionally, the study concluded that MRI was important in both the detection and management of musculoskeletal disorders.

Disadvantages of MRI include cost, which may be prohibitive (63–67) and the protracted imaging time required for obtaining coronal and sagittal sections (67). Furthermore, MRI has been suggested to be insensitive to soft-tissue calcifications and soft-tissue gas (66) and has not been proven to accurately differentiate malignant from benign neoplasms.

In conclusion, although none of the previously discussed modalities, with the possible exception of MRI, is specific for fibrous soft-tissue neoplasms, each may contribute to the detection and subsequent management of such lesions.

TUMORS AND TUMOR-LIKE LESIONS OF FIBROUS TISSUE

To facilitate further discussion of fibrous soft-tissue tumors of the lower extremity, we will use the classification of Enzinger and Weiss.

Benign

Generally, these entities represent a group of well-defined reactive rather than neoplastic lesions (3).

NODULAR FASCIITIS

Synonyms are proliferative fasciitis, infiltrative fasciitis (3, 68), pseudosarcomatous fasciitis (69–73), and pseudosarcomatous fibromatosis (68, 69).

Nodular fasciitis is a fairly common benign disorder (68, 71–73) that displays rapid growth. Males and females are equally affected, with most individuals being young adults 20–35 years of age. However, Chung and Enzinger (74) noted a median age of 54 years.

Clinically, one notes a firm palpable mass or nodule situated subcutaneously, with lower extremity involvement noted rarely (74).

Histologically, plump, immature fibroblasts are noted, with frequent mitotic figures and the virtual absence of atypical mitosis (74).

Local excision is the treatment of choice for this benign lesion, with a recurrence rate of only 1–2% (74).

The etiology of this lesion has been suggested to be local trauma (74–76).

Due to the diffuse infiltrative appearance, both clinically and histologically, the possible diagnoses range from sarcoma (3) to necrotizing fasciitis (74).

FIBROMA

Synonyms are acrochordon, cutaneous tag (3). Lever (77) states there are three forms: (a) small, furrowed papule, (b) a filiform variety, and (c) a pedunculated form. Each has its own characteristic histologic features. The literature does not cite anatomic predilection of fibroma.

Proliferative Fasciitis

Enzinger and Weiss (3) state that this entity does not always arise from fascia; hence the term "proliferative fasciitis" may be misleading.

Proliferative fasciitis is a fairly common benign lesion (77–79), occurring primarily in adults 40–70 years of age, without race or gender predilection (77). It has not been identified in children (3, 77).

Clinically, the lesion is noted as a thickening in the subcutaneous tissue, with an infiltrative growth pattern over a short period of time. Approximately two-thirds of the cases are seen in the upper extremities. Because of its infiltrative nature, it is often referred to as pseudosarcomatous fasciitis. It is closely related clinically and histologically to proliferative myositis and may be the cutaneous counterpart of proliferative myositis (3).

Histologically, proliferative fasciitis contains immature fibroblasts and cells thought by Kern (80) to be "rhabdomyoblasts" but later redefined by Enzinger and Dulcey (81) as modified fibroblasts. Additionally, large, characteristic ganglion-like giant cells are noted.

Unlike nodular fasciitis, which is focal, proliferative fasciitis may be poorly circumscribed and multifocal. However, as with nodular fasciitis, proliferative fasciitis is thought to be a benign, self-limiting reactive process that may result from trauma and that responds well to local excision.

Proliferative Myositis

Proliferative myositis is considered the deep or intramuscular counterpart of proliferative fasciitis (3, 74).

Kern (80) first described it in 1960 and noted its rapid growth and unusual histologic appearance.

The clinical presentation of proliferative myositis is that of a discrete nodule, usually affecting the flat muscles of the trunk or, occasionally, the thigh, with a duration sometimes as short as 3 weeks. Women are affected as frequently as men, and there is no racial predilection. Patients may be in their 40s or 50s.

Histologically, proliferative myositis exhibits two characteristic features: (a) poor demarcation with involvement of perimysium, epimysium, and endomysium and (b) large, basophilic cells resembling ganglion or rhabdomyoblasts (3).

As with nodular and proliferative fasciitis, proliferative myositis is considered by many to be a reactive rather than neoplastic lesion that may be cured by local excision. Proliferative myositis may also be designated pseudosarcomatous proliferative lesions of soft tissue and bone, as Dahl et al. (82) prefer, because of its infiltrative nature.

Although the precise etiology of this disorder is not known, trauma has been implicated, through possible local vascular impairment (74).

Fibroma of Tendon Sheath

This lesion, first described by Chung and Enzinger (83) in 1979, is a benign process, however, it is a reactive fibrosing disorder (3). Clinically, fibroma of tendon sheath resembles giant cell tumor of tendon sheath, but the former has distinct histologic and ultrastructural features (3, 82).

Fibroma of tendon sheath presents as a firm, dense, slow-growing nodule firmly adherent to tendon sheath (83). It is encountered most frequently in the extremities, particularly the hands and feet, with one series asserting that 86% of all reported cases are in the upper extremity (3). Patients may be of any age; however, most are between 20 and 50 years old, with males affected twice as frequently as females (84).

Histologically, fibroma of tendon sheath is hypocellular and collagenous, containing neither giant cells nor xanthoma cells (3, 85).

Ultrastructurally, this entity exhibits both fibroblasts and myofibroblasts (85).

Treatment entails complete resection of the lesion. A recurrence rate of 24% (3) has been noted, attributable to incomplete initial resection rather than to the aggressive nature of this lesion (85).

The etiology of fibroma of tendon sheath is unclear; however, trauma has been reported in a small percentage of patients (3, 86).

Elastofibroma

Elastofibroma is an unusual benign tumor-like entity initially reported by Jarvi and Saxen in 1961 (3, 13, 87). The vast majority are encountered on the trunk, in the connective tissue of the latissimus dorsi; hence, the term elastofibroma dorsi was originally designated for it (87).

Elastofibromas are seen primarily in elderly individuals, with a 2:1 female predominance (87).

Clinically, the lesion is an ill-defined, slow-growing, fibroelastic nodule which may infiltrate muscle or periosteum. It may be tender, painful, or restrictive to motion (88).

Histologically, elastofibromas are sparsely cellular, containing both fibrous and elastic fibers (3).

Treatment is surgical excision.

Repetitive trauma has been suggested as the etiology in many of the reported cases (87).

Keloid

Keloid is a benign overgrowth of scar tissue (3). Initially, both keloids and hypertrophic scars have the same clinical appearance—that of a raised, smooth, firm surface (77). With time, however, the latter flatten out, whereas the former persist as raised surfaces.

The occurrence of keloids is more frequent in dark-skinned individuals (3), especially Blacks (77). Familial tendencies for keloid formation have also been reported (3, 77, 91). Some genetic disorders, in which spontaneous keloid formation is a feature, have been cited (90).

Females outnumber males, and most individuals are young, between 15 and 45 (3).

Histologically, keloids and hypertrophic scars are indistinguishable in their initial phases (89, 90). They contain hyalinized collagen fibers that are randomly arranged with sparse fibroblasts. Peripheral vascularity is seen early, with increasing hyalinization noted with greater duration (3). Myofibroblasts, which are found in normal granulation tissue and are responsible for nonpathologic wound contracture as noted by Majno et al. (92), are numerous in hypertrophic scars and early keloids but diminish in mature keloids.

Orientation of collagen fibers is responsible for nodularity or flattening of the lesion. Keloids characteristically demonstrate persistence of a whorl-like arrangement of hyalinized collagen fibers, whereas hypertrophic scars exhibit parallel orientation of fibers (77).

Treatment of keloid ranges from pressure pads, dry ice, surgical excision, and topical corticosteroids to low-dose radiation therapy (3). Intralesional injections of triamcinolone acetate, as reported by Ketchum et al. (93), may yield acceptable results.

As trauma is an etiologic factor in the vast majority of keloid, elective surgical procedures should be carefully considered in individuals with tendencies toward keloid or hypertrophic scar formation.

Fibrous Tumors of Infancy and Childhood

Collectively, fibrous proliferations in infancy and childhood may be categorized into two divisions: (a) those seen in infants and children, with clinical and microscopic findings similar to their analogous counterparts in adults and (b) those fibrous proliferative disorders, unique to infants and children, that have distinct morphologic and histologic features and are peculiar to this age group.

The latter classification of disorders will be discussed. Since this text is concerned with neoplasms of the foot and lower extremities, we will concentrate on the fibrous proliferative disorders encountered in the lower extremities of infants and children.

FIBROUS HAMARTOMA OF INFANCY

Reye (94) first described this lesion in 1956 as subdermal fibromatous tumor of infancy. In 1965, Enzinger (95) reviewed additional cases filed at the Armed Forces Institute of Pathology and recommended the term fibrous hamartoma of infancy.

Generally, the lesion develops during the first year of life and is a small, rapidly growing mass in the lower dermis or cutis. Up to one-fifth of the cases are noted at birth, with males affected twice as frequently as females (3, 94).

The most common site of involvement is reported to be the anterior or posterior axillary fold, with 70% of the cases noted in this area of the upper extremity (94, 95). Several authors state that fibrous hamartoma of infancy never occurs in the hands or feet (93, 95). This helps distinguish it from digital fibromatosis and calcifying aponeurotic fibroma (3).

Histologically, the lesion contains fibrous trabeculae, whorls of immature-appearing spindle cells in a mucoid matrix, and mature adipose (96). Mitosis is not a prominent feature (97).

The prognosis is excellent after local surgical excision, with rare reports of recurrence (3).

INFANTILE DIGITAL FIBROMATOSIS

As the name implies, this disorder is characterized by solitary or multiple minute nodules occurring exclusively in the digits (3, 77, 97). The lesions are further characterized by a tendency toward local recurrence in approximately 60–75% of the cases.

Females may be affected more frequently than males (98). Sparing of the thumbs and halluces has been cited (98, 99).

Histologically, the dermis contains multiple spindle-shaped fibroblasts and collagen bundles in interlacing fascicles (97). The presence of eosinophilic inclusion bodies in many of the fibroblasts is a characteristic diagnostic finding (3).

The ultimate prognosis is excellent, despite a high recurrence rate. There are no reports of aggressive behavior or malignant transformation. MacKenzie (96) actually reported several cases of spontaneous regression.

INFANTILE MYOFIBROMATOSIS; SOLITARY AND MULTICENTRIC TYPES

Synonyms are generalized hamartomatosis (101), multiple congenital mesenchymal hamartomas (102, 103), and multiple vascular leiomyomas (3). Because of the histologic similarities of this lesion to smooth muscle tissue, the designations of infantile myofibroma for a solitary lesion and of myofibromatosis for multicentric lesions are more precise (101).

This disorder, in the multicentric form, consists of multiple nodules in the soft tissue, myocardium, lung or other viscera, muscle, and/or bone in an infant that are present at birth or noted shortly thereafter. The solitary form is approximately twice as common as the multicentric form, according to the Armed Forces Institute of Pathology (104).

The clinical course of the disorder is determined largely by the extent of involvement, with a poor prognosis for infants with multiple visceral lesions.

Histologically, there is a striking eosinophilia of tumor cells resembling that of leiomyoma. Fibroblasts and myofibroblasts are noted.

The clinical course of this disorder is dependent on the extent and location of lesions (215). Alteman et al. (105) noted flaccid paralysis resulting from spinal cord compression by a myofibroma, while Dimmick and Wood (106) reported respiratory distress and quadraparesis in a case of infantile myofibromatosis, with ultimate neurologic improvement following regression of the lesions.

Spontaneous remission of bone, soft-tissue, and visceral lesions have been noted by numerous authors.

Infantile myofibromatosis in the isolated or multicentric forms is a benign, self-limiting disorder of hamartomatous origin (109, 110).

The etiology of this disorder has not been fully elucidated; however, the occurrence of myofibromatosis in several members of one family suggests a possible inherited nature, with onset in utero (104, 111, 112).

JUVENILE HYALIN FIBROMATOSIS

Juvenile hyalin fibromatosis is an exceedingly rare, recessive, inherited disorder characterized by multiple nodules on the scalp, trunk, and extremities with predilection for the ears, scalp, back, and knees (3, 77).

The disorder may be first noted in infancy by the appearance of multiple nodules that may gradually increase in size. There is an associated tendency toward dwarfism and poorly developed musculature (3, 77). Males and females are equally affected.

Histologically, the tumors consist of spindle-shaped cells in a homogeneous eosinophilic matrix. Small, newly developed nodules contain proportionately more cells, while larger tumors contain more ground substance (77).

Nodules and/or tumors that develop in childhood may gradually increase in size or persist into adulthood without change. Surgical excision may be attempted for cosmetic or functional purposes. Radiotherapy yields unimpressive results, whereas cortisone and ACTH improve joint function (3, 77).

GIANT CELL FIBROBLASTOMA

This lesion originally described in 1982 by Enzinger and Shmookler (113) has been more recently reviewed by others (114, 115) and found to be a slow-growing solitary nodule in the dermis and subcutis of children. The histologic similarity between giant cell fibroblastoma and dermatofibrosarcoma protuberans is noteworthy and strongly suggests that the two are related.

Anatomical sites of occurrence are back, thigh, chest wall, and inguinal region. Patients are from 4 months to 31 years, with the vast majority being younger than 10 years of age.

The tumor is poorly circumscribed and histologically exhibits loosely arranged spindle cells with moderate nuclear pleomorphism (3). Giant cells are also noted within the prominent myxoid matrix.

Absence of lipoblasts, lack of characteristic capillary patterns, and superficial location of giant cell fibroblastoma allow for differentiation from liposarcoma (3).

Although giant cell fibroblastoma demonstrates some cellular atypism, there is no suggestion that it behaves clinically as a malignant neoplasm (3).

Surgical excision may be advocated, with the Armed Forces Institute of Pathology reporting a 50% recurrence rate. Reexcision of recurrent giant cell fibroblastoma renders the patient disease-free.

CALCIFYING APONEUROTIC FIBROMA

Keasbey (116) initially described this disorder in 1953 and noted its resemblance to giant cell tumor of tendon sheath. On initial description, Keasbey does not preclude the existence of a malignant counterpart to this entity. Since then, various authors (3, 116–119) have reported additional cases and further elucidated its clinical, histologic, and prognostic features.

Clinically, juvenile aponeurotic fibroma presents as a firm, dense nodule firmly adherent to the underlying palmar or plantar aponeurosis. Enzinger reports 70% of cases occur in the palmar region and 13% plantarly (3), with a male predominance.

Microscopically, plump fibroblasts are noted, and in older lesions, typically exhibited in adults, usually *not* those of infants and young children, a central focus of calcification and cartilage formation is frequently exhibited (120). Mitotic figures are sparse.

Two phases in the development of calcifying aponeurotic fibromas have been reported (120). The initial phase noted in infants and small children is associated with increased activity of the tumor. The second, or late phase, is characterized by decreased tumorous activity, with focal calcification exhibited in older lesions in older children.

Approximately 50% of calcifying aponeurotic fibromas recur locally following local surgical excision; however, there are no reported instances of malignant transformation or metastasis (119).

Fibromatosis

In 1954, A. P. Stout (120) introduced the term, "fibromatoses," initially used to designate "all fibrous growth that cannot be assigned to any other category" (97).

At present, fibromatoses are collectively regarded as nonmetastasizing, fibroblastic tumors that may be invasive. They may also recur following surgical excision. The fibromatoses may be multiple as familial and are characterized as having an initial rapid growth phase. Some may resolve spontaneously. They should not be referred to as low-grade fibrosarcomas, as they do not metastasize (120), nor should the term fibromatoses be used for nonspecific reactive fibrous proliferations.

The fibromatoses may be classified as either superficial or deep. The former consists of fascial fibromatoses; palmar fibromatosis (Dupuytren's contracture), plantar fibromatosis (Ledderhose's disease), penile fibromatosis (Peyronie's disease), and knuckle pads. The latter consists of musculoaponeurotic, extraabdominal (extraabdominal desmoid), abdominal (abdominal desmoid), and intraabdominal (intraabdominal desmoid) fibromatoses (97).

As we are limiting our discussion to fibrous neoplasms encountered on the lower extremity, we will confine evaluation of the fibromatoses to the superficial (fascial) classification.

Generally, the superficial (fascial) fibromatoses are slow-growing and small in size. They arise from fascia or aponeurosis with involvement of deeper structures rarely demonstrated (3). The lesions have a propensity to recur following surgical excision.

PALMAR FIBROMATOSIS (DUPUYTREN'S CONTRACTURE)

As its name implies, the lesion is encountered in the upper extremity and will not be discussed here.

PLANTAR FIBROMATOSIS (LEDDERHOSE'S DISEASE)

Plantar fibromatosis is a benign, nodular fibrous proliferation emanating from the middle band of plantar aponeurosis. The nodules are firm, dense, and may be characterized by an initial rapid growth period (See Fig. 5.45).

Unlike palmar fibromatosis, which frequently causes digital contracture, flexural digital deformity is rarely encountered as a result of plantar fibromatosis (97, 121). This may be attributable to anatomic differences between palmar and plantar fibromatosis. It has been suggested that the plantar aponeurosis has a much less well-developed extension distally to the digits than does the palmar aponeurosis (3, 121).

Historically, plantar fibromatosis, with its clinical presentation of rapid, frequently infiltrative growth, combined with a highly cellular histologic appearance, is frequently misdiagnosed as fibrosarcoma. This confusion had in the past prompted amputation in some cases (121–128). Since its description in 1897 by Ledderhose (129), many authors have examined the pathophysiology, clinical course, ultrastructure, and hereditary influence associated with plantar fibromatosis.

Plantar fibromatosis (Ledderhose's disease) may be referred to as Dupuytren's disease or Dupuytren's of the plantar fascia as it is believed that palmar and plantar fibromatoses are very similar clinically, microscopically, and ultrastructurally (3, 122–126).

The incidence of plantar fibromatosis in males is much greater than that in females; some authors cite a 2:1 male predominance (126) and others assert a mere 20% female incidence for this and related fibrosing disorders (128, 129). In a series by Aviles et al. (123), no sex predilection was noted.

Age incidence is also variable. Allen et al.'s series (124) reports that 35% of their subjects were 30 years of age or younger; Enzinger and Weiss' (3) review of 200 cases at the Armed Forces Institute of Pathology reports that 55% were less than 30 years of age. Aviles et al. (123) however, report that 77% of the patients

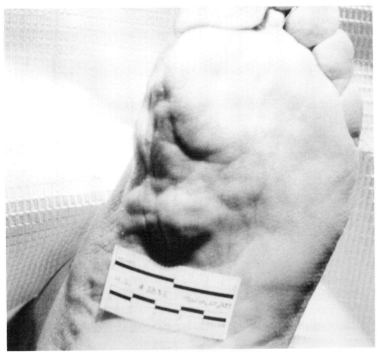

Figure 5.45. Plantar fibromatosis in a male patient.

in their series were older than 45. It is generally accepted that there is an increased incidence of plantar fibromatosis with advancing age (3).

The coexistence of plantar fibromatosis with one or more of the related superficial (fascial) fibromatoses has been well-documented (3, 97, 134). Reports of palmar and plantar fibromatoses occurring in the same individual vary from 5 to 20%, although the appearance of one may antedate the other by 5–10 years (3). The association between plantar fibromatosis and Peyronie's penile fibromatosis has also been cited and is less commonly encountered. Knuckle pads and keloids coexisting with plantar fibromatosis have also been recorded (124, 128, 134).

Histologically, the appearance of plantar fibromatosis is quite similar to that of its palmar analogue. The specimen is exceedingly cellular, with interlacing bundles of fibroblasts (3, 127, 133). Mitotic figures range from 2–3/high power field to more numerous in other areas of the specimen. Loss of polarity of cells, nuclear pyknosis, and occasional atypical mitosis may be encountered (136, 137, 138). This atypia, combined with the consistent lack of capsule and recurrence after local excision could certainly substantiate a misdiagnosis of fibrosarcoma. Hence, thorough histologic evaluation, corroborated by clinical presentation, is essential at operation.

Gelberman et al. (137) in 1980 and Kiryu et al. (138) in 1985 detail the appearance of myofibroblasts. Modified fibroblasts in plantar fibromatosis correlate with the stages of development of this plantar lesion. The data suggest that myofibroblasts may be responsible for clinical recurrence subsequent to local surgical excision (138).

Luck (139) in 1959 described histologic changes noted in each of his three proposed stages of development of Dupuytren's (palmar fibromatosis) contracture. He asserted the amount of clinical deformity could be predicted and suggested specific surgical intervention based on the stage of the disorder. As yet, it appears that this examination and stage-specific surgical correction of plantar fibromatosis has not been performed. Perhaps, in the near future, an enthusiastic and innovative colleague will do so.

The etiology of plantar fibromatosis is poorly understood. Hereditary factors (121, 128, 134, 135, 140) have been established, particularly when it occurs with other related fibrosing disorders. Trauma (3) has also been suggested. However, occupational predilection has not been noted (3). Other etiologic factors have been proposed (e.g., neuropathy, gout and rheumatism, endocrinopathy, atavistic development, local infection, and chronic intoxication) (141).

Treatment of Ledderhose's disease is symptomatic with some authors advocating conservative therapy (127, 141). Others recommend fasciectomy (3, 127, 128) to eliminate discomfort. The high recurrence rate following surgical intervention is thought to result from inadequate resection on initial operation (123, 137, 138, 143).

As plantar fibromatosis most frequently responds favorably to localized excision and does not metastasize, it is considered a benign, self-limiting disorder.

KNUCKLE PADS

Knuckle pads are fibrous noninflammatory thickenings on the dorsa of the proximal interphalangeal joints of the digits. The term was introduced by Jones (144) in 1923. These lesions may be found in association with palmar and/or plantar fibromatoses (128, 139, 144).

A male predilection is seen with patients in their fourth, fifth, or sixth decades (3, 145).

Histologically, knuckle pads resemble palmar fibromatosis (133) and probably plantar fibromatosis. However, as digital lesions are infrequently excised, comprehensive evaluation is lacking.

Several authors state that knuckle pads are never encountered on the foot (3). However, if trauma is accepted as an etiologic agent in the development of other superficial fascial fibromatoses, I (Stewart) suggest that nonkeratotic soft-tissue hypertrophy overlying proximal, middle, or distal interphalangeal joints in flexible or "swing-phase" hammer digits may represent the pedal analogue of knuckle pads on the fingers.

Malignant Fibrous Tumors

FIBROSARCOMA

True fibrosarcomas are the malignant analogues of fibromas (97, 146). The lesions are derived from fibroblasts, contain collagen and are characterized by invasive, infiltrative growth, a propensity to metastasize, and local recurrence (3, 9, 147, 148). Histologically, fibrosarcomas demonstrate pleomorphism and mitotic activity (3, 147).

In the past, the terms giant cell sarcoma, recurrent fibroids, spindle-cell sarcoma, myxofibrosarcoma, myxosarcoma malignant myxoma, and neurofibrosarcoma (3) were used to denote fibrosarcomas. The designation fibrosarcoma was also assigned to entities now regarded as spindle-cell sarcomas, mesatheliomas, metaplastic carcinomas, liposarcomas, rhabdomyosarcomas, and synovial sarcomas (148). Thus, confusion as to nature and origin of fibrosarcomas is well-documented. Clarification of the term fibrosarcoma and its restriction to only those tumors "composed of cells and fibers derived from fibroblasts" was strongly urged by Stout and Lattes in 1967 (149).

As the histologic appearance, clinical presentation, and behavior of adult sarcomas are fairly consistent regardless of etiology, we will only discuss adult and infantile/childhood forms as proposed by Enzinger and Weiss (3).

ADULT FIBROSARCOMA

Fibrosarcoma is encountered in young adults ranging from 25 to 55 years (3, 15, 132, 148–152) of age, with a median range of 39.4–47.7 years (149, 153). Most of these series consider soft-tissue sarcomas rather than fibrosarcomas exclusively. Many of the reports do not identify fibrosarcoma confined to the lower extremity.

Sex incidence is conflicting (152–154); several authors describe a higher incidence in females (3) whereas others report a male predominance (155–157).

Sites of occurrence within the lower extremity vary somewhat; however, the thigh and knee (3, 143, 147) are reported as the most common areas of involvement. Several case studies have also documented fibrosarcoma arising from structures of the foot (3, 148, 158–160, 182).

The clinical presentation is a firm nodular or tumorous lesion emanating most frequently from deeper structures such as the intermuscular or intramuscular fibrous septa, aponeurosis, or tendons of the lower extremity. The mass may be lobulate and demonstrate infiltrative, destructive growth to surrounding structures (162). Pain may not be a subjective complaint until the lesion reaches considerable magnitude. Overlying skin is generally intact; however, in cases of extremely rapid growth or trauma, ulceration may occur (3).

The excised specimen generally is fleshy to firm and solitary with a white-gray to tan-yellow appearance. It has been noted that smaller tumors tend to be well circumscribed and partially or completely encapsulated, while larger ones appear to be less well-defined, with multiple processes (3), and may exhibit a "pseudocapsule" (3, 162, 163).

Systemic findings are rare; however, weight loss associated with advanced tumor and widespread metastasis have been cited (164), as have infrequent reports of hypoglycemia (3, 165, 167) attributed to increased peripheral utilization of glycogen (167).

The histologic appearance forms the basis for the grading system for most malignant tumors (158, 168, 169). That of fibrosarcoma is one of fusiform fibroblasts, which may contain scant cytoplasm, arranged in fascicular patterns. Collagen fibers are present and parallel in orientation (3, 15).

Low-grade fibrosarcomas are those which are well-differentiated, with relatively uniform fibroblast size and shape, abundant cytoplasm (3, 15, 153, 154, 158), and normochromic nuclei. Few mitoses are noted.

High-grade fibrosarcomas (grades III and IV) demonstrate a higher cell-to-matrix ratio and have less collagen than low-grade lesions (158, 169). Cellular arrangement has been described as a "herringbone pattern" (10, 164). Nuclei may be hyperchromic with frequent mitotic figures. Giant cells may also be present. Furthermore, anaplasia and less differentiation are exhibited in the higher-grade tumors (5, 77).

Numerous studies have clearly shown that lower-grade fibrosarcomas have a better prognosis, in terms of survival rate and local recurrence, than do high-grade lesions of equal magnitude (3, 15, 77, 152, 154, 169–174).

Primary tumor size, as the time of detection has also been shown to be of prognostic significance (162, 175–176).

Factors such as necrosis noted within the tumor (177), location of the primary tumor (156, 169), patient's age (178), and perioperative blood transfusion (168) have all been cited as influencing prognosis.

Management of fibrosarcoma entails prevention of local recurrence following surgical intervention and prevention of distant metastases (176). Both recurrence and metastasis, which is primarily to the lungs via the hematogenous route, reduce survival (179, 180) of the patient.

Treatment of fibrosarcoma is wide surgical

excision, which may be accomplished by local, radical, or amputative means (163, 181, 182). Histologic grade and stage of the primary tumor (183), size of the lesion, and anatomic location determine the surgical margins. Radiotherapy, pre- and postoperatively, may be administered as well (174). Current research indicates increased survival rates and decreased local recurrence rates with the use of various chemotherapeutic agents (184–186).

A combined effort by the pathologist, oncologist, surgeon, and other health professionals is required in the treatment, in an attempt to reduce disease-associated morbidity and mortality and to preserve function for the patient.

Various etiologic factors (i.e., trauma (152, 162), thermal injury (182), previous irradiation (188), and hereditary influences (189) have been documented in the development of fibrosarcomas. However, the vast majority of the lesions arise de novo.

CONGENITAL AND INFANTILE FIBROSARCOMA

Congenital and infantile fibrosarcoma occurring in the lower extremity are well-documented (10, 189).

Clinically, they usually appear as well-circumscribed masses noted at birth or within the first months of life (10, 77).

The microscopic appearance of the lesions closely parallels those in adults. However, the prognosis for infantile and congenital fibrosarcomas for children to age 10 is better than that in adults for a comparable grade of lesion (3, 10, 77).

Treatment of infantile and childhood fibrosarcoma is wide excision. Adjuvant chemotherapy and/or radiation therapy may also be employed as indicated by stage, grade, and location of the lesion.

As noted earlier, fibrous tumors can be classified into those of fibroblastic origin and those that are fibrohistiocytic. Thus far, we have discussed those of fibroblastic origin. In the remainder of this chapter, we will address fibrohistiocytic tumors.

FIBROHISTIOCYTIC TUMORS

Fibrous histiocytoma, in general, is considered a benign tumor (3, 10). It is composed of a mixture of fibroblastic and histiocytic cells. However, its histogenesis, at this time, is still controversial. A simplified approach has been adapted by Enzinger and Weiss (3). They divide fibrous histiocytoma into cutaneous fibroma

histiocytoma (i.e., tumors found superficially on the skin) and fibrous histiocytoma (i.e., those tumors in the subcutaneous and deep structures) (3).

Cutaneous fibrous histiocytoma presents as elevated pedunculated lesions found to be slow-growing and usually solitary. They measure a few millimeters to a few centimeters in diameter (3). Color varies from red to brown and, in some cases, black (most commonly due to hemosiderin deposition). In this situation, the clinician may mistake it for malignant melanoma (192). It is most commonly found during the ages of 20–40, although it can occur at any age (193). (See Fig. 5.46.)

Fibrous histiocytoma of the subcutaneous and deep tissues are less common than the superficial type. It, too, presents during the same early-to-midadult life span. Usually found on the extremities, it occurs as painless masses that tend to be larger than their cutaneous counterparts (3). Grossly, they are circumscribed yellow or white areas of hemorrhage (3).

The benign nature of the tumor is most appreciated histologically. The cells appear well-differentiated, contain little mitotic activity, and have a small degree of pleomorphism. An increase in pleomorphic or mitotic activity should alert the clinician to suspect malignancy (3).

Histochemical, immunohistochemical, and electron microscopic studies have failed to contribute to the precise diagnosis of these tumors. Lysosomal and oxidative enzymes can consistently be found within the tumors. Between one-quarter and three-quarters of cutaneous fibrous histiocytomas contain immunoreactive α-1-antitrypsin which has been used to support histiocytic origin (3).

Electron microscopic studies have demonstrated cells resembling fibroblasts (194) and histiocytes, and transitions between the two have also been documented. This raises questions as to whether the origin is truly fibroblastic or histiocytic (195).

Fibrous histiocytomas must be differentiated from other benign tumors such as nodular vasculitis neurofibroma or leiomyoma. Histologically, nodular vasculitis is distinguished from fibrous histiocytoma by its loosely arranged bundles of fibroblasts. Nodular vasculitis appears much more cellularly active and contains increased mitotic activity (195). Neurofibroma have a more uniform orientation and are found in bundles which contain ser-

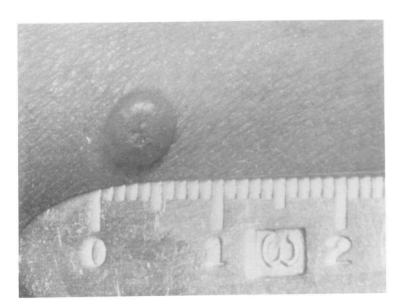

Figure 5.46. A cutaneous fibrous histiocytoma on the anterior surface of the leg in a 28-year-old female.

pentine nuclei, which is characteristic of Schwann cells (3), and thick bundles of collagen. The main difference is the lack of any storiform pattern or significant inflammation, usually seen in fibrous histiocytoma. Sclerotic forms of leiomyoma may mimic fibrous histiocytoma; however, smooth muscle tumors have a more distinct fascicular growth pattern. They contain blunt-ended nuclei and striations found in the cytoplasm but not found in fibrous histiocytoma.

It is of paramount importance to differentiate this tumor from malignant aggressive tumors such as dermatofibrosarcoma protuberans or malignant fibrous histiocytoma. Dermatofibrosarcoma protuberans lacks giant cells, inflammatory cells, and xanthomatous elements found in fibrous histiocytoma. Its margins are infiltrative and contain larger fasciculations of fibroblasts arranged in storiform patterns. Malignant fibrous histiocytoma is pleomorphic and deeply situated, with many atypical mitotic figures and large areas of hemorrhage and necrosis not seen in fibrous histiocytoma (195).

Treatment is usually by wide local excision. Enzinger and Weiss (3) report a 10% recurrence rate of cutaneous and soft-tissue fibrous histiocytomas following conservative therapy. It appears that greater depth and overall size suggest an increased risk for recurrence (3, 196). Histologic features play a small role in determining recurrence. The most controversial aspect of this lesion is whether it is fibroblastic

or histiocytic. Lysosomal and proteolytic enzymes found within the lesion favor a histiocytic origin (3); however the primarily fibroblastic appearance and lack of Langerhans' granules support a fibroblastic origin (197).

Juvenile xanthogranuloma is a regressing form of fibrous histiocytoma occurring during infancy that presents with one or more cutaneous nodules (198). It may occur in either deep or soft tissue. It commonly develops shortly after birth, with two-thirds of patients developing lesions by age 6. Males and females are equally affected. There is no underlying lipid abnormality nor familial tendency (199).

Cutaneous lesions are usually found on the head, neck, and extremities. The primary lesions are red papules, whereas older lesions are brown to yellow. After a period of growth, the nodules spontaneously regress, leaving a depressed hyperpigmented area of skin. Generally, all lesions subside by adolescence (200).

Microscopically, the lesion presents with sheets of histiocytes invading the dermis but sparing the epidermis. The histiocytes are well-differentiated, exhibit little pleomorphism, and show slight mitosis. Primary lesions have minimal amounts of lipid, whereas older lesions give the appearance of finely vacuolated xanthomatous cytoplasm (3). Touton giant cells are typical. A modest amount of inflammatory cells are present, especially eosinophils (206).

Electron microscopic studies reveal cells to have characteristic histiocytes. They contain numerous pseudopodia, lipid droplets, and lysosomes (3). The lesion must be differentiated from histiocytosis X involving skin. Whereas juvenile xanthogranuloma does not generally invade the epidermis, histiocytosis X does. It has greater cellular cohesion and fewer eosinophils. Histiocytosis X does not have these characteristics. Touton giant cells are prominent features of juvenile xanthogranuloma and are absent from histiocytosis X (202).

Juvenile xanthogranulomas need to be differentiated from other xanthomatous tumors. Usually, xanthomatous lesions contain more foamy cells and lack the characteristic Touton giant cells (203).

The prognosis of this disease is excellent (3). However, cutaneous lesions may be accompanied by similar lesions in other sites such as eyes, lungs, epicardium oral cavity, and testes (204). The eye is the most common extracutaneous site (3). Conservative therapy is generally indicated in these cases. However, no treatment is usually indicated in cases of cutaneous manifestations, as lesions are usually self-limiting.

Localized histiocytic tumors, experimentally induced in monkeys following injection, spontaneously regressed after a period of growth (3). It has been postulated that this is not a true neoplasm but may represent a response to some viral infection (200, 201).

Atypical fibroxanthoma is a pleomorphic spindle-cell tumor that occurs on actinic-damaged skin of the head and neck of elderly persons. It is also termed pseudosarcoma of the skin (3), paradoxical fibroxanthoma (207), pseudosarcomatous dermatofibroma (208), and pseudosarcomatous reticulohistiocytoma (209). Helwig and May (211) was the first to describe a nodular ulcerative lesion found in actinic radiation affected skin (210). It is generally benign and classified as a benign fibrohistiocytic tumor because of its excellent prognosis following conservative therapy (211). Atypical fibroxanthoma most closely resembles malignant fibrous histiocytoma, both histologically and ultrastructurally (211, 212).

The difference between atypical fibroxanthoma and malignant fibrous histiocytoma appears to be depth rather than histologic variation. Enzinger and Weiss regard atypical fibroxanthoma as a superficial or early form of malignant fibrous histiocytoma (3).

Reticulohistiocytoma may present as part of two separate clinical settings (3). One is a purely cutaneous manifestation, and the other contains systemic manifestations (213). The cutaneous form appears as a slow-growing solitary nodule on the upper portion of the body. It is benign and self-limiting (214). The systemic manifestation presents with mucocutaneous nodules, destructive arthritis, pyrexia, and weight loss. The systemic condition is also termed multicentric reticulohistiocytosis and lipodermatoid arthritis. The patient is left with a disfiguring and crippling arthritis, most severely affecting the distal interphalangeal joint (215). The etiology is unknown; however, both conditions are thought to be processes reactive to an unknown stimulus rather than true neoplasms (216). Orken et al. (216) associate a coincidence with tuberculosis, thyroid disease, and diabetes (214).

The cutaneous lesions present as small nodules ranging in size from a few millimeters to a few centimeters. The color ranges from red to brown or yellow. The surface epithelium may be crusted or ulcerated (216). The disseminated form poses few diagnostic problems for the clinician as the clinical history is enormously helpful. The differential diagnosis must include malignant melanoma and superficial malignant fibrohistiocytoma (3).

Xanthomas are tumors characterized by collections of foamy histiocytes. They occur equally in all races, both sexes, and in association with familial or acquired disorders leading to hyperlipidemia (3). Xanthomas also occur in relation to malignancy, especially lymphoproliferative and myeloproliferative types (217). In many individuals, they arise without any underlying disorder. On the basis of their clinical appearance and location, xanthomas are classified into five types: eruptive, tuberous, tendon xanthoma, plane xanthoma, and xanthelasma (218).

Eruptive xanthomas usually occur as numerous small, soft, yellow papules that come and go as triglycerides and lipid levels increase and decrease. They have a predilection for the buttocks, posterior thighs, knees, and elbows. Histologically, they appear as foamy and nonfoamy histiocytes. Tuberous and tendinous xanthomas appear as yellow nodules. The latter are usually found on the exterior surface of the feet and hands and also the Achilles tendon (214, 220). The typical appearance is that of sheets of xanthomatous histiocytes with large amounts of extracellular cholesterol deposits. A considerable amount of fibrosis with occasional inflammatory cells is also seen. Xanthelasma refers to soft, yellow plaques on the eyelids. Plane xanthomas occur in skin folds, especially palmar creases. Both plane xanthomas and xanthelasmas are characterized by sheets of foamy histiocytes and a small amount of inflammation and fibrosis (221).

These lesions usually present little if any problem for the clinician to diagnose and manage. However, xanthomas of tendon sheaths may present a challenge as the deep location and slow progression may be mistaken for a sarcoma. Giant cell tumors of tendon sheaths and diffuse villonodular synovitis may resemble this lesion as well (77).

The prognosis of these lesions is excellent. Conservative therapy is usually the treatment of choice. However, radiation therapy has also been employed.

So how do these xanthomas receive classification within the benign fibrohistiocytic tumors? The fibrous characteristic of mature long-standing xanthomas is believed to be related to the fibrogenic properties of extracellular cholesterol (3).

INTERMEDIATE

Dermatofibrosarcoma protuberans is an uncommon, slow-growing and locally aggressive tumor of the dermis (222). The condition was first described in 1924 by Darrier and Ferrand (224). One year later, Hoffman (495) coined its current name, dermatofibrosarcoma protuberans (225). Clinically, lesions consist of solitary or multiple nodules often arising within an indurated plaque. They are most frequently found on the trunk, but the extremities, head, neck, scalp, and face may be affected as well. Although locally invasive, only a small percentage have been documented to metastasize. The lesion usually presents with a reddish-brown or blue tint and, occasionally, are yellow-brown or skin-colored. The lesions are painless and the fact that they are slow-growing leads to a delay in the patient seeking treatment. If the lesion is left untreated, it may reach enormous proportions. This lesion seldom occurs in children.

The diagnosis must be made on the basis of history, clinical findings, and, most important, histopathology. The histologic appearance is that of a nonencapsulated, cellular, dermal neoplasm composed of fusiform cells mixed with collagen and, frequently, having a storiform pattern (3).

Lesions of this tumor need to be differentiated from dermatofibromas, fibrosarcomas, malignant melanomas, schwannomas, and Kaposi's sarcoma.

The treatment of choice is wide surgical excision, deep enough to include the deep fascia, because these tumors can recur in up to 50% of the patients. Prompt wide local excision can reduce the recurrence rates to 1.75%. If local recurrence occurs it usually happens within 3 years from the initial surgery (226). The lesions are known to re-present more aggressively on recurrence. The highly recurrent nature of this tumor makes close follow-up of the patient imperative (3).

BEDNAR'S TUMORS

Tumors that resemble dermatofibrosarcoma protuberans but that possess a melanin pigment are termed Bednar's tumors. These tumors are uncommon (3). According to Enzinger and Weiss, they account for less than 5% of all cases of dermatofibrosarcoma protuberans. Bednar suggested they may represent neural lesion. However S-100 protein has not yet been identified (3, 227).

They are slow-growing, cutaneous masses which extend to the epidermis and advance to the deep dermis. Recurrence is extremely rare. Enzinger and Weiss state that 1 out of 9 reported cases recurs. They state that, considering the similarity to dermatofibrosarcoma protuberans, the biologic behavior is probably identical.

MALIGNANT FIBROUS HISTIOCYTOMA

The malignant fibrous histiocytoma, according to Enzinger and Weiss, is the most common soft-tissue tumor in adult life (3). Because it presents histologically in many different ways, Enzinger and Weiss divided it into five categories: storiform-pleomorphic, myxoid (myxofibrosarcoma), giant cell, inflammatory, and angiomatoid (228).

The storiform-pleomorphic type is morphologically highly variable (229). The cells frequently undergo transition from storiform type patterns to pleomorphic type patterns. In its most common form, microscopically, plump spindle cells are arranged in the pathognomonic storiform or cartwheel-like pattern. Modest numbers of lymphocytes and plasma cells are seen in many tumors. There is usually a predominance of either acute or chronic inflammatory cells, as opposed to equal mixtures of both. Enzinger and Weiss state that the significance of these inflammatory cells is not clear. They think that it may contribute to a better prognosis than those with little or no inflammatory cells (228).

The diagnosis of these tumors requires excellent tissue sampling and evaluation of hematoxylin and eosin-stained sections. Immunohistochemistry and electron microscopy do not play a role in the primary diagnosis but may be used as supplemental techniques to rule out other lesions appearing similar to malignant fibrous histiocytomas. There has been evidence to suggest that the tumors are of fibroblastic origin rather than of monocyte or macrophage origins (230). Histiocytic origins can also reasonably be ruled out by the fact that the histiocytic markers, Lev-3 and Lev-M3, have not been identified (231). There are three cell types that can be identified in these tumors: fibroblastic cells with elongated nuclei, prominent nucleoli, and abundant lamellae of rough endoplasmic reticulum (232). Langerhans' granules, almost always absent, are most common in tumors of histiocytic origin.

The differential diagnosis of the storiform-pleomorphic type of malignant fibrous histiocytoma entails distinguishing it from other neoplasms exhibiting various degrees of cellular pleomorphism. The basis of diagnosis is to discern whether a tumor contains the storiform pattern and, most importantly, the specific cellular differentiation. To distinguish this tumor from the benign fibrous type is easy, as the benign tumor conspicuously exhibits the storiform pattern but not the pleomorphic cells and necrosis seen in the malignant type. Enzinger and Weiss caution, however, that when benign tumors are deeply situated they should be regarded as potentially malignant (3).

Enzinger and Weiss (3) state that this tumor is a fully malignant sarcoma, with 44% developing local recurrence, and 42% developing metastasis. The depth of the tumor correlates best with metastatic disease (3). Tumors of the distal extremities have a better prognosis than those of the proximal extremities; those that exhibit some degree of inflammation have a slightly better prognosis than those that do not (3).

MYXOID TYPE

In order for a malignant fibrous histiocytoma to be classified as this type, at least half of it should contain myxoid areas. These areas should contain small foci, blending with adjacent cellular areas (3). The difference between the myxoid areas and the cellular areas is the presence of hyaluronidase-sensitive mucopolysaccharide. The storiform pattern becomes less evident. Cells within the myxoid areas contain well-differentiated fibroblasts, pleomorphic areas, mitotic areas, and multinucleation. Vessels form arcs along which the tumor and inflammatory cells condense (3).

This tumor must be differentiated from benign myxoid lesions such as nodular fasciitis and myxomas. The sarcoma most nearly resembling this tumor is liposarcoma. Nodular vasculitis and myxomas do not exhibit the orderly vasculature bizarre cells and atypical mitotic figures. Myxomas have relatively small cells and few, if any, mitotic figures. The liposarcoma contains a more uniform population of spindle cells, bizarre cells are absent, and few mitotic figures are present. Lipoblasts are also present (234).

The myxoid variant is thought to have a better prognosis than the storiform pleomorphic type. Enzinger and Weiss (3) state that this tumor recurs in almost two-thirds of cases but metastasizes in only one-fourth. It is treated by wide local excision or amputation. The significance of the myxoid change is not clear. The reason for the better prognosis may be that the cells multiply more slowly and produce mucoid matrix as a form of differentiation (234).

GIANT CELL TYPE

The giant cell type of malignant fibrous histiocytoma is multinodular and exhibits a mixture of histiocytes, fibroblasts, and, most important, osteoclast-type giant cells (3). Dense fibrous bands containing vessels encircle the nodules. Secondary hemorrhage and necrosis are also seen. As in the other forms of malignant fibrous histiocytoma, the fibroblasts and histiocytes exhibit pleomorphism, mitotic activity, and, according to Guccion and Enzinger (235), sometimes contain ingested material (i.e., lipid and hemosiderin) (235). The key cell is the giant cell and, in approximately half the cases, osteoid or mature bone is present. The question has been raised as to whether this tumor is one of bone-forming mesenchyme. One study described a population of cells with features of primitive osteoblasts and chondroblasts and matrix similar to osteoid (3). Enzinger and Weiss state that this tumor has more in common with malignant fibrous histiocytoma than those of bone-forming mesenchyme (3), as long as the osteoid is relatively focal. When the osteoid is prominent, a diagnosis of extraosseous osteosarcoma seems justified. In the differential diagnosis, the concern to verify giant cell tumors of bone is recognized. This tumor has a degree of multinodularity not encountered in giant cell tumors of bone, and no osseous defects are seen, as would be expected in bone tumors (3).

Treatment is by wide radical excision. As mentioned previously, superficial tumors have a much better prognosis, as exhibited by the fact that two-thirds of superficial tumors recur and one-quarter metastasize, whereas in deep tumors, 40% recur and one-half metastasize (3).

INFLAMMATORY TYPE

Alternately named retroperitoneal xanthogranuloma, these tumors are bulky, infiltrating, retroperitoneal masses which contain inflammatory and xanthoma cells. Secondarily, they are seen in the lower extremity. The most important feature is the xanthoma cell, which helps establish the diagnosis. The first description was by Oberling in 1935 (237). He concluded that the lesions were not malignant but variants of Hand-Schüller-Christian disease (237).

The inflammatory component usually consists of both acute and chronic inflammatory cells, with the emphasis on the acute cells. Overall metastasis resembles the parent lesion; however, in those instances, the tumors are less xanthomatous and more fibroblastic.

The differential diagnosis concerns itself with the nonneoplastic xanthomatous process. This tumor, however, is extremely aggressive, as evidenced in a study where all patients suffered severe local effects and four developed metastasis (238). It is not clear how the degree of malignancy compares with other forms of malignant fibrous histiocytoma. However, as stated earlier, the prominent inflammatory presence would confer an improved prognosis. Enzinger and Weiss feel that it has a lower metastatic rate than the storiform-pleomorphic type. However, its deep location and surgical inaccessability usually leads to a delay in treatment that adversely affects the prognosis. Radical excision is indicated and radio- and chemotherapy have been used as adjunctive measures (239).

ANGIOMATOID TYPE

This is a rare tumor that combines features of both fibrohistiocytic and vascular tumors (3). It has a predilection for the very young and is less aggressive than conventional malignant fibrous histiocytic tumors. It presents as a slow-growing, nodular, multinodular, or cystic mass, at the hypodermis or subcutaneous level. Most occur on the extremities, with the majority of patients less than 20 years old. The tumors form circumscribed lesions that measure a few centimeters in diameter and vary in color from gray-tan to brown-red. Irregular blood-filled cystic spaces are one of the most characteristic features of the tumor on cross-section.

The lesions are characterized by three major features: irregular solid masses of histiocytic type cells, cystic areas of hemorrhage, and chronic inflammation. Multifocal hemorrhage is a striking feature in all cases. Pain and tenderness is uncommon, but systemic symptoms are often encountered (240). Anemia, pyrexia, and weight loss may be out of proportion to the size of the tumor. Enzinger and Weiss state that, in their experience, two-thirds of patients develop local recurrence and one-fifth develop metastasis. They have limited data on this variant, and the biologic potential of this neoplasm cannot be fully appreciated at this time. However, they feel that wide local excision is the treatment indicated at the present time (241, 242).

REFERENCES

1. Berlin SJ. A review of 2,720 lesions in the foot. J Am Podiatr Assoc 1980;70:318–324.
2. Berlin SJ. A laboratory review of 67,000 foot tumors and lesions. J Am Podiatr Assoc 1984;74:341–347.
3. Enzinger FM, Weiss SW, eds. Soft tissue tumors. 2nd ed. St. Louis: CV Mosby, 1988: 1–222.
4. Robbins SL, Cotran RS, eds. Pathologic basis of disease. 2nd ed. Philadelphia: WB Saunders, 1979:141–212.
5. Rydholm G, Berg N. Size, site and clinical incidence of lipoma. Acta Orthop Scand 1983; 928–981.
6. Rantakko V, Ekfors TO. Sarcomas of the soft tissue in the extremities and limb girdles: Analysis of 240 cases diagnosed in Finland in 1960–69. Acta Chir Scand 1979;145: 383–395.
7. Lever W, ed. Histopathology of the skin. 6th ed. Philadelphia: Lippincott, 1983:597–622.
8. Samitz MH. Cutaneous disorders of the lower extremities. Philadelphia: Lippincott, 1981: 203–221.
9. Campbell CJ. Tumors of the foot. In: Jahss MH, ed. Disorders of the foot, vol 1. Philadelphia: WB Saunders, 1982:979–1013.
10. Hajdu SI. Pathology of soft tissue tumors. Philadelphia: Lea & Febiger, 1979: 1–164.
11. Madwell JE, Moser RP. Radiologic evaluation of

soft tissue tumors. In: Enzinger FM, Weiss SW, eds. Soft tissue tumors. 2nd ed. St. Louis: CV Mosby, 1988:41–63.

12. Chung EB, Enzinger FM. Proliferative fasciitis. Cancer 1975;36:1450–1458.

13. Cross DL, Mills SE, Kulund DN. Elastofibroma arising in the foot. South Med J 1984; 77:1194–1196.

14. Seale KS, Lange TA, Monson D, Hackbarth DA. Soft tissue tumors of the foot and ankle. Foot Ankle 1988;9:19–27.

15. Broders AC, Hargrave R, Meyerding HW. Pathological features of soft tissue fibrosarcoma with special reference to the grading of its malignancy. Surg Gynecol Obstet 1939;69: 267–280.

16. Norman A, Dorfman HD. Juxtacortical circumscribed myositis ossificans: evaluation and radiographic features. Radiology 1970;96:301.

17. Frantzell A. Soft tissue radiography: technical aspects and applications in the examination of limbs. Acta Radiol [Suppl] 1951; 85:5–30.

18. Martel W, Abell MR. Radiographic evaluation of soft tissue tumors. Cancer 1973; 32: 351–359.

19. Melson GL, Staple TW, Evens RG. Soft tissue radiographic technique. Semin Roentgenol 1973;8:18–26.

20. Pirkey EL, Hurt J. Roentgen evaluation of the soft tissues in orthopedics. AJR 1959; 82:271–278.

21. Bernadino ME, Jing BS, Thomas JL, Lindell MM, Zornoza J. The extremity soft tissue lesion: a comparative study of ultrasound, computed tomography and xeroradiography. Radiology 1981;139:53–59.

22. Melson GL, Staple TW, Evens RG. Soft tissue radiographic technique. Semin Roentgenol 1973;8:18–26.

23. Otto RC, Pouliadis GP, Kumpe DA. The evaluation of pathologic alterations of juxtaosseous soft tissue by xeroradiography. Radiology 1976;120:195–201.

24. Wolfe JN. Xeroradiography of the bones, joints and soft tissues. Radiology 1969;93:583–587.

25. Heiken JP, Lee JKT, Smathers RL, Toffy WG, Murphy WA. CT of benign soft tissue masses of the extremities. AJR 1984;142:575–580.

26. Blatt CJ, Hayt DB, Desai M. Soft tissue sarcomas imaged with technetium-99m pyrophosphate. NY State J Med 1977; 77:2118–2119.

27. Desai A, Eymontt M, Alavi A. ^{99m}Tc-MDP uptake in nonosseous lesions. Radiology 1980;135:181–183.

28. Kaufman JH, Cedermark BJ, Parthasarthy KL, et al. The values of ^{67}Ga scintigraphy in soft tissue sarcoma and chondrasarcoma. Radiology 1977;123:131–139.

29. Matsui K, Yamada H, Chiba K. Visualization of soft tissue malignancies by using ^{99m}Tc polyphosphate, pyrophosphate and diphosphonate ([99m]TcP). J Nucl Med 1973;14:632–637.

30. Shiu MH, Castro EB, Hajdu SI, Fortner JG. Surgical treatment of 297 soft tissue sarcomas of the lower extremity. Ann Surg 1975;182: 597–602.

31. Deleted in proof.

32. Hunter JC, Johnston WH, Genant HK. Computed tomography evaluation of fatty tumors of the somatic soft tissues: clinical utility and radiologic-pathologic correlation. Skeletal Radiol 1979;4:82–86.

33. Broder MS, Leonidas JC, Mitty HA. Pseudosarcomatous fasciitis: an unusual cause of soft tissue calcification. Radiology 1973;107: 173–175.

34. Goldman AB. Myositis ossificans circumscripta: a benign lesion with malignant differential diagnosis. AJR 1976;126:32–34.

35. Richman LS, Gumerman LW, Lewine G, et al. Localization of Tc-99m polyphosphate in soft tissue malignancies. AJR 1975;124:577–579.

36. Rosenthal L. ^{99m}Tc-Methylene diphosphonate concentration in soft tissue malignant fibrous histiocytoma. Clin Nucl Med 1978;3:59–62.

37. Thrall JH, Ghaed N, Geslien GE. Pitfalls in Tc-99m polyphosphate skeletal imaging. AJR 1974;121:739–743.

38. Madwell JE, Moser RP. Radiographic evaluation of soft tissue tumors. In: Enzinger FM, Weiss SW, eds. Soft tissue tumors. 2nd ed. St. Louis: CV Mosby, 1988:64–79.

39. Enneking WF, Chew FS, Springfield DS, Hudson TM, Spanier SS. The role of radionucleotide bone-scanning in determining resectability of soft tissue sarcomas. J Bone Joint Surg (Am) 1981;63:249–257.

40. Burrows PE, Muciken JB, Fellows KE. Childhood hemangiomas and vascular malformations: angiographic differentiation. AJR 1983;141:486–491.

41. Cockshott WP, Evans KT. The place of soft tissue arteriography. Br J Radiol 1964; 37: 367–372.

42. Finck EJ, Moore TM. Angiography for mass lesions of bone, joint and soft tissue. Orthop Clin North Am 1977;8:999–1004.

43. Herzberg DL, Schreiber MH. Angiography in mass lesions of the extremities. AJR 1971; 111:541–548.

44. Jaffee N. Hemangiopericytoma. Angiographic findings. Br J Radiol 1960;33:614–619.

45. Lagergren C, Lindblom A. Angiography of peripheral tumor. Radiology 1962;49:371–375.

46. Lagergren C, Lindblom JA, Soderberg G. Vascularization of fibromatous and fibrosarcomatous tumors. Histopathologic, microangiographic and angiographic studies. Acta Radiol 1960;53:1.

47. Levin DC, Watson RC, Baltaxe HA. Arteriography of peripheral hemangiomas. Radiology 1976;121:628–633.

48. Levine E, Lee KR, Neff JR, et al. Comparison of computed tomography and other imaging modalities in the evaluation of musculoskeletal tumors. Radiology 1979;131:431–439.

49. Hudson TM, Haas G, Enneking WF, Hawkins IF. Angiography in the management of musculoskeletal tumors. Surg Gynecol Obstet 1975;141:139–143.

50. Viamonte M, Roen S, Lepage J. Nonspecificity of abnormal vascularity in the angiographic di-

agnosis of malignant neoplasms. Radiology 1973;106:59–64.

51. Neifeld JP, Walsh JW, Lawrence W. Computed tomography in the management of ST tumors. Surg Gynecol Obstet 1982;155:535–540.

52. Egund N, Ekelund L, Sako M, Persson B. CT of soft tissue tumors. AJR 1981;137:725–729.

53. Lange TA, Austin CW, Seibert JJ, Angtuaco TA, Yandow DR. Ultrasound imaging as a screening study for management of soft tissue tumors. J Bone Joint Surg (Am) 1987; 63:100–105.

54. Alpern MB, Thorsen MK, Kellman GM, et al. CT appearance of hemangiopericytoma. J Comput Assist Tomogr 1986;10:263–268.

55. Berger PE, Kuhn JP. Computed tomography of tumors of the musculoskeletal system in children. Radiology 1978;127:170–175.

56. Dooms GC, Hricak H, Sotlitto RA. Lipomatous tumors with fatty components: MR imaging potential and comparison of MR and CT results. Radiology 1985;157:479–483.

57. Heelan RT, Watson RC, Smith J. Computed tomography of lower extremity tumors. AJR 1979;132:936–942.

58. Hermann G, Rose JS. Computed tomography in bone and soft tissue pathology of the extremities. J Comput Assist Tomogr 1979;3:66–69.

59. Hunter JC, Johnston WH, Genant HK. Computed tomography evaluation of fatty tumors of the somatic soft tissues: clinical utility and radiologic-pathologic correlation. Skeletal Radiol 1979;4:80–84.

60. Lee KR, Cox GG, Neff JR. Cystic masses of the knee: arthrographic and CT evaluation. AJR 1987;148:334.

61. Levitt RG, Sagel SS, Stanley RJ, et al. Computed tomography of the pelvis. Semin Roentgenol 1978;13:193.

62. Weekes RG, McLeod RA, Reiman HM, et al. CT of soft tissue neoplasms. AJR 1985;144: 355–359.

63. Petasnick JP, Turner DA, Charters JR, Gitelis S, Zacharias CE. Soft tissue masses of the locomotor system: comparison of MR imaging with CT. Radiology 1986;160:125–133.

64. Neifeld JP, Walsh JW, Lawrence W. Computed tomography in the management of ST tumors. Surg Gynecol Obstet 1982;155:535–540.

65. Chang AE, Motory YL, Dwyer AJ, Hill SC, Girton M, Steinberg SM, et al. Magnetic resonance imaging versus computed tomography in the evaluation of soft tissue tumors of the extremities. Ann Surg 1987;205:340–348.

66. Totty WG, Murphy WA, Lee JKT. Soft tissue tumors: MR imaging. Radiology 1986; 160: 135–141.

67. Moon KL, Genant HK, Helms CA, Chafetz NI, Crooks LE, Kaufman L. Musculoskeletal application of NMR. Radiology 1983;147:161–171.

68. Sherwin RP, Friedell GH. Pseudosarcomatous fibromatosis (infiltrative fasciitis): report of two cases. Boston Med Q 1959;10:49.

69. Bono JA. Nodular pseudosarcomatous fasciitis. Ann Surg 1974;40:601.

70. Culberson JD, Enterline HT. Pseudosarcoma-tous fasciitis; a distinctive clinical-pathologic entity: report of five cases. Ann Surg 1960; 151:235.

71. Stout AP. Pseudosarcomatous fasciitis in children. Cancer 1961;14:1216.

72. Wallace RT, Wilson RS, Cain JR. Pseudosarcomatous fasciitis. South Med J 1962; 55:475–480.

73. Phelan JT, Jurado J. Pseudosarcomatous fasciitis. N Engl J Med 1962;266:645.

74. Chung EB, Enzinger FM. Proliferative fasciitis. Cancer 1975;36:1450.

75. Hutter RVP, Stewart FW, Foote FW Jr. Fasciitis: a report of 70 cases with follow up proving the benignity of the lesion. Cancer 1962;15:992.

76. Price EB, Silliphant WM, Shuman R. Nodular fasciitis: a clinico-pathologic analysis of 65 cases. Am J Clin Pathol 1961;35:122.

77. Lever W, ed. Histopathology of the skin. 6th ed. Philadelphia: Lippincott, 1983:600–635.

78. Hutter RVP, Stewart FW, Foote FW Jr. Fasciitis: a report of 70 cases with follow up proving the benignity (sic) of the lesion. Cancer 1962;15:992.

79. Price EB Jr. Silliphant WM, Shuman R. Nodular fasciitis: a clinicopathological analysis of 65 cases. Am J Clin Pathol 1961;35:251–259.

80. Kern WH. Proliferative myositis—a pseudosarcomatous reaction to injury. Arch Pathol 1960;69:209–212.

81. Enzinger FM, Dulcey F. Proliferative myositis—a report of 33 cases. Cancer 1967; 20:2222.

82. Dahl I, Agerwall L, Magnusson S. Classical and cystic nodular fasciitis. Pathol Europ 1972;7: 211–215.

83. Chung EB, Enzinger FM. Fibroma of tendon sheath. Cancer 1979;44:1945–1954.

84. Sarma DP, Townsend GH, Rodriquez FH. Fibroma of tendon sheath. J Foot Surg 1987; 26:422–424.

85. Sarma DP, Weilbaechert G, Rodriquez FH. Fibroma of tendon sheath. J Surg Oncol 1986;32:230.

86. Cooper PH. Fibroma of tendon sheath. J Am Acad Dermatol 1984;11:628.

87. Jarvi OH, Saxen E. Elastofibroma dorsi. Acta Pathol Microbiol Scand 1961;51:83–85.

88. Deleted in proof.

89. Murray JC, Pollack SV, Pinnel SR. Keloids: a review. J Am Acad Dermatol 1981;4:461–468.

90. Kurwa AR. Rubinstein-Taybi syndrome and spontaneous keloids. Clin Exp Dermatol 1978; 4:254–257.

91. Bloom D. Heredity of keloids: review of the literature and report of a family with multiple keloids in five generations. NY State J Med 1956;56:511–516.

92. Majno G, Gabbiani G, Hirschel B. Contraction of granulation tissue in vitro: similarity to smooth muscle. Science 1971;548.

93. Ketchum LD, Cohen KI, Masters FW. Hypertrophic scars and keloids. Plast Reconstruct Surg 1974;53:140–143.

94. Reye RDK. Consideration of certain subdermal

"fibromatous tumors" of infancy. J Pathol Bacteriol 1956;72:149–153.

95. Enzinger FM. Fibrous hamartoma of infancy. Cancer 1965;18:241.

96. MacKenzie DH. The fibromatoses—a clinicopathologic concept. Br Med J 1972;4:277–281.

97. Allen PW. The fibromatoses—a clinicopathologic classification based on 140 cases, part II. Am J Surg Pathol 1977;314–322.

98. Makagasw K, Maruo M, Yeda K, Ose C. Infantile digital fibromatosis. J Cutan Pathol 1980; 7:431–433.

99. Santa Cruz DJ, Reiner DB. Recurrent digital fibroma of childhood. J Cutan Pathol 1978; 5:339–346.

100. Deleted in proof.

101. Morettin LB, Mueller E, Schreiber M. Generalized hamartomatosis (congenital generalized fibromatosis). Am J Roentgenol Radium Ther Nucl Med 1972;114:722.

102. Bartlett RC, Otis RD, Laakso AO. Multiple congenital neoplasms of soft tissue—report of 4 cases in one family. Cancer 1961;14:913.

103. Lin JJ, Svoboda DJ. Multiple congenital mesenchymal tumors—multiple vascular leiomyomas in several organs of a newborn. Cancer 1971;28:1046.

104. Chung EB, Enzinger FM. Infantile myofibromatosis. A review of 59 cases with localized and generalized involvement. Cancer 1981; 48:1807.

105. Alteman AM, Amstalden EL, Filho JM. Congenital generalized fibromatosis causing spinal cord compression. Hum Pathol 1985;16:1063.

106. Dimmeck JE, Wood WS. Congenital multiple fibromatosis. Am J Dermatopathol 1983;5:289.

107. Bartlett RC, Otis RD, Laakso AO. Multiple congenital neoplasms of soft tissue. Report of 4 cases in one family. Cancer 1961;14:913.

108. Benjamin SP, Mercer RD, Hawk WA. Myofibroblastic contraction in spontaneous regression of multiple congenital mesenchymal hamartomas. Cancer 1977;40:2343.

109. Shnitka TK, Asp DM, Horner HR. Congenital generalized fibromatosis. Cancer 1958; 11:627.

110. Walts AE, Asch M, Raj C. Solitary lesion of congenital fibromatosis. Am J Surg Pathol 1982;6:255.

111. Baird PA, Worth AJ. Congenital generalized fibromatosis—an autosomal recessive condition. Clin Genet 1976;9:488.

112. Jennings T, Duray PH, Collins FS, et al. Infantile myofibromatosis—evidence for an autosomal-dominant disorder. Am J Surg Pathol 1984;8:529.

113. Shmookler BM, Enzinger FM. Giant cell fibroblastoma: a peculiar childhood tumor. Lab Invest 1982;46:302–307.

114. Abdul-Karim FW, Evans HL, Silva EG. Giant cell fibroblastoma: a report of three cases. Am J Clin Pathol 1985;83:165–169.

115. Barr RJ, Young EM, Liao S. Giant cell fibroblastoma: an immunohistochemical study. J Cutan Pathol 1986;13:301–305.

116. Keasbey LE. Juvenile aponeurotic fibroma (calcifying fibroma): a distinctive tumor arising in the palms and soles of young children. Cancer 1953;6:3–7.

117. Goldman RL. The cartilage analogue of fibromatosis (aponeurotic fibroma)—further observation based on seven new cases. Cancer 1970; 26:1325–1327.

118. Keasbey LE. Juvenile aponeurotic fibroma (calcifying fibroma): a distinctive tumor arising in the palms and soles of young children. Cancer 1953;6:338–346.

119. Keasbey LE, Fanselau HA. The aponeurotic fibroma. Clin Orthop 1961;19:115–120.

120. Stout AP. Juvenile fibromatosis. Cancer 1954;7:953–960.

121. Pickren JW, Smith AG, Stevenson TW. Fibromatosis of the plantar fascia. Cancer 1951; 846–856.

122. Pederson HE, Day AJ. Dupuytren's disease of the foot. J Am Med Assoc 1954;154:33–36.

123. Aviles E, Arlen M, Miller T. Plantar fibromatosis. Surgery 1971;69:117–120.

124. Allen RA, Woolner LB, Ghormley RK. Soft tissue tumors of the sole with special reference to plantar fibromatosis. J Bone Joint Surg (Am) 195;37:14–26.

125. Janssen P. Zur Lehre von der Dupuytrenschen Fingercontractur, mit besonderer Berücksichtigung der operativen Beseitigung und der pathologischen Anatomie des Leidens. Arch F Klin Chir 1902;67:789–791.

126. Kiryu H, Tsuneyoshi M, Enjoji M. Myofibroblasts in fibromatoses—an electron microscopic study. Acta Pathol Jpn 1985;35: 543–547.

127. Samitz MH, ed. Cutaneous disorders of the lower extremities. Philadelphia: Lippincott, 1981:206–230.

128. Campbell CJ. Tumors of the foot. In: Jahss MH, ed. Disorders of the foot, vol 1. Philadelphia: WB Saunders, 1982:985–990.

129. Ledderhose. Zur Pathologic der Aponeurose des Fusses und der Hand. Arch F Klin Chir 1897;55:694–670.

130. Allen PW. The fibromatoses: a clinicopathologic classification based on 140 cases, part I. Am J Surg Pathol 1977;255–270.

131. Ushijima M, Tsuneyoshi M, Enjoji M. Dupuytren's type fibromatoses. A clinicopathologic study of 62 cases. Acta Pathol Jpn 1984; 34:991–1001.

132. Chen KTK, Van Dyne TA. Familial plantar fibromatosis. J Surg Oncol 1985;29:240.

133. Kiryu H, Tsuneyoshi M, Enjoji M. Myofibroblasts in fibromatoses—an electron microscopic study. Acta Pathol Jpn 1985;35: 533–537.

134. Wooldrige WE. Four related fibrosing diseases. Postgrad Med 1988;84:269–274.

135. Legge JW. Dupuytren's disease. Surg Ann 1985;17:355–362.

136. Hueston JT. Dupuytren's contracture. Edinburgh: E & S Livingstone, Ltd., 1963.

137. Gelberman RH, Amiel D, Rudolph RM, Vance RM. Dupuytren's contracture—an electron microscopic biochemical and clinical correla-

tive study. J Bone Joint Surg (Am) 1980; 62:425–432.

138. Kirju H, Tsuneyoshi M, Enjoji M. Myofibroblasts in fibromatoses—an electron microscopic study. Acta Pathol Jpn 1985; 35: 533–547.

139. Luck JV. Dupuytren's contracture—a new concept in pathogenesis correlated with surgical management. J Bone Joint Surg (Am) 1959; 41:635–664.

140. Chen KTK, Van Dyne TA. Familial plantar fibromatosis. J Surg Oncol 1985;29:240–241.

141. Skoog T. Dupuytren's contraction with special reference to aetiology and improved surgical treatment. Its occurrence in epileptics. Note on knuckle pads. Acta Chir Scand 1948;96(Suppl 139): 183–189.

142. Allen RA, Woolner LB, Ghormley RK. Soft tissue tumors of the sole with special reference to plantar fibromatosis. J Bone Joint Surg (Am) 1955;37:14–28.

143. Curtin JW. Fibromatosis of the plantar fascia surgical technique and design of skin incision. J Bone Joint Surg (Am) 1965;47:1605–1608.

144. Jones HW. Two cases of "knuckle pads." Br Med J 1923;1:759–760.

145. Mikkelson OA. Knuckle pads in Dupuytren's disease. Hand 1977;9:301–303.

146. Robbins SL. Pathology. Philadelphia: WB Saunders, 1968:122–150.

147. Young C, Ketai NH. Fibrosarcoma differentiated: a case report. J Foot Surg 1972;11:33–35.

148. Hajdu SI. Pathology of soft tissue tumors. Philadelphia: Lea & Febiger, 1979:135–201.

149. Stout AP, Lattes R. Tumors of the soft tissues. In: Atlas of tumor pathology. 2nd series. Washington, DC: Armed Forces Institute of Pathology, 1967.

150. Bizer LS. Fibrosarcoma, a report of 64 cases. Am J Surg 1971;121:586–587.

151. Simon MA, Enneking WF. The management of soft tissue sarcomas of the extremities. J Bone Joint Surg (Am) 1976;58:321–330.

152. Brindley HH, Phillips C, Fernandez JN. Fibrosarcoma of the extremities. J Bone Joint Surg (Am) 1955;37:602–609.

153. Pack GT, Ariel IM. Fibrosarcoma of the soft somatic tissues. A clinical and pathologic study. Surgery 1952;31:443.

154. Pritchard DJ, Soule EH, Taylor WF, Ivins JC. Fibrosarcoma—a clinicopathologic and statistical study of 199 tumors of the soft tissues of the extremities and trunk. Cancer 1974; 33:888–897.

155. Stout AP. Fibrosarcoma. The malignant tumor of the fibroblasts. Cancer 1948;1:30–63.

156. Meyerding HW, Broder AC, Hargrave RL. Clinical aspects of fibrosarcoma of the soft tissue of the extremities. Surg Gynecol Obstet 1936; 62:1010–1021.

157. Simon MA, Enneking WF. The management of soft tissue sarcoma of the extremities. J Bone Joint Surg (Am) 1976;58:320–331.

158. Wu K. Fibrosarcoma of the foot. J Foot Surg 1987;26:530–534.

159. Collins NC, Anspach WE. Fibrosarcoma of plantar tissues. Am J Cancer 1940;40: 465–470.

160. Young C, Ketai NH. Fibrosarcoma differentiated: a case report. J Foot Surg 1972;11:33–34.

161. Deleted in proof.

162. Shiu MH, Castro EB, Hajdu SI, Fortner JG. Surgical treatment of 297 soft tissue sarcomas of the lower extremity. Ann Surg 1975; 182:597–602.

163. Enneking WF. Staging of musculoskeletal neoplasms. Skeletal Radiol 1985;13:183–194.

164. Simon MA, Enneking WF. The management of soft tissue sarcoma of the extremities. J Bone Joint Surg (Am) 1976;58:317–327.

165. McLeak CJ, Papaionnau AN. Nonpancreatic tumors associated with hypoglycemia. Arch Surg 1966;93:1019.

166. Deleted in proof.

167. Porter MR, Frantz VK. Tumor associated with hypoglycemia; pancreatic and extrapancreatic. Am J Med 1956;21:944.

168. Markhede G, Angervale L, Steiner B. A multivariate analysis of the prognosis after surgical treatment of malignant soft tissue tumors. Cancer 1982;49:1721–1733.

169. Costa J, Wesley RA, Glatstein E, Rosenberg SA. The grading of soft tissue sarcomas— results of a clinicohistopathologic correlation in a series of 163 cases. Cancer 1984;53: 530–541.

170. Castro EB, Hajdu SI, Fortner JG. Surgical therapy of fibrosarcoma of the extremities. Arch Surg 1973;107:284–296.

171. Ivins JC, Dockerty MB, Ghormley RK. Fibrosarcoma of the soft tissues of the extremities. A review of 78 cases. Surgery 1950;28:495–503.

172. Pack GT, Ariel IM. Fibrosarcoma of the soft somatic tissues—a clinical and pathologic study. Surgery 1952;31:443–451.

173. Phelan JT, Nigogasyan G. Fibrosarcoma of superficial soft tissue origin. Arch Surg 1963; 86:276–280.

174. Rosenberg SA, Tepper J, Glatstein E, Costa J, Baker A, Brennan M. The treatment of soft tissue sarcomas of the extremities—prospective randomized evaluation of 1) limb sparing surgery plus radiation therapy compared with amputation & 2) the role of adjuvant chemotherapy. Ann Surg 1982;196:305–315.

175. Suit HD, Russell WO, Martin RG. Management of patients with sarcoma of the soft tissue in an extremity. Cancer 1973;31:1247–1255.

176. Potter DA, Kinsella T, Glatstein E, Wesley R, White DE, Seipp CA, et al. High grade soft tissue sarcoma of the extremities. Cancer 1986;58:203–210.

177. Abbas SS, Holyoke ED, Moore MS, Kara Kousis CP. The surgical treatment outcome of soft tissue sarcomas. Arch Surg 1981;116:765–769.

178. Sears HF, Hopson R, Inouye W, Rizzo T, Grotzinger PJ. Analysis of staging and management of patients with sarcoma—a 10-year experience. Ann Surg 1980;191:488–493.

179. Van der Werf-Messing B, Van Unnik Jam. Fibrosarcoma of the soft tissues—a clinicopathologic study. Cancer 1965;18:1123–1130.

180. Simon MA, Enneking WF. The management of soft tissue sarcoma of the extremities. J Bone Joint Surg (Am) 1976;58:317–328.
181. Brennhovd IO. The treatment of soft tissue sarcomas—a plea for a more urgent and aggressive approach. Acta Chir Scand 1966;131:438.
182. Scale KS, Lange TA, Monson D, et al. Soft tissue tumors of the foot and ankle. Foot Ankle 1983;9:24.
183. Bizer LS. Fibrosarcoma, a report of 64 cases. Am J Surg 1971;121:586.
184. Suit HD, Russell WO, Martin RG. Sarcoma of soft tissue: clinical and histopathologic parameters and response to treatment. Cancer 1975;35:1483.
185. Krementz ET, Carter RD, Sutherland CM, et al. Chemotherapy of sarcomas of limbs by regional perfusion. Ann Surg 1977;185:564–570.
186. Morton DL, Eilber FR, Townsend CM, et al. Limb salvage from a multidisciplinary treatment approach for skeletal and soft tissue sarcomas of an extremity. Ann Surg 1976;184:268–278.
187. Deleted in proof.
188. Wilson H, Brunschwig A. Irradiation sarcoma. Surgery 1937;2:607–610.
189. Gray GR. Fibrosarcoma: a complication of interstitial radiation therapy for a benign hemangioma occurring after 18 years. Br J Radiol 1974;47:60–70.
190. Deelman HT. Heredity and cancer. Ann Surg 1931;93:34–37.
191. Niemi KM. The benign fibrohistiocytic tumors of the skin. Acta Dermatoren 1970;50(Suppl 63):1–14.
192. Newman DM, Walter IB. Multiple dermatofibromas in patients with systemic lupus erythematosus on immunosuppressive therapy. N Engl J Med 1973;289:842–865.
193. Fitzpatrick TB, Gilchrest BA. Dimple sign to differentiate benign from malignant pigmented cutaneous lesions. N Engl J Med 1977;296:1518–1532.
194. Klaus SN, Winkelmann AK. The enzyme histochemistry of nodular subepidermal fibrosis. Br J Dermatol 1966;78:389–410.
195. Fine G, Morales MD, Pardov. Ultrastructure of histiocytomas. Am J Clin Pathol 1977;67:214–222.
196. Hakimi M, Pair, Fine G. Fibrous histiocytoma of the trachea and chest. Am J Clin Pathol 1975;68:367–371.
197. Mihatsch-Konz B, Schaumburg-Lever G, Lever WR. Ultrastructure of dermatofibroma. Arch Derm Forsch 1973;246:181–192.
198. Katenkamp D, Stiller D. Cellular composition of the so-called dermatofibroma. Pathol Anat 1975;367:325–331.
199. Webster SB, Reister HC, Harman LE. Juvenile xanthogranuloma with extracutaneous lesions. A case report and review of the literature. Arch Dermatol 1966;93:71–76.
200. Sonoda T, Hashimoto H, Enjoji M. Juvenile xanthogranuloma, clinicopathologic analysis and immunohistochemical study of 57 patients. Cancer 1985;56:2280–2330.
201. Gonzalez-Crussi F, Campbell RJ. Juvenile xanthogranuloma ultrastructural study. Arch Pathol 1970;89:65–76.
202. Esterly NB, Sahihi T, Medenica M. Juvenile xanthogranuloma: an atypical case with a study of ultrastructure. Arch Dermatol 1972;105:99–110.
203. Sonoda T, Hashimoto H, Enjoji M. Juvenile xanthogranuloma, clinicopathologic analysis and immunohistochemical study of 57 patients. Cancer 1985;56:2280–2330.
204. Eller JL, Limmer BL. Roentgen therapy for visceral: juvenile xanthogranuloma including a case with involvement of the heart. AJR 1965;95:52–65.
205. Niven JSF, Armstrong JA, Andrews CH. Subcutaneous growth in monkeys produced by pox virus. J Pathol Bacteriol 1961;81:1–10.
206. Sproul EE, Metzgar RS, Grace JT Jr. The pathogenesis of Yaba virus-induced histiocytomas in primates. Cancer Res 1963;23:671–683.
207. Finlay-Jones LR, Nicoll P, Seldam R. Pseudosarcoma of the skin. Pathology 1971;3:215–236.
208. Bourne RB. Paradoxical fibrosarcoma of the skin (pseudosarcoma): a review of thirteen cases. Med J Aust 1963;50:504–524.
209. Levan NE, Hirsch P, Kwong MQ. Pseudosarcomatous dermatofibroma. Arch Dermatol 1963;88:2908–2929.
210. Gordon HW. Pseudosarcomatous reticulohistiocytoma: a report of 4 cases. Arch Dermatol 1964;90:319–331.
211. Helwig EB, May D. Atypical fibroxanthoma of the skin with metastasis. Cancer 1986;57:368–379.
212. Fretzin DF, Helwig EB. Atypical fibroxanthoma of the skin. Cancer 1973;31:1541–1560.
213. Montgomery H, Polley HF, Pugh DG. Reticulohistiocytoma. Arch Dermatol 1958;77:61–77.
214. Barrow MV, Holvbark. Multiantric reticulohistiocytosis. Medicine 1969;48:287–301.
215. Purvis WE, Helwig EB. Reticulohistiocytic granuloma of the skin. Am J Clin Pathol 1954;24:1005–1015.
216. Orkin M, Goltz RW, Good RA. Reticulohistiocytic granuloma of the skin. Am J Clin Pathol 1954;24.
217. Crocker AC. Skin xanthomas in childhood. Pediatrics 1951;8:573–581.
218. Hamilton WC, Ramsey PL, Hanson SM. Osseous xanthoma and multiple hand tumors as a complication of hyperlipidemia. Circulation 1965;31:321–332.
219. Fredrickson DS, Lees RS. A system for plenotyping hyperlipoproteinemia. Circulation 1965; 31.
220. Friedman MS. Xanthoma of Achilles tendon. J Bone Joint Surg 1947;29:760–779.
221. Galloway JOB, Broders AC, Ghormley RK. Xanthoma of tendon sheaths and synovial membranes. Arch Surg 1940;40:485–499.
222. Adams CWM, Bayliss LB, Ibrahim MZM. Phos-

pholipids in atherosclerosis: the modification of the cholesterol granuloma by phospholipid. J Pathol Bacteriol 1963;86:43–61.

223. Riznyk PJ, Hugar DW. Dermatofibrosarcoma protuberans. J Am Podiatr Med Assoc 1987; 26:2–36.

224. Darrier S, Ferrand M. Dermatofibromes progressifs et ricidivantes. Ann Dermatol Syph 1924;5:545–581.

225. Hoffman E. Uberdas Knollentreibende Fibrosarkom der Haut. Dermatol Ztschr 1925; 43:1–30.

226. Taylor HB, Helwig EB. Dermatofibrosarcoma protuberans—a study of 115 cases. Cancer 1962;115:717–739.

227. Bednar B. Storiform neurofibromas of the skin: pigmented and nonpigmented. Cancer 1978; 41:2250–2271.

228. Weiss SW, Enzinger FM. Malignant fibrous histiocytoma: an analysis of 200 cases. Cancer 1978;41.

229. Weiss SW. Malignant fibrous histiocytoma: a reaffirmation. Am J Surg Pathol 1982; 6: 773–781.

230. Weiss SW, Enzinger FM. Myxoid variant of malignant: fibrous histiocytoma. Cancer 1977; 39:1672–1690.

231. Brecher ME, Franklin WA. Absence of mononuclear phagocyte antigens in malignant fibrous histiocytoma. Am J Clin Pathol 1986; 86:344–360.

232. Wood GS, Beckstead JH, Turner RR. Malignant fibrous histiocytoma tumor cells resembling fibroblasts. Am J Surg Pathol 1986;10: 323–352.

233. Taxy JB, Battifora H. Malignant fibrous histiocytoma: a clinicopathologic and ultrastructural study. 1977;40:254–260.

234. Leak LV, Caulfield JB, Burke JF. Electronmicroscopic studies on a human fibromyxosarcoma. Cancer Res 1967;27:261–273.

235. Guccion JG, Enzinger FM. Malignant giant cell tumor of soft parts. An analysis of 32 cases. Cancer 1972;29:1518–1531.

236. Algvacil-Garcia A, Unni KK, Goellner JR. Malignant giant cell tumor of soft parts: ultrastructural study of 4 cases. Cancer 1977;40: 244–266.

237. Oberling C. Retroperitoneal xanthogranuloma. Am J Cancer 1935;23:477–489.

238. Waller JI, Hellwig CA, Barboga E. Retroperitoneal xanthogranuloma associated with visual eosinophilic granuloma. Cancer 1957;10: 388–401.

239. Kyriakos M, Kempson RL. Inflammatory fibrous histiocytoma—an aggressive and lethal lesion. Cancer 1976;37:1584–1601.

240. Enzinger FM. Angiomatoid malignant fibrous histiocytoma: a distinct fibrous histiocytic tumor of children and young adults stimulating a vascular neoplasm. Cancer 1979; 41: 2147–2163.

241. Sun CC Jr, Toker C, Breitenecker R. An ultrastructural study of angiomatoid fibrous histiocytoma. Cancer 1982;49:2103–2120.

242. Enzinger FM. Angiomatoid malignant fibrous histiocytoma: a distinct fibrous histiocytic tumor of children and young adults stimulating a vascular neoplasm. Cancer 1979; 41:2147–2169.

Part F/ **Lower Extremity Soft-tissue Tumors of Adipose Tissue**
—Arthur Steinhart

Lipomas are the most common soft-tissue tumors (1), with more than 50% of soft-tissue neoplasms of the extremities diagnosed as such (2). Although they may occur anywhere, lipomas arise most often in areas where there is much adipose tissue. This may be why they are reported to occur twice as frequently in women than in men. They usually occur on the back of the neck, trunk, abdomen, axilla, forearm, buttocks, thighs, and it is not unusual to find lipoma just anterior to the lateral malleolus in middle-aged obese women. Lipomas are considered to be unusual on the foot and very rare in the digits, with only a few cases reported in the literature (2–10). Lipomas found in areas where fat is not normally found are thought to result from misplacement of adipose or preadipose tissue (11), from the fatty degeneration of other cells, or from metaplasia of muscle cells (12). Although they can occur at any age, approximately 40% are reported to arise during the fourth and fifth decades. The average age of onset is 41 (13).

Lipomas appear as soft, subcutaneous, nontender masses with normal overlying skin. They are generally asymptomatic. Symptoms, however, may be produced due to pressure on adjacent structures. Steroid-induced fat deposition in the popliteal fossa has been reported to be the cause of compression-induced peroneal and tibial nerve palsies (14). Growth and pressure from lipomas have even been reported to cause death (15).

Lipomas are self-limited in size and are reported to grow even in emaciated patients. It is thought that this is the result of differences in the metabolic behavior of lipoma tissue. Fatty acid precursors have been found to be more rapidly incorporated into lipoma fat than other fat, and the activity of lipoprotein lipase is diminished in lipoma (16).

Lipomas may occur either singly (solitary lipoma) in infiltrating or noninfiltrating forms, or multiply as multiple familial lipomatosis or multiple systemic lipomatosis (Madelung's disease, benign symmetric lipomatosis, Lanois-Bensaude) adenolipomatosis, symmetric adenolipomatosis, diffuse symmetric lipomatosis, or lipomatosis simplex indolens (17, 19).

Histologically, lipomas are composed of lobules of mature fat cells separated by connective tissue, all within a fibrous capsule. Other mesenchymal components can be found within the tumor, and, based on the type and amount, lipomas are also classified as angiolipoma, spindle-cell lipoma, fibrolipoma, myxolipoma, lipoblastoma, or pleomorphic lipoma. In addition, the growth may be benign or malignant.

SOLITARY LIPOMA

Lipomas may be infiltrating or noninfiltrating. The infiltrating type grows between striated muscle fibers and into the surrounding tissue. It tends to be unencapsulated, whereas the noninfiltrating type tends to be well-defined and encapsulated (19). Infiltrating lipomas may arise as intramuscular or intermuscular masses, usually affecting the large muscles of the extremities. They are most commonly found in the shoulder girdle, groin, buttocks, or thigh (20). They occur more often in men between the ages of 30–60 than in other groups. It is thought that intermuscular infiltrating lipomas arise from the septa between muscles.

Infiltrating lipomas tend to be slow-growing and painless. Histologically, mature fat cells are seen infiltrating the muscle, with the muscle cells demonstrating atrophic changes. The growth can be differentiated from a well-differentiated liposarcoma by the absence of lipoblasts and the absence of atypical cells in the infiltrating lipoma, etc. The infiltrating type is likely to recur after excision, since its borders are more obscure. It is suggested that, when the tumor is removed, a generous border of normal muscle be included to reduce chances of recurrence (21).

Several forms of solitary lipoma, based on the presence of other mesenchymal tissue, have been described.

(a) Angiolipoma (vascular lipoma, lipoma telangiectaticum, lipoma cavernosum) (16). This growth develops shortly after puberty, arising as small painful bumps under the skin that increase in number by two or three each year, over a period of several years (22). Clinically, the tumors look and feel like a typical subcutaneous lipoma. However, since these tumors are more vascular than the ordinary lipoma, they appear red when cut. It is thought that angiolipomas begin as simple lipomas that subsequently undergo capillary and fibrous proliferation (16). Pathologists, based on the proportions of fat, capillary, and stroma found, have referred to these growths as angiolipoma, angiofibrolipoma, or benign mesenchymoma (22). Howard and Helwig (22) reported the results of a study of 288 angiolipomas removed from 248 patients ranging in age from 16 to 58 (average age of onset, 17), in which only 39 (13.5%) were found on the lower extremity and none on the sole. There were 149 (51.7%) removed from the upper extremity.

This tumor has also been described as infiltrating or noninfiltrating. In one study, 5–17% of all lipomas were found to be noninfiltrating angiolipomas (19). Although the infiltrating type is rare, 52% have been reported on the lower extremity (19). Infiltrating angiolipomas are more common in children than simple lipomas (21). These tumors tend to recur after excision (23).

(b) Spindle-cell lipoma. This tumor was first described in 1975 by Enzinger and Harvey (as cited in Brady et al. (13)) as containing undifferentiated spindle cells, eosinophilic collagen bundles, and mature fat cells. It arises more commonly in men, at an average age of 56. Its usual location is the shoulder, back, or posterior of the neck. There are no reports of it occurring on the foot.

(c) Fibrolipoma. Much fibrous tissue present.

(d) Myxolipoma.

(e) Lipoblastoma. Most of these rare tumors, developing in infants and children, are reported to occur on the extremities. Most arise during the first 3 years of life and are reported to occur on the extremities (24). These tumors are composed of mature fat cells arranged in distinct lobular fashion and interspersed with spindle- and stellate-shaped mesenchymal cells. They are reported to resemble myxoid liposarcoma. The term "lipoblastomatosis" is used to refer to these tumors when they develop as deep, poorly circumscribed growths. The more superficial ones are considered lipoblastoma.

(f) Pleomorphic lipoma (giant cell lipoma).

This is a solitary growth, occasionally recurring, which tends to affect middle-aged and elderly men. Clinically, these growths appear as solitary, asymptomatic, mobile masses. Although usually arising in the subcutaneous and muscular fat of the neck, shoulder, and back, the growths are also reported on the lower extremity (25). A case of a pedunculated pleomorphic lipoma arising in the dermis of the thigh has been reported (26). They have been described as appearing completely or partially circumscribed, ovoid, or spherical in shape, sometimes lobulated, with a soft to firm consistency, and a yellow, yellowish-gray, or yellow-tan color. The tumor, which histologically resembles several forms of liposarcoma, contains many floret-like multinucleated giant cells, which are more numerous than lipoblasts, in a myxoid stroma of dense bundles of mature collagen, interspersed with mature fat cells. It differs from liposarcoma in that the sarcoma contains more lipoblasts, fewer multinucleated giant cells, and displays more uniform delicate collagen fibrils.

MULTIPLE SYMMETRIC LIPOMATOSIS

Multiple symmetric lipomatosis was first described in 1898 by Launoise and Bensaude (as cited in Enzi et al. (27)). This condition, which generally affects middle-aged men of Mediterranean descent, is characterized by the development of unencapsulated subcutaneous symmetric fat masses and the accumulation of fat in the deep tissue. The subcutaneous fat accumulation most often occurs about the neck and shoulders in a cape-like distribution (29). The face, distal extremities, hands, and feet are always spared (17). Many of these patients are found to demonstrate somatic and autonomic neuropathy as well as a significant increase in the plasma high-density lipoprotein fraction and a decrease in the low-density fraction (27).

FAMILIAL MULTIPLE LIPOMATOSIS

This rare condition is characterized by the development of multiple, often symmetric, encapsulated lipomas among several generations in a family. The condition may involve an autosomal dominant inheritance. The growths tend to affect the forearms and thighs, as well as the trunk and arms; the neck and shoulders are rarely affected. The masses usually appear in the third decade and, after an initial period of

rapid growth, tend to remain stable, typically reaching 5–6 cm.

TREATMENT

Treatment of cutaneous lipoma, other than for cosmetic effect, is usually unnecessary. However, treatment may be necessary to relieve the symptoms caused by the pressure exerted by deep lipomas. Tender angiolipomas may be excised, as are "bothersome" simple lipomas. Excision of a simple lipoma is accomplished by making an incision extending over the length of the tumor. The mass is then bluntly dissected out (16). This "shelling out" technique may not be appropriate for all lipomas but is best when reserved for small superficial growths (29). Surgical excision must be performed with care taken to obliterate the dead spaces resulting after removal of the mass. Care must also be taken to avoid disruption of the neurovascular bundle when excising a growth on a digit. There is usually no recurrence of the tumor after excision, although some have been reported (9).

Recently, two modifications of the traditional excision procedure have been described. Rubenstein et al. (30) described the use of liposuction for the removal of large lipomas. Their technique involved making a small incision over the center of the tumor, inserting a cannula and suctioning out the fat. Scissors and forceps were then used to remove the fibrous stroma of the growth. The authors stated that this technique permitted the use of local anesthesia rather than general, avoided the large incision needed for excision, and resulted in better healing.

The second technique, described by Powell and McLean (31) as the "squeeze" technique, involved removing the lipoma by squeezing it through a small incision.

LIPOSARCOMA

Liposarcoma is the most common malignant soft somatic tissue tumor in adults (32). It is rare in children. When it does occur in a child, the prognosis is good, since the type that arises in many children (myxoid liposarcoma) tends not to metastasize (24). This type comprises between 7 and 15% of all soft-tissue tumors (33). Some reports have described the tumor as occurring with equal frequency in men and women (33), whereas others report a male:female ratio of 7:2 (34). Liposarcomas tend to arise most commonly in the intermuscular fascia of the lower extremity, especially the thigh, buttock, and retroperitoneal region. It is rare on the foot, although several cases of pedal liposarcoma are reported (9, 32, 35–38). They present as painless, slowly growing, non-tender, well-circumscribed masses located deep in the soft tissue. Symptoms are related to the presence of the mass. The tumors do not appear to arise out of preexisting lipoma but arise de novo and are not related to trauma (35). Theories regarding liposarcomas arising from preexisting lipomas and the effect of trauma in inducing malignant transformation have been proven inaccurate. Metastases occurs through the bloodstream rather than the lymphatics and is to the lungs, liver, and bone. In general, the prognosis is better when the tumor is on the lower extremity, which is probably the result of easier early detection and accessibility (39). A liposarcoma appears grossly as a soft, lobulated mass surrounded by a pseudocapsule. Its color varies from white to yellow, orange, tan, and brownish-red to dark red and black in areas of degeneration and hemorrhage. Virchow (as cited in Kimbrough and Soule (33)), in 1857, is thought to have presented the first authoritative histologic description of a malignant tumor derived from fatty tissue (33). Since then, several histologic types of liposarcoma have been described.

(a) Myxoid. The myxoid liposarcoma is the most common type of liposarcoma (22). The lipoblasts in the tumor are seen in different stages of maturity and differentiation. The growth consists of a myxomatous intercellular matrix and a delicate plexiform capillary network. Stellate fibroblasts are seen but rarely display thick mature collagen bundles or floret-like multinucleated giant cells.

(b) Pleomorphic. This tumor is highly cellular, with many of the cells showing atypical mitotic figures. The cells within the tumor include extremely large anaplastic cells and multivacuolated lipoblasts. This type has the poorest prognosis (39).

(c) Sclerosing. This form displays a uniform network of delicate collagen fibrils, numerous lipoblasts, and occasionally shows a few multinucleated giant cells.

(d) Round cell (adenoid type). The tumor cells of this growth are round, relatively uniform lipoblasts with a centrally located nucleus and a foamy cytoplasm in which there are lipid-filled vacuoles. The cells are arranged in branching rows with strands along the capillaries. This is an aggressive tumor with frequent metastases and, therefore, has a poor prognosis.

(e) Well-differentiated. The well-differentiated liposarcoma displays mature adipose tissue with some pleomorphism. It has an aggressively infiltrating growth pattern and may have a high local recurrence rate, but otherwise follows a relatively benign course (32).

It has been suggested (33) that when a biopsy is performed, it be done after double tourniquets are applied so that amputation, if needed, can be performed between the tourniquets to prevent leaving behind any malignant emboli of tumor cells which may resulted from the biopsy procedure. During biopsy procedures, transverse sectioning of tissue planes may allow extension of the mass and seeding of the tumor that may occur as a result of incision into the tumor or bleeding.

The treatment of choice for liposarcoma is excision, which should extend well beyond the palpable borders of the tumor. Although a pseudocapsule usually surrounds the sarcoma, the tumor frequently perforates this and invades the surrounding tissue. Wide excision, therefore, is necessary. If such excision is not possible, the amputation is suggested. Simon and Enneking (40) suggest that the local excision be "radical," that is, the zone of surrounding normal tissue should extend to one anatomic plane beyond the tissue of origin. The resected tissue would, therefore, include any muscles, neurovascular structures, and bone in the involved compartment. Irradiation has been used when local excision is performed in order to reduce the incidence of recurrence or when the mass is not removable (35). Routine use of post-excision radiation therapy is controversial, with some thinking that the only time for postsurgical radiation therapy is when a cure is not expected (33).

It has been suggested that palpation alone is sufficient to correctly diagnose a superficial lipoma (41). Palpation alone, however, cannot be used to differentiate between a deep benign infiltrating lipoma and a liposarcoma. Among the diagnostic procedures used to distinguish these two tumors are plain radiography, technetium-99m scanning, computed tomography scanning, and angiography. Plain radiographs of a lipoma reveal a mass demonstrating a density similar to normal fat. Calcifications may also be seen within the mass (42). The mass visualized in a liposarcoma may show areas of varying densities, including calcifications. Technetium-99m radionuclide imaging better assists in distinguishing between benign and malignant tumors because, if there is no activity, the mass is not a liposarcoma. The presence of activity is, however, not pathognomonic of malignancy, since there will be activity when calcification is present, regardless of the benign nature of the growth (42).

Computed tomography (CT) is considered the test of choice in differentiating between lipoma and liposarcoma. On CT studies, a benign lipoma is visualized as a sharply demarcated, well-delineated growth, with homogeneous low density equal to or less than the patient's normal fat, that shows no tumor contrast enhancement. Liposarcomas tend to be less well-delineated, demonstrate an inhomogeneous CT appearance with higher CT numbers than lipomas, and show contrast enhancement due to their vascularity. It should be noted that angiolipomas are reported to be difficult to differentiate from liposarcoma because, as a result of their vascularity, they show areas of high density interspersed with areas of normal fat density. They may also show poorly defined margins (42). CT studies can also be used to differentiate between lipoma and old hematoma. Another method of differentiating liposarcomas from lipomas is magnetic resonance when short and long repetition times are used (44). However, it is difficult to distinguish between lipoma and old hematoma using magnetic resonance.

Liposarcoma reveals increased vascularity, as well as enlarged draining veins, on angiography in addition to demonstrating poor definition of its margins and displacement and/or tumor encasement of major vessels (42). Peripheral angiography and technetium polyphosphate bone scans are used as part of the preoperative evaluation. The relationship of the tumor to major vessels, the extent of the tumor, and its venous drainage are all demonstrated through arteriography. Bone scanning helps to indicate bone involvement. Amputation, rather than excision, is indicated when arteriography indicates displacement of a major vessel or when bone scan demonstrates involvement of "nonexpendable" bone (40).

MISCELLANEOUS CONDITIONS

Lipoma arborescens, also known as villous lipomatous proliferation of the synovial membrane, is characterized by slowly progressive painless swelling of a joint with intermittent effusions. The knee is usually affected, although other joints, including the ankle, are reported to be affected (45). The subsynovial tissue is completely replaced by mature fat cells, and there is villous hypertrophy of the synovial membrane. Laboratory tests, including blood studies, joint aspiration for crystals, and cultures are all negative. Treatment has been synovectomy. The differential diagnosis includes any condition causing painless effusion and synovial thickening with only local involvement (e.g., synovial chondromatosis, pigmented villonodular synovitis, and synovial hemangiomatosis) (45).

Nevus lipomatosus superficialis is a nevoid anomaly in which ectopic fat cells, derived from perivascular mesenchymal tissue, are found in the dermis. The lesions develop during the first two decades and appear as groups of soft, flattened papules or nodules, usually on the buttock. The growths may extend to the adjacent skin of the back or thigh.

Adiposis dolorosa (Dercum's disease) is a variant of multiple lipomatosis in which painful, tender, tumor-like masses overgrow the subcutaneous fat (46). The condition occurs bilaterally and most commonly affects the medial sides of the knee. The cardinal signs of this disorder are adiposity, asthenia, pain, and psychologic disturbances (47).

Piezogenic papules were first described by Shelly and Rawnsley in 1968. The disorder involves herniations of the subcutaneous fat tissue through defects in the dermal connective tissue. The masses are generally asymptomatic, but some patients may complain of pain when standing. They respond well to orthotics; cases requiring surgical intervention have been reported.

Angiomyolipoma is an uncommon tumor most frequently found in the kidney, but cases of it appearing on the foot are presented by Moien and Giltman (16) and Krolick and Black (7). The growth consists of various proportions of nodules of blood vessels (either single or multiple), smooth muscle, and fat tissue. They are considered to be hamartomas or focal malformations resulting from faulty development in an organ.

Lipofibromatous hamartoma is a rare neoplasm, usually present at birth and often associated with digital enlargement on the hand but not the foot. It most commonly affects the median nerve, but the plantar nerve has also been described as involved (46). Treatment includes excision of the involved nerve and microsurgical intraneural dissection of the neoplastic elements. Histologic findings consist of the presence of peripheral nerve bundles within fibrofatty tissue.

REFERENCES

1. Hart JAL. Intraosseous lipoma. Bone Joint Surg 1973;55B:624–626.
2. Lisch M, Mittleman M, Albin R. Digital lipoma of the foot: an extraordinary case. J Foot Surg 1982;21:330–331.
3. Greenberg GS. Lipomas: discussion and report of an unusual case. J Foot Surg 1980;19:68–69.
4. Kerman BL, Foster LS. Lipoma of the foot: a large and unusual case. J Foot Surg 1985; 24: 345–346.
5. Bartis JR. Massive lipoma of the foot—a case report. J Am Podiatr Assoc 1974;64:874–875.
6. Moien AJ, Giltman LI. Angiomyolipoma of the foot. J Am Podiatr Assoc 1978;68:773–775.
7. Krolick WD, Black JR. Angiomyolipoma in the foot—a case report. J Am Podiatr Med Assoc 1987;77:290–292.
8. Chagares WE, Cornell DE, Garoufalis MG, Kessler RL. Lipoma and fibroma occurring in the same foot. J Am Podiatr Med Assoc 1986; 75:34–35.
9. Booher RJ. Lipoblastic tumors of the hands and feet. J Bone Joint Surg 1965;47A:727–731.
10. Cristofaro RL, Maher JO. Digital lipoma of the foot in a child. J Bone Joint Surg 1988; 70A:128–129.
11. Wells HG. Adipose tissue, a neglected subject. J Am Med Assoc 1940;114:2284–2289.
12. Truhan AP, Garden JM, Caro WA, Roenigk HH Jr. Facial and scalp lipomas: case reports and study of prevalence. J Dermatol Surg Oncol 1985;11:981–985.
13. Brody HJ, Meltzer HD, Someren A. Spindle cell lipoma—an unusual dermatologic presentation. Arch Dermatol 1978;114:1065–1066.
14. Rawlings CE, Bullard DE, Caldwell DS. Peripheral nerve entrapment due to steroid induced lipomatosis of the popliteal fossa. 1986; 64:666–668.
15. Adair FE, Pack GT. Lipomas. Am J Cancer 1932;16:110–112.
16. Osment LS. Cutaneous lipomas and lipomatosis. Surg Gynecol Obstet 1968;129:129–132.
17. Ruzicka T, Vieluf D, Landthaler M, Braun-Falco O. Benign symmetrical lipomatosis Lanoise-Bensaude. J Am Acad Dermatol 1987; 17:663–665.
18. Economides NG, Liddell HT. Benign symmetric lipomatosis (Madelung's disease). South Med J 1986;79:1023–1025.
19. Matsuoka Y, Kurose K, Nakagawa O, Katsuyama J. Magnetic resonance imaging of infiltrating angiomyolipoma of the neck. Surg Neurol 1986; 29:62–68.
20. Leffert P. Lipomas of the upper extremity. J Bone Joint Surg 1972;54A:375–379.
21. Winkler M, Petrelli N, Cohen A. Pediatric infiltrating lipomas: case report and review of the literature. Surg Oncol 1987;35:59–62.
22. Howard WR, Helwig EB. Angiolipoma. Arch Dermatol 1960;82:924–928.
23. Kaminsky CA, De Kaminsky AR, Chajchir A, Constantini S. Palmar subcutaneous lipoma. Cutis 1987;40:29–31.
24. Hanada M, Tokuda R, Ohnishi Y, Takahashi T, Kimura M. Benign lipoblastoma and liposarcoma in children. Acta Pathol Jpn 1986; 36:605–609.
25. Shmoolker BM, Enzinger FM. Pleomorphic lipoma: a benign tumor simulating liposarcoma. Cancer 1981;47:126–128.
26. Nigro MA, Chieregato GC, Della Rovere GQ. Pleomorphic lipoma of the dermis. Br J Dermatol 1987;116:713–715.
27. Enzi G, Angelini C, Negrin P, Pierobon S, Fedele D. Sensory, motor, and autonomic neuropathy in patients with multiple symmetric lipomatosis. Medicine 1986;64:388—389.
28. Leffell DJ, Braverman IM. Familial multiple lipomatosis—report of a case and a review of the literature. 1986;15:275–279.
29. Halldorsdottir A, Ekelund L, Rydholm A. CT-diagnosis of lipomatous tumors of the soft tissues. Arch Orthop Trauma Surg 1982; 100:211–218.
30. Rubenstein R, Roenigk HH, Garden JM, Goldberg NS, Pinski JB. Liposuction for lipomas. J Dermatol Surg Oncol 1985;11:1070–1072.
31. Powell B, McLean NR. The treatment of lipomas by the "squeeze" technique. J R Coll Surg Edinb 1985;30:391–392.
32. Wu K. Liposarcoma of the ankle. J Foot Surg 198;27:276–279.
33. Kimbrough RF, Soule EH. Liposarcoma of the extremities. Clin Orthop 1961;19:40–43.
34. Rossouw DJ, Cinti S, Dickerson GR. Liposarcoma. Am J Cell Pathol 1986;85:649–653.
35. Kelly PC, Shramowiat M. Liposarcoma of the foot: a case report. J Foot Surg 1978;17:27–30.
36. Eisenberg LA. Myxoid liposarcoma—a case report. J Am Podiatr Assoc 1968;58:267–271.
37. Pack GT, Pierson JC. Liposarcoma. Surgery 1964;36:687–695.
38. Wilson G, Adelman KA, Gventer M. Radiation osteitis in the foot. A case report. 1989; 79:146–149.
39. Sarkar K, Buckley C, Uhthoff HK. Liposarcoma simulating a Baker's cyst: a case study. Arch Orthop Trauma Surg 1986;105:316–315.
40. Simon MA, Enneking WF. The management of soft-tissue sarcomas of the extremities. J Bone Joint Surg 1976;58A:317–321.
41. Caprio F, Lanza R, Amoroso L, Manzotti M, Cerioni M, Fabbri M, Nicolini S. Computed tomographic findings and clinicopathologic features of intramuscular lipoma. Rays 1985; 10:39–41.
42. Chew FS, Hudson TM. Radionuclide imaging of lipoma and liposarcoma. Radiology 1980; 136:741–743.
43. Varma DGK, Muchmore JH, Mizushima A. Computed tomography of infiltrating benign lipoma. 1987;11:45–49.
44. Dooms GC, Hricak H, Sollitto RA, Higgins CB. Lipomatous tumors and tumors with fatty com-

ponent: MR Imaging potential and comparison of MR and CT results. Radiology 1985; 157: 479–483.

45. Hallel T, Lew S, Bansal M. Villous lipomatous proliferation of the synovial membrane (lipoma arborescens). J Bone Joint Surg 1988; 70A:264–266.

46. Berlin SJ. Soft somatic tumors of the foot. Philadelphia: Futura Publishing Company, 1975.

47. Amadio PC, Reiman HM, Dobyns JH. Lipofibromatous hamartoma of nerve. J Hand Surg 1988;13A:67–71.

Part G/ **Cutaneous Neoplasms of the Foot and Leg**

—Christopher W. Sciales

Robert A. Schwartz

W. Clark Lambert

There are a number of cutaneous neoplasms of the foot. Almost any skin neoplasm may be seen there, from benign appendageal ones to premalignancies and both primary and metastatic cancers (1). However, there are a few tumors in the above categories which merit special attention, as they have a predilection for the foot.

NONMELANOCYTIC CUTANEOUS TUMORS OF THE LEG AND FOOT
Benign Cutaneous Tumors
EPIDERMAL

Stucco keratoses are small grayish stuck-on papules which appear symmetrically on the distal legs and ankles (Fig. 5.47). They are best considered a special type of seborrheic keratoses. The more common seborrheic keratosis is a well-demarcated papule or nodule that begins to appear on patients after age 30. It has a characteristic "stuck-on" appearance with a verrucous surface. Although most common on the face, shoulders, and back, it is known to appear on the lower extremities. It may, at times, be difficult to distinguish from the common wart.

Multiple punctate hyperkeratoses of the palms and soles (Fig. 5.48) is a relatively common, autosomal dominant condition which may require distinction from precancerous arsenical keratosis (2). These lesions present as multiple, discrete, hyperkeratotic papules, gradually enlarging with age that, when picked, form a punctate depression which may appear somewhat reminiscent of common pitted keratolysis, a condition caused by a gram-positive filamentous bacteria (3). Punctate hyperkeratosis of the palms and soles may be seen in a wide variety of disease, including the basal cell nevus syndrome and Cowden's disease, the latter being a marker for thyroid and breast cancer (2, 4).

The eccrine poroma is a somewhat common epidermal tumor with a predilection for the soles and sides of the feet in patients over the age of 40. It usually presents a solitary, firm, erythematous nodule or papule which may occasionally ulcerate at points of pressure (5). Porokeratotic eccrine ostial and dermal duct nevus, a rare congenital type of eccrine duct tumor, must also be considered. It classically presents in young patients as multiple, pruritic, keratotic papules and comedo-like pits on the medial border of the foot. An adult-onset form has been described (6). These

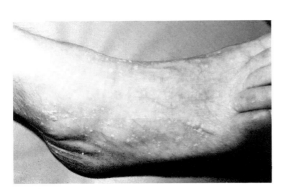

Figure 5.47. Stucco keratoses, foot.

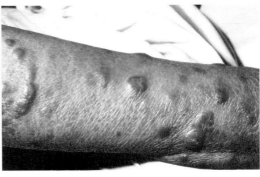

Figure 5.48. Nodules of histoid leproma (lepromatous leprosy).

cutaneous neoplasms must be distinguished from granulomas and other processes affecting the feet, such as lepromas (Fig. 5.49) (7, 8).

The keratoacanthoma is a common, benign, cutaneous tumor found most often on sun-exposed areas of the skin of older individuals. The lesion presents as a rapidly growing, yet spontaneously resolving, dome-shaped nodule with a central keratotic core (Fig. 5.50). It may histologically and clinically resemble a squamous cell carcinoma (9, 10). This common neoplasm may be solitary or multiple and is best viewed as a failed squamous cell carcinoma. Malignant transformation is very rare. Keratoacanthomas usually spontaneously involute, although they may be best handled with an incisional biopsy. Total excision, intralesional 5-fluorouracil, and curettage and electrodesiccation are therapeutic options.

Other benign foot alterations include cysts and acanthosis nigricans. Cutaneous cysts of the foot may also be seen, usually the common epidermal inclusion cyst and, rarely, the cutaneous ciliated cyst (11). These lesions are slow-growing, firm, dome-shaped nodules occurring most commonly on the scalp, face, neck, and back. Occasionally, a widespread neoplastic growth of epidermis of the foot may be seen, with velvety and hyperpigmented hyperplasia. This special type of acanthosis nigricans, called acral acanthotic anomaly, is not associated with an underlying malignancy (12). Acanthosis nigricans itself may be associated with a diffuse hyperkeratosis of the palms and soles. It is an important marker for internal disease, usually endocrinologic or malignant in nature.

Several modalities may be employed in the treatment of benign epidermal tumors. Curettage, cyrosurgery, laser surgery, local excision, electrodesiccation, and other procedures have all been employed successfully; choice of treatment is dependent upon size, location, and type of tumor.

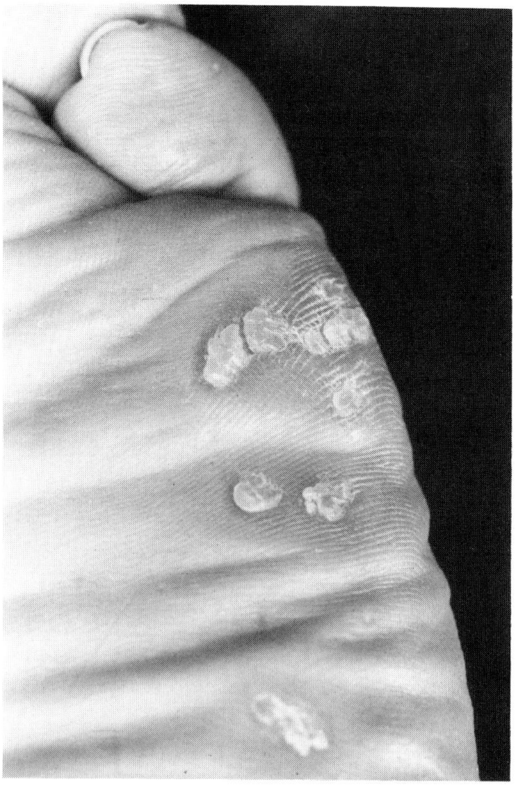

Figure 5.49. Punctate hyperkeratoses of the sole. (From Rubenstein DJ, Schwartz RA, Hansen RC, Payne CM. Punctate hyperkeratosis of the palms and soles: an ultrastructural study. J Am Acad Dermatol 1980;3:43.)

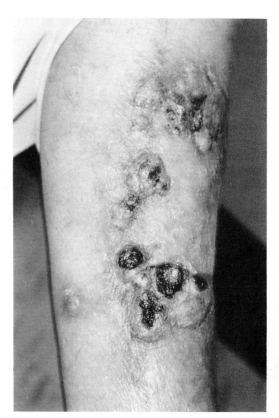

Figure 5.50. Multiple keratoacanthomas. (From Schwartz RA. Skin cancer: recognition and management. New York: Springer-Verlag, 1988;49.)

DERMAL

Benign dermal neoplasms of the foot include benign growths of any of the dermal elements. As a possible result of gravitational forces, vascular neoplasms seem to be well-represented in this category and are discussed first.

The most common tumors of the foot associated with blood vessels are angiokeratoma circumscriptum, pyogenic granuloma, capillary hemangiomas, and the glomus tumor. Appearing as solitary or clustered violaceous small papules on the feet, angiokeratoma circumscriptum may resemble melanoma (13, 14). The lesions tend to enlarge and become more keratotic with advancing age.

The glomus tumor is a benign soft-tissue proliferation of epithelioid cells surrounding blood vessels. The glomus cells are thought to originate from smooth muscle cells. Although its typical location is beneath the fingernails, it may occur on the toes as well (15). The solitary glomus tumor is usually a small violaceous nodule which may be associated with attacks of paroxysmal pain. The pain may be initiated by pressure, temperature changes, or other environmental alterations. Multiple glomus tumors are less common and not as likely to be associated with pain. They may be inherited in an autosomal dominant fashion. Complete relief of symptoms usually follows after simple excision. Recurrence occurred in 4 of 35 patients in one series (15). Like the pyogenic granuloma, the glomus tumor may be a reactive proliferation rather than a true neoplasm.

The pyogenic granuloma is neither pyogenic nor a granuloma. Rather, it is a proliferating benign tumor that tends to appear in younger patients as a single polypoid or sessile red nodule. This nontender nodule may develop superficial ulceration and crusting over its smooth surface and may bleed with mild trauma (16). Cavernous hemangiomas are large subcutaneous masses that may be seen in solitary form or may be associated with a number of syndromes (17). In the Kasabach-Merritt syndrome, extensive hemangiomas sometimes associated with glomus tumors are associated with thrombocytopenia and purpura, representing a consumption coagulopathy (18). In Maffucci's syndrome the cavernous hemangiomas are associated with dyschondroplasia, bone fragility, and osteochondromas (19).

Other benign dermal tumors of the foot vary widely. Giant cell tendon sheath tumors, dermatofibromas, angioleiomyomas, neurofibromas, lipomas, dermatofibromas, and digital mucous cysts are among the most common in this category. We will also discuss dermatomal digital papillary adenomas, clear cell acanthomas, and multicentric reticulohistiocytomas.

The angioleiomyoma tends to appear as a painful cutaneous nodule of the lower extremities, often of the lower leg and ankle (20). Digital papillary adenomas appear as solitary painless masses on the toes adjacent to the soles (21). The giant cell tumor of tendon sheath appears as a solitary nodule usually adherent to tendons, tendon sheaths, and joint capsules (22). This benign tumor is probably best classified as a type of fibrous histiocytoma. The dermatofibroma, or histiocytoma of the leg, is also very common, appearing as solitary or multiple dome-shaped cutaneous nodules, frequently on the lower extremities of women (23). Multiple dermatofibromas may be associated with systemic lupus erythematosus. Neurofibromas usually appear as soft, often compressible, skin-colored cutaneous nodules; patients with these should be evaluated for neurofibromatosis, the most common form of which is von Recklinghausen's disease (24). Multicentric reticulohistiocytosis may involve the foot as multiple nonpruritic reddish-brown or violaceous nodules up to 1 cm in diameter. Patients with this syndrome of cutaneous neoplasms and arthritis have an increased risk of internal malignancy (25, 26). The lipoma appears as solitary or multiple subcutaneous nodules varying in size from small and imperceptible to huge and disfiguring (27). The clear cell acanthoma is an unusual benign tumor with a predilection for the lower legs (28). It appears as a dome-shaped, sharply delineated, erythematous plaque or nodule with fine stippling and a wafer-like adherent scale at the periphery. This characteristic presentation suggests the diagnosis.

Once biopsy-proven, most benign dermal tumors may be treated with many of the common dermatologic and surgical modalities available. Effective modes of treatment include simple excision, cryosurgery, laser surgery, electrodesiccation, and curettage.

Premalignant Cutaneous Tumors

Premalignant cutaneous tumors of the foot are uncommonly observed and include arsenical keratoses and scar keratoses (1, 29). Arsenical keratoses (Fig. 5.51) appear as corn-like, hard, yellowish papules which may

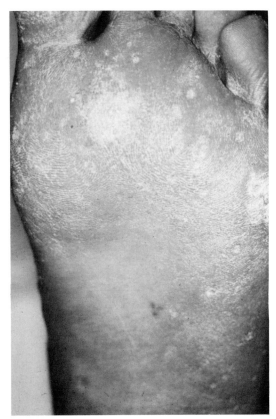

Figure 5.51. Arsenical keratoses, sole. (From Schwartz RA. Skin cancer: recognition and management. New York: Springer-Verlag, 1988;12.)

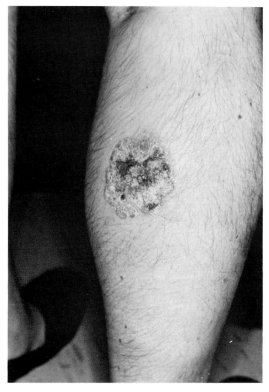

Figure 5.52. Bowen's disease of the leg. (From Holland JF, Frei E. Cancer and the skin. In: Cancer medicine, 2nd ed., Philadelphia: Lea & Febiger, 1982;2057–2108.)

progress into verrucous plaques (30). These must be distinguished from the various benign forms of hyperkeratoses of the palms and soles. Lesions may evolve into carcinoma in situ, or Bowen's disease (Fig. 5.52); however, the majority of arsenical dermatoses persist for years without progressing to invasive squamous cell carcinoma. Scar keratoses appear with the same cutaneous morphology, usually at the site of a scarring process, such as an old osteomyelitis scar, or a chronic genodermatosis, such as epidermolysis bullosa dystrophica (Fig. 5.53) (31). These lesions also have significant malignant potential. Treatment options for arsenical and scar keratoses are numerous and depend on the location, size, and type of lesion involved. Laser surgery, cryosurgery, electrodesiccation, and curettage, as well as simple excision, have all been successfully employed. Favorable results in patients with arsenical keratoses have been obtained with oral retinoid therapy (32).

Malignant Cutaneous Tumors of the Foot

There are many cutaneous cancers affecting the foot. We will discuss primary epidermal carcinomas, sarcomas, lymphomas, metastatic cancers, and melanomas.

EPIDERMAL

Most epidermal carcinomas can affect the leg and foot. As solar exposure at this site may be less important than other carcinogenic stimuli, these cancers tend to result from chronic scars (scar carcinomas) or other factors including, most likely, human papillomavirus infection (verrucous carcinoma) (1).

Squamous cell carcinoma is one of the most common skin cancers and usually arises within solar keratoses on sun-exposed skin. However, on the lower extremities, this malignancy mostly arises from chronic scars, ulcers, and points of constant irritation. These scar carcinomas tend to be more aggressive than those that are solar-induced. The interval between

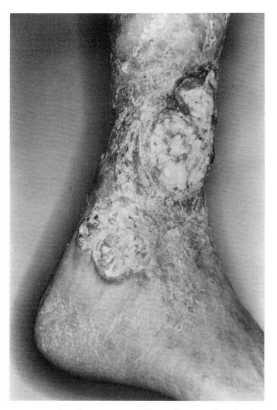

Figure 5.53. Squamous cell carcinoma developing in patient with autosomal dominant epidermolysis bullosa. (From Schwartz RA. Skin cancer: recognition and management. New York: Springer-Verlag, 1988;38.)

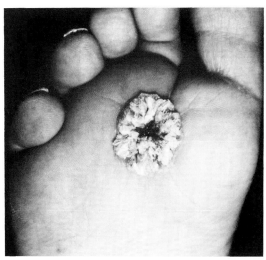

Figure 5.54. Verrucous carcinoma of the foot. (From Schwartz RA. Skin cancer: recognition and management. New York: Springer-Verlag, 1988;41.)

onset of the initial condition and onset of malignancy is, on average, 23 years (33). Lesions can present in a variety of ways, sometimes as ulcerations with raised edges or as hyperkeratotic nodules (31). Any chronic process may be affected, from epidermolysis bullosa acquisita and linear porokeratosis of Mibelli to leprous neurotrophic ulcers (31, 34). Metastatic potential in such lesions is real.

Verrucous carcinoma of the sole (epithelioma cuniculatum) is a well-differentiated type of squamous cell carcinoma that rarely metastasizes but can be locally invasive (35, 36). It typically appears on the sole or heel as an expansile, sharply demarcated tumor, with multiple, foul-smelling crypts (Fig. 5.54). Often, these tumors are mistakenly treated as a recalcitrant wart for many years before the correct diagnosis is made. The tumor may, at times, cause significant morbidity, including pain with ambulating. Its cause is unclear, al-

though it has been postulated to be related to a human papilloma virus. The clinical differential diagnosis includes amelanotic melanoma, basal cell carcinoma, and eccrine poroma. Once the correct diagnosis is made, a wide excision is usually the most effective treatment. Radiation therapy is contraindicated since it has a tendency to convert tumor into a more malignant form with an increased likelihood of metastasis.

The basal cell carcinoma is the most common sun-induced tumor of light-complected persons. It may also arise on the legs and feet, sometimes without solar exposure as a likely carcinogenic stimulus. Basal cell carcinomas may be seen in chronic lymphedematous legs or may present in the legs or feet without apparent predisposing factors or as part of the basal cell nevus syndrome (37, 38).

DERMAL

There are a number of dermal sarcomas of the foot and leg. The most important one is Kaposi's sarcoma, which will be covered in depth after the less common ones are discussed. We limit our comments to malignant angioendotheliomatosis, synovial sarcoma, epithelioid sarcoma, malignant eccrine poroma, digital papillary adenocarcinoma, and neurofibrosarcoma. Patients with extremity soft-tissue tumors may be evaluated by magnetic resonance imaging, computed tomography, and other techniques (39); however, one should recall that the diagnosis of a malignancy is always a histologic one.

Malignant angioendotheliomatosis is a rare condition characterized by a multifocal proliferation of malignant mononuclear cells found within the lumen of venules, arterioles, and capillaries. Originally thought to be a neoplasm of endothelial cells, recent immunofluorescent and immunochemical studies confirm its lymphoid origin and, thus, it has been reclassified as an angiotropic lymphoma (40, 41). Malignant angioendotheliomatosis typically presents as erythematous or violaceous macules, nodules, or plaques. Constitutional symptoms and fever are often present and multisystem involvement is common. Chemotherapy may mitigate symptoms, but the prognosis remains poor.

Epithelioid sarcoma, a malignant soft-tissue tumor that affects the extremities of young adults, often arises near tendons and may present as a firm, slow-growing subcutaneous nodule with a central depression and surrounding ulceration. Unfortunately, this malignancy is frequently misinterpreted, clinically and histologically, as a benign condition, usually as some type of granuloma. This may further delay the diagnosis. Distant metastases occur frequently, and prognosis is poor (43). This must be distinguished from synovial sarcoma, a rare neoplasm that also affects the lower extremities of young adults where it may present as a tender subcutaneous mass (44).

Malignant eccrine poroma, also known as eccrine porocarcinoma, is a rare malignancy that is thought to arise either de novo or from an existing benign eccrine poroma. It tends to occur on the lower extremities of older individuals as a solitary, occasionally ulcerated, polypoid nodule or plaque with a verrucous surface. These lesions metastasize widely and respond poorly to therapy (45, 46). Digital papillary adenocarcinoma, another eccrine malignancy, may present as a solitary, painless mass on the toes and adjacent sole. In one series, 47% recurred locally after treatment, and 41% had metastases, most commonly to the lung (47).

Neurofibrosarcoma is a malignant transformation of existing neurofibromas usually seen in patients with von Recklinghausen's disease, a form of neurofibromatosis. It commonly occurs between 20 and 50 years of age, and has a predilection for the lower extremities. Lesions present as a rapid growth of a preexisting lesion, and metastasize widely. Prognosis is poor (48).

Kaposi's Sarcoma

Kaposi's sarcoma (KS), also known as idiopathic, multiple, pigmented sarcoma of the skin, is a form of angiosarcoma first described by Kaposi in 1872 (49). It classically affects older men of Jewish or Mediterranean descent with skin lesions having a predilection for the lower extremities. In this form, it is quite rare, with a reported incidence of 0.021–0.061/100,000 population (50, 51). Recently KS has been increasingly reported in patients receiving immunosuppressive therapy, particularly in renal transplant recipients. The prevalence of KS among these patients is reported in one study to be 2.4%, a greater than fifty-fold increase over the general population (52). Since 1979, KS has been reported with increasing frequency in patients afflicted with acquired immune deficiency syndrome (AIDS), particularly in male homosexuals. A 1985 survey of AIDS patients revealed that 36% of male homosexuals had KS, compared with only 4.3% of intravenous drug abusers (53).

The lesions of "classic" KS are usually distributed symmetrically over the lower extremities, including the feet. Lesions of KS in AIDS show a preferential distribution on the head, neck, and trunk. In either presentation, the lesions may begin as flat, discrete, violaceous patches (Fig. 5.55), nodules (Fig. 5.56), or plaques (54). They may also appear as pink, translucent, and telangiectatic (55), as keratotic cutaneous hornlike lesions, or as dark purple or black, suggestive of a melanoma. Rarely, KS is reported to be bullous (56). The clinical classification of KS is characterized as follows: localized nonaggressive, which includes (a) patch stage KS and (b) localized (nondestructive) nodular KS; locally aggressive, which includes (a) exophytic KS and (b) infiltrative KS; and disseminated, which includes (a) generalized lymphadenopathic KS with widespread cutaneous nodules and (b) widespread visceral disease.

Locally aggressive KS may be firmly adherent to underlying anatomic structures, including bone. It may also occur as a large infiltrating mass (infiltrative KS) or as multiple cone-shaped friable tumors (exophytic). KS can disseminate, spreading to the lymph nodes, internal organs, and bone. Most patients have multiple lesions. Thus, a lesion on the foot may be a sign of other cutaneous and visceral ones.

The etiology of KS is unknown. Cytomegaloviruses have been implicated, although the

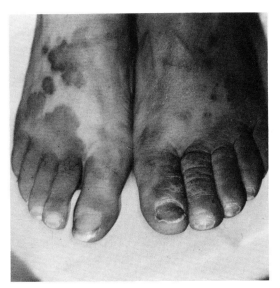

Figure 5.55. Patch stage Kaposi's sarcoma. (From Schwartz RA. Skin cancer: recognition and management. New York: Springer-Verlag, 1988;85.)

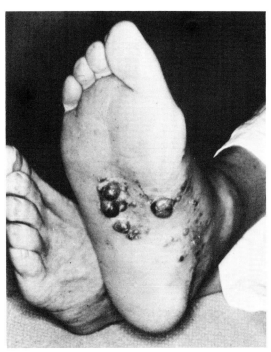

Figure 5.56. Kaposi's sarcoma, nodular stage. (From Schwartz RA. Skin cancer: recognition and management. New York: Springer-Verlag, 1988;85.)

human immunodeficiency virus itself may be the cause. Lymphedema may also be interrelated with KS formation (57). It is well-established that chronic lymphedema predisposes to the induction of an angiosarcoma similar to KS (58). This type of lymphangiosarcoma most often develops in women with chronic lymphedema after mastectomy and is called the Stewart-Treves syndrome (59). It also may occur in patients with congenital lymphedema of the legs (Milroy's disease), chronic varicose leg ulcerations (60), or chronic leg lymphedema from trauma or surgery (61). This is rarely a complication of superficial node dissection of the groin, but is an important complication of deep dissection of the groin.

Histopathologic examination of KS usually reveals a normal epidermis and replacement of the reticular dermis with an increase in vascular structures and spindle cells (Fig. 5.57). The vascular spaces are lined by swollen endothelial cells, and lesions may contain numerous extravasated erythrocytes and an increased amount of hemosiderin pigment. Hyperkeratosis may be seen on plantar lesions. Immunohistochemistry techniques are useful to confirm the endothelial origin of KS tumor cells (62).

In immunocompetent individuals, KS tends to run an indolent course, and the patient usually dies from other unrelated medical problems. In immunosuppressed patients, particularly those with AIDS, KS is often an aggressive

malignancy that quickly leads to the patient's demise. In a study conducted on Ugandan patients, those with localized nodular disease had the best prognosis with no reported deaths to KS; those with locally aggressive disease had a 64% three-year survival rate. The generalized pattern had a 0% 3-year survival rate (63). It is this latter form which appears to be prevalent in AIDS patients.

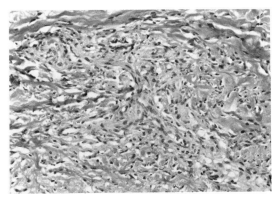

Figure 5.57. Histologic view of nodular stage Kaposi's sarcoma, showing a normal epidermis and a dermis filled with spindle cells. Vascular slits and extravasated red blood cells are evident.

Treatment of KS is dependent upon the extent of the disease and the general health of the patient. In patients with AIDS, one must evaluate the benefits of treatment with the risks of further compromising immune function (64). In non-AIDS associated KS, specific therapy may not be indicated in the early stages of the disease. In advanced local disease, cutaneous lesions may be removed with laser or conventional surgery, radiotherapy, or chemotherapy. In the latter modality, success with systemic and intralesional vinblastine has been reported. Systemic treatment may be advantageous in that it also attacks covert visceral lesions (65).

Cutaneous Lymphoma

Lymphoma and leukemia involve the skin, including cutaneous surfaces of the foot and leg. Cutaneous lymphomas may be preceded by a widespread papular eruption called lymphomatoid papulosis (66), or by large patches of erythema and scaling called large plaque parapsoriasis (67). As the lymphoma or leukemia progresses, plaque or tumor formation with or without ulceration occurs whether the lymphoma is of T cell type, (i.e., mycosis fungoides (68)), or of B cell origin (69).

Cutaneous Metastatic Disease

Cutaneous metastasis occur in up to 9% of all cancer patients and is occasionally the initial presenting complaint of the primary cancer. In one recent series of cancer patients who had cutaneous skin involvement at presentation, 64% had not yet been diagnosed of their underlying malignancy (70a). After treatment, skin lesions may also represent the first sign of recurrence. The frequency of metastases largely depends upon the type of cancer. In women, breast and colon cancer, respectively, were the most common types associated with cutaneous disease. In men, lung, colon, and melanoma cancers were the most common.

Clinically, cutaneous metastases do not have any specific clinical description, although many appear as nonspecific painless subcutaneous nodules, papules, or indurated plaques. They can be flesh-colored or hyperpigmented, and rock-hard when palpated. The morphology and distribution of the metastases do not necessarily reflect the primary malignancy. Lesions of the lower extremities that are suspicious for metastatic disease must be differentiated from primary skin cancers and benign growths, e.g., dermatofibromas or granu-lomas. Metastatic lesions usually respond to systemic chemotherapy, although local excision or radiotherapy may be palliative.

MELANOCYTIC TUMORS OF THE LEG AND FOOT
Benign Cutaneous Tumors

Lentigo simplex, a benign lentigo, is a symmetrical, light-brown oval macule that is usually 5–10 mm in diameter. These spots can appear anywhere on the skin, and histologically are characterized by increased numbers of melanocytes in the basal layers of elongated rete ridges. They are usually acquired during childhood and do not have malignant potential. However, when present on the volar surfaces, the lesion may be indistinguishable from acral melanoma. Rarely, widespread lentiginosis may be part of a variety of syndromes, including Peutz-Jeghers syndrome, leopard syndrome, and inherited patterned lentiginosis in Blacks (71). Lentigo-like lesions of the sole have also been reported to be acral lentiginous melanoma in situ (72).

Acquired melanocytic nevi, or common moles, are the most frequently encountered pigmented lesions. These lesions are small, pigmented macules or papules that are acquired after 6 months of age and reach their maximum number in the second decade. Nevi are well-circumscribed and uniform in color, size, and symmetry. In one study, nevi were the lesions most frequently confused with melanoma (73).

There are three types of common melanocytic nevi: junctional, compound, and intradermal. All may appear on the lower leg and the foot. Junctional nevi are the common mole of childhood and present as flat, hyperpigmented macules which may remain the same size, or grow very slowly over many years. Histologically, one sees nests of melanocytes above the dermoepidermal junction. Compound nevi are small, dome-shaped papules that appear most often in adults. They may be flesh-colored or pigmented, and are thought to develop from junctional nevi as the nevus cells drop down into the dermis. Malignant degeneration is very rare. Intradermal nevi are well-circumscribed, flesh-colored papules that frequently contain hairs. Histologically, nevus cells are located only in the dermis. These lesions commonly occur on the head and neck; they are not known to occur on the volar surfaces.

The blue nevus is a dark blue or black papule that measures approximately 5 mm. It is most commonly located on the dorsum of the hand and foot, and may be seen on the head, neck, and buttocks as well. Histologically, one sees numerous dendritic and spindle-shaped cells in the middle and deep dermis. The cellular blue nevus is usually a bit larger, and tends to occur in the deep dermis and internal structures. It is known to spread to lymph nodes and has, therefore, on occasion, been confused with metastatic melanoma (74).

The spitz nevus, or spindle-cell and epithelioid cell nevus, occurs most commonly in children and young adults, and, histologically, may be difficult to distinguish from melanoma. It usually appears as a pink, red, or darkly pigmented dome-shaped nodule on the face or trunk. Spitz nevi may attain a diameter greater than 1 cm and extend into surrounding subcutaneous adipose tissue and nearby lymph nodes. This aggressive variant is called a malignant spitz nevus and, in a recent study, most commonly occurred on the legs. However, further metastases are very unusual and the tumor is generally considered benign (75).

Premalignant Cutaneous Tumors

Congenital melanocytic nevi appear at birth or shortly thereafter, affecting about 1% of newborns. These lesions are usually larger than acquired nevi and present as brown to black macules which, over time, become raised and typically hairy. Although the lesions appear infrequently on the foot, they are known to be precursors to melanoma and, therefore, must be considered whenever a large, pigmented macule or plaque appears on the lower extremities. Risk of malignant transformation is known to occur at a rate of 2–5% in large or giant congenital melanocytic nevi of over 20 cm (76). Early excision is recommended before adulthood.

Dysplastic nevi are acquired melanocytic nevi which serve as markers for melanoma susceptibility. These lesions may appear sporadically in individuals or may be familial. In the latter, the risk of melanoma is increased tremendously. Thus, a thorough family history of the patient may be valuable. Clinically, the lesions appear as ill-defined, hyperpigmented macules or papules, with variegated pigmentation and irregular borders. They are generally a bit larger than ordinary nevi (5–10 mm) and may show evidence of surrounding erythema.

They should be excised and confirmed by histologic examination. These patients require close follow-up care (77). In the full blown presentation, the dysplastic nevus syndrome, occurring as an autosomal dominant condition with partial penetrance, may present with too many dysplastic nevi to excise. These patients must be followed closely, and those nevi that appear to change are to be removed at each visit.

Malignant Cutaneous Tumors
MELANOMA

Melanoma is a malignancy of the pigment-producing cells that are derived from neural crest tissue. Although it represents only 3% of all skin cancers, melanoma accounts for almost three-fourths of all deaths due to cutaneous malignancies (78). When recognized early, melanoma is nearly always curable; thus, it is imperative for the podiatrist to clinically and histologically evaluate all suspicious pigmented skin lesions.

The incidence of melanoma increases with age and most commonly affects the sun-exposed skin of fair-complected individuals. However, melanoma may arise on areas that receive little or no sun exposure, e.g., the foot and soles. In Blacks and Asians, melanoma is extremely rare, but when present most frequently appears on the foot. In a recent survey of Japanese patients, melanoma of the foot occurred in 34.5% of melanoma cases (79); in Black patients, 81% of melanoma cases were of the foot (80). This contrasts to Whites, in which melanoma is more prevalent overall, but only 5% of cases are located acrally. It must be pointed out that the absolute incidence of acral melanoma is similar in all races; it is only the distribution pattern that varies (1).

A patient's history of a sudden change in size or color of an existing mole or nevus, or complaints of pruritus, bleeding, or even pain of a skin lesion may be indicative of melanoma. Clinically, there are many features which help to differentiate melanoma from a benign tumor. Grossly, melanoma may present as an irregularly shaped, hyperpigmented macule, papule, nodule, or plaque. Notching of the border and areas of ulcerations, crusts, and inflammation may be noted. Close inspection may reveal hues of red, white, and blue, in addition to brown and black. Areas of tumor regression may be seen within the lesion. Verrucous changes in melanoma are also reported

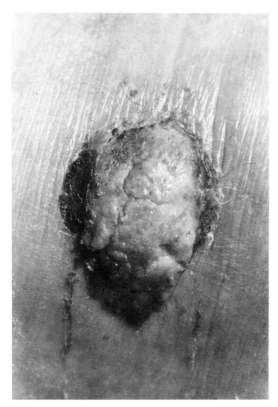

Figure 5.58. Verrucous melanoma, leg. (From Schwartz RA, Hill WE, Hansen RC, Fleishman JS. Verrucous malignant melanoma. J Dermatol Surg Oncol 1980;6:719.)

(Fig. 5.58), and it may be clinically difficult to distinguish from benign growths such as seborrheic keratoses (81).

There are four major clinicopathologic types of melanoma: (a) superficial spreading melanoma, (b) nodular melanoma, (c) lentigo maligna melanoma, and (d) acral lentiginous melanoma. Each type of melanoma carries a different incident rate and prognosis. All may appear on the lower extremities; however, it is the acral lentiginous melanoma that has a predilection for the volar surfaces and is the most common type found on the foot (82).

Superficial spreading melanoma is the most common and has a predilection for the lower extremities in women. This lesion presents as a flat, hyperpigmented macule or plaque, with irregular borders. Superficial spreading melanoma has a relatively good prognosis. Nodular melanoma accounts for about 15–20% of all melanoma and is particularly aggressive. The presenting lesion progresses rapidly to form a hyperpigmented nodule that may ulcerate. It

has a poor prognosis. Lentigo maligna melanoma accounts for less than 5–10% of all melanoma and arises from a preexisting macule known as a lentigo maligna. This lesion, characteristically, appears on the face and other sun-exposed areas as a large pigmented macule. It may spread slowly over years or even decades before becoming invasive (79).

Acral lentiginous melanoma is the most common clinicohistologic type of melanoma in dark-complected individuals, occurring most often on the sole and less frequently on the palm and subungual areas (83). Of those appearing on the sole, about half involve the heel (Fig. 5.59). Acral lentiginous melanoma may initially appear as a hyperpigmented macule with variegated colors and notched borders. Flat lesions may have an unexpectedly deep invasion. After an initial radial growth phase of months to years, nodules or papules may appear in the central part of the lesion, signifying the onset of the vertical growth phase (84).

An uncommon type of acral melanoma is that which occurs in the subungual areas; these make up from 1 to 3% of all melanomas in Whites and up to 25% among Chinese (85). When involving the foot, the great majority of these tumors appear on the large toe (86). Subungual melanoma may present on the nail as a longitudinal, hyperpigmented streak, as a split nail, or with ulceration and crusting. Variegated colors within the nail bed should be cause for concern. Leaching of pigment from the nail bed to the proximal or lateral nail folds is characteristic of subungual melanoma and is known as Hutchinson's sign (87). Subungual melanoma must be distinguished from trau-

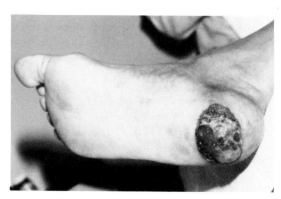

Figure 5.59. Acral lentiginous melanoma affecting the heel of a 57-year-old Japanese male.

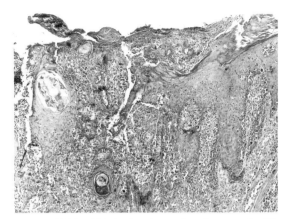

Figure 5.60. Histologic view of melanoma in Fig. 5.60 showing malignant melanocytes streaming into the dermis.

matic nail injury, foreign body, melanocytic and congenital subungual nevi, various infections of the nail, and other benign conditions (88, 89).

The histopathologic appearance of melanoma reveals an increased number of atypical melanocytes that may invade and distort the epidermis and dermoepidermal junction (Fig. 5.60). Nests of melanocytes may vary greatly in size and be confluent. The nuclei of melanocytes are enlarged and pleomorphic and do not exhibit normal maturation as they descend into the dermis. Prominent nucleoli may be noted. Acral lentiginous melanoma may show a distinctive lentiginous pattern in which there is elongation of the rete ridges with hyperpigmentation and increased numbers of melanocytes. Melanocytes of acral lentiginous melanoma are reported to possess particularly prominent dendritic processes as seen in benign volar lesions, thus further confusing the diagnosis (90, 91).

Melanoma is most often clinically staged as locally invasive lesions (stage I), regional nodal disease (stage II), or disseminated disease (stage III); the latter carries a consistently poor prognosis. For stage I disease, the metastatic potential increases dramatically upon entering the vertical growth phase, in which the tumor invades the deep dermis and subcutaneous fat. One can estimate prognosis by determining level of tumor invasion, known as Clark's levels of invasion (92), and tumor thickness, which was described by Breslow (93). Clark's levels of invasion are correlated directly with incidence of nodal metastases and subse-

quently, survival of the patient. Breslow's thickness of melanoma is measured by the use of an ocular micrometer and is also directly correlated with incidence of lymph node metastases and prognosis (94, 95). A depth of less than 0.85 mm measured from the stratum granulosum to the deepest portion of the tumor carries a very good prognosis if adequate local excision is carried out.

Any suspicious lesion of the foot or toenail should be biopsied and examined histologically. Biopsy-proven lesions must be staged. Wide local excision of the primary tumor is usually performed and regional lymph node dissection may be indicated depending on the degree of invasion and location of tumor. Melanoma of the sole is usually, unfortunately, quite advanced, and, as a substitute for amputation, local excision of the tumor along with limb perfusion employing a chemotherapeutic agent may be employed by those familiar with the technique (96). Small superficial lesions, however, are adequately removed with a 1–2-cm margin on all sides with careful follow-up for local recurrence. Mutilating surgery for small superficial lesions should be avoided if possible.

REFERENCES

1. Schwartz RA. Skin cancer: recognition and management. New York: Springer-Verlag, 1988.
2. Rubenstein DJ, Schwartz RA, Hansen RC, Payne CM. Punctate hyperkeratosis of the palms and soles: an ultrastructural study. J Am Acad Dermatol 1980;3:43–50.
3. Stanton RL, Schwartz RA, Aly R. Pitted keratolysis: a clinicopathological review. J Am Podiatr Assoc 1982;72:436–439.
4. Shapiro SD, Schwartz RA, Lambert WC. Cowden's disease: a marker of internal malignancy. Int J Dermatol 1988;27:232–237.
5. Moeller CA, Welch RH, Kaplan DL. Enlarging tumor of foot. Arch Dermatol 1987;123:653–654.
6. Stoof TJ, Starink TM, Nieboer C. Porokeratotic eccrine ostial and dermal duct nevus. Report of a case of adult onset. J Am Acad Dermatol 1989;20:924–927.
7. Robertozzi C, Aronson L, Schwartz RA. Localized granuloma annulare involving the feet. J Am Podiatr Assoc 1982;72:94–97.
8. Janniger CK, Kapila R, Schwartz RA, Lewis WR, Lambert WC. Histoid lepromas in lepromatous leprosy. Int J Dermatol, in press.
9. Schwartz RA. The keratoacanthoma: a review. J Surg Oncol 1979;12:305–317.
10. Schwartz RA. Multiple persistent keratoacanthomas. Oncology 1979;36:281–285.
11. Ross AJ, Schwartz RA. Ciliated cutaneous cyst of the foot. J Surg Oncol 1983;24:90–93.

12. Schwartz RA. Acral acanthotic anomaly (AAA). J Am Acad Dermatol 1981;5:345–346.
13. Goldman L, Gibson SH, Richfield DF. Thrombotic angiokeratoma circumscriptum simulating melanoma. Arch Dermatol 1981;117:138–139.
14. Rossi A, Bozzi M, Barra E. Verrucous hemangioma and angiokeratoma circumscriptum: clinical and histologic differential characteristics. J Dermatol Surg Oncol 1989;15: 88–91.
15. Tsuneyoshi M, Enjoji M. Glomus tumor. A clinicopathologic and electron microscopic study. Cancer 1982;50:1601–1607.
16. Bucci FA Jr, Wiener BD. The pyogenic granuloma. Ariz Med 1984;41:794–796.
17. Mihara M, Kambe N, Shimao S. Superficial spreading capillary hemangioma. A peculiar type of capillary hemangioma. Dermatologica 1986;172:116–119.
18. Phillippe M, Acker D, Frigoletto FD Jr. Pregnancy complicated by the Kasabach-Merritt syndrome. Obstet Gynecol 1980;56:256–258.
19. Anderson IF. Maffucci's syndrome: report of a case with review of the literature. S Afr Med J 1967;39:1066–1067.
20. Hachisuga T, Hashimoto H, Enjoji M. Angioleiomyoma. A clinicopathologic reappraisal of 562 cases. Cancer 1984;54:126–130.
21. Kao GF, Helwig EB, Graham JH. Aggressive digital papillary adenoma adenocarcinoma. A clinicopathological study of 57 patients, with histochemical, immunopathological, and ultrastructural observations. J Cutan Pathol 1987;14: 129–146.
22. Schwartz RA, Southwick GJ. Solitary multinodular giant cell tumor of tendon sheath. J Surg Oncol 1979;12:191–197.
23. Soini Y. Cell differentiation in benign cutaneous fibrous histiocytomas: an immunohistochemical study with antibodies to histiomonocytic cells and intermediate filament proteins. Am J Dermatopathol 1990;12:134–140.
24. Sanchez CMJ, Herrera SA. Segmental neurofibromatosis. J Am Acad Dermatol 1989; 20:681–682.
25. Coupe MO, Whittaker SJ, Thatcher N. Multicentric reticulohistiocytosis. Br J Dermatol 1987; 116:245–247.
26. Giknsburg WW, O'Duffy JD, Morris JL, Huston KA. Multicentric reticulohistiocytosis: response to alkylating agents in six patients. Ann Intern Med 1989;111:384–388.
27. Spinowitz AL. The treatment of multiple lipomas by liposuction surgery. J Dermatol Surg Oncol 1989;15:538–540.
28. Naeyaert JM, de Bersaques J, Geerts M-L, Kint A. Multiple clear cell acanthomas. A clinical, histological, and ultrastructural report. Arch Dermatol 1987;123:1670–1673.
29. Schoolmeester WL, White DR. Arsenic poisoning. South Med J 1980;73:198–208.
30. Southwick GJ, Schwartz RA. Arsenically associated cutaneous squamous cell carcinoma with hypercalcemia. J Surg Oncol 1979;12:115–118.
31. Schwartz RA, Birnkrant AP, Rubenstein DJ. Squamous cell carcinoma in dominant type epidermolysis bullosa dystrophica. Cancer 1981;47: 615–620.
32. Thianprasit M. Chronic cutaneous arsenicism treated with aromatic retinoid. J Med Assoc Thai 1984;67:93–100.
33. Stromberg BV, Keiter JE, Wray RC, Weeks PM. Scar carcinoma: prognosis and treatment. South Med J 1977;70:821–822.
34. Lozinski AZ, Fisher BK, Walter JB, Fitzpatrick PJ. Metastatic squamous cell carcinoma in linear porokeratosis of Mibelli. J Am Acad Dermatol 1987;16:448–451.
35. Schwartz RA. Verrucous carcinoma of the skin. In: Demis DJ, ed. Clinical dermatology. 11th ed. New York: Harper & Row, 1984;Unit 21–22, pp. 1–6.
36. Fugate DS, Romash MM. Carcinoma cuniculatum (verrucous carcinoma) of the foot. Foot Ankle 1989;9:257–259.
37. Benson PM, Pessoa CM, Lupton GP, Winton GB. Basal cell carcinomas arising in chronic lymphedema J Dermatol Surg Oncol 1988;14:781–783.
38. Southwick GJ, Schwartz RA. The basal cell nevus syndrome: disasters occurring among a series of 36 patients. Cancer 1979;44: 2294–2305.
39. Chang AE, Matory YL, Dwyer AJ, Suvimol CH, Girton ME, Steinberg SM, et al. Magnetic resonance imaging versus computed tomography in the evaluation of soft tissue tumors of the extremities. Ann Surg 1987;205:340–348.
40. Petroff N, Koger OW, Fleming MG, Fishleder A, Bergfeld WF, Tuthill R, et al. Malignant angioendotheliomatosis: an angiotropic lymphoma. J Am Acad Dermatol 1989;21:727–733.
41. Drobacheff C, Blanc D, Zultak M, Humbert P, Carbillet JP, Dupond JL, et al. Malignant angioendotheliomatosis. Int J Dermatol 1989; 28:454–456.
42. Gupta AK, Lipa M, Haberman HF. Proliferating angioendotheliomatosis. Arch Dermatol 1986; 122:314–319.
43. Manivel JC, Wick MR, Dehner LP, Sibley RK. Epithelioid sarcoma: an immunohistochemical study. Am J Clin Pathol 1987;87:319–326.
44. Abenoza P, Manivel JC, Swanson PE, Wick MR. Synovial sarcoma: ultrastructural study and immunohistochemical analysis by a combined peroxidase-antiperoxidase/avidin-biotin peroxidase complex procedure. Hum Pathol 1986;17: 1107–1115.
45. Puttick L, Ince P, Comaish JS. Three cases of eccrine porocarcinoma. Br J Dermatol 1986; 115:111–116.
46. Baril A, Claudy A, Boucheron S, Garcier F, Elbaz N. Le carcinome eccrine epidermotrope: a propos d'une observation avec etude ultra-structurale. Ann Pathol 1984;4:203–209.
47. Kao GF, Helwig EB, Graham JH. Aggressive digital papillary adenoma and adenocarcinoma. A clinicopathological study of 57 patients, with histochemical, immunopathological, and ultrastructural observations. J Cutan Pathol 1987;14:129–146.
48. Coleman BG, Arger PH, Dalinka MK, Obringer AC, Raney BR, Meadows AT. CT of sarcomatous degeneration in neurofibromatosis. AJR (Am J Roentgenol) 1983;140:383–387.
49. Kaposi M. Idiopathisches multiples pigmentsar-

kom der Haut. Arch Dermatol Syphilol 1872;4:265–273.

50. Laor Y, Schwartz RA. Epidemiologic aspects of American Kaposi's sarcoma. J Surg Oncol 1979;12:229–303.

51. Schwartz RA, Volpe JA, Lambert MW, Lambert WC. Kaposi's sarcoma. Semin Dermatol 1984;3:303–315.

52. Shmueli Z, Shapira A, Yussim R, Nakache R, Ram Z, Shaharabani E. The incidence of Kaposi sarcoma in renal transplant patients and its relation to immunosuppression. Transplant Proc 1989;21:3209–3210.

53. Haverkos HW, Drotman DP. Prevalence of Kaposi's sarcoma among patients with AIDS [Letter]. N Engl J Med 1985;312:1518.

54. Schwartz RA, Burgess GH, Hoshaw RA. Patch stage Kaposi's sarcoma. J Am Acad Dermatol 1980;2:509–512.

55. Synder RA, Schwartz RA. Telangiectatic Kaposi's sarcoma: occurrence in a patient with thymoma and myasthenia gravis receiving long term immunosuppressive therapy. Arch Dermatol 1982;118:1020–1021.

56. Recht B, Nickoloff BJ, Wood GS. A bullous variant of Kaposi's sarcoma in an elderly female. J Dermatol Surg Oncol 1986;12:1192–1197.

57. Warner TFCS, O'Loughlin S. Kaposi's sarcoma: a byproduct of tumor rejection. Lancet 1975;2:687–689.

58. Schwartz RA. Stewart-Treves syndrome. In: Demis DJ ed. Clinical dermatology. 16th rev. Philadelphia: Harper & Row, 1989; Unit 7–77, pp. 1–6.

59. Stewart FM, Treves N. Lymphangiosarcoma in postmastectomy lymphedema. Cancer 1948;1:64–81.

60. Stromberg BV, Keiter JE, Wray RC, Weeks PM. Scar carcinoma: prognosis and treatment. South Med J 1977;70:821–822.

61. Troy JL, Grossman ME, Walther RR. Squamous-cell carcinoma arising in a leprous neurotrophic ulcer. Report of a case. J Dermatol Surg Oncol 1980;6:659–661.

62. Muksi K, Rosai J. Application of immunoperoxidase techniques in surgical pathology. Prog Surg Pathol 1980;1:15–49.

63. Templeton AC, Bhana D. Prognosis in Kaposi's sarcoma. J Natl Cancer Inst 1975;5:1301–1304.

64. Lane HC, Falloon J, Walker RE, Deyton L, Kovacs JA, Masur H, et al. Zidovudine in patients with human immunodeficiency virus (HIV) infection and Kaposi sarcoma. Ann Intern Med 1989;111:41–50.

65. Klein E, Schwartz RA, Laor Y, Milgrom H, Burgess GH, Holtermann OA. Treatment of Kaposi's sarcoma with vinblastine. Cancer 1980;45:427–431.

66. Macaulay WL. Lymphomatoid papulosis update: a historical perspective. Arch Dermatol 1989;125:1387–1389.

67. Lambert WC, Schwartz RA. Dermatitic precursors of mycosis fungoides. In: Schwartz RA. Skin cancer: recognition and management. New York: Springer-Verlag, 1988:152–161.

68. Zackheim HS. Cutaneous lymphoma, leukemia, and related disorders. In: Schwartz RA. Skin cancer: recognition and management. New York: Springer-Verlag, 1988;162–184.

69. Wilkel CS, Grant-Kels JM. Cutaneous B-cell lymphoma. An unusual presentation. Arch Dermatol 1987;123:1362–1367.

70. Spencer PS, Helm TN. Skin metastases in cancer patients. Cutis 1987;39:119–121.

70a. Lookingbill DP, Spangler N, Sexton FM. Skin involvement as the presenting sign of internal carcinoma. J Am Acad Dermatol 1990;22:19–26.

71. O'Neill JF, Jame WD. Inherited patterned lentiginosis in blacks. Arch Dermatol 1989;125:1231–1235.

72. Kato T, Tanita Y, Takematsu H, Tagami H. Pigmented freckles on the soles as acral lentiginous melanoma in situ. J Dermatol (Tokyo) 1985;12:263–266.

73. Cohen PJ, Lambert WC, Hill GJ, Schwartz RA. Melanoma. In: Schwartz RA. Skin cancer: recognition and management. New York: Springer-Verlag, 1988:152–161.

74. Lambert WC, Brodkin RH. Nodal and subcutaneous cellular blue nevi: a pseudometastasizing pseudomelanoma. Arch Dermatol 1984;120:367–370.

75. Smith KJ, Barrett TL, Skelton HG, Lupton GP, Graham JH. Spindle cell and epitheloid cell nevi with atypia and metastasis (malignant spitz nevus). Am J Surg Pathol 1989;13:931–939.

76. Kaplan EN. The risk of malignancy in large congenital nevi. Plast Reconstruct Surg 1974;53:421–428.

77. Kelly JW, Crutcher WA, Sagebiel RW. Clinical diagnosis of dysplastic melanocytic nevi. A clinicopathologic correlation. J Am Acad Dermatol 1986;14:1044–1052.

78. Becker JK, Goldberg LH, Tschen JA. Differential diagnosis of malignant melanoma. Am Fam Physician 1989;39:203–214.

79. Ikeda S, Kiyohara Y, Mizutani H. Comparative aspects of melanoma and non-melanoma skin cancers in Japan. J Invest Dermatol 1989;92:204S–209S.

80. Isaacson C, Spector I. Malignant melanomas in the Eur-African-Malay population of South Africa. Am J Dermatopathol 1987;9:109–110.

81. Schwartz RA, Hill WE, Hansen RC, Fleishman JS. Verrucous malignant melanoma. J Dermatol Surg Oncol 1980;6:719–724.

82. Jimbow K, Ikeda S, Takahashi H, Kukita A, Miura S. Biological behavior and natural course of acral malignant melanoma: clinical and histologic features and prognosis of palmoplantar, subungual, and other acral malignant melanomas. Am J Dermatopathol 1984; 6(suppl 1):43–53.

83. Kukita A, Ishihara K. Clinical features and distribution of malignant melanoma and pigmented nevi on the soles of the feet in Japan. J Invest Dermatol 1989;92:210S–213S.

84. Milton GW, Balch CM, Shaw HM. Clinical characteristics. In: Balch CM, Milton GW, eds. Cutaneous melanoma: clinical management and treatment results worldwide. Philadelphia: Lippincott, 1985:13–28.

85. Collins RJ. Melanoma in the Chinese of Hong

Kong: emphasis on volar and subungual sites. Cancer 1984;54:1482–1488.

86. Klausner JM, Inbar M, Gutman M, Weiss G, Skornick Y, Chaichik S, et al. Nail-bed melanoma. J Surg Oncol 1987;34:208–210.

87. Hutchinson J. Melanosis often not black: melanotic whitlow. Br Met J 1886;1:491.

88. Baron R, Kechijian P. Longitudinal melanonychia (Melanonychia Striata): diagnosis and management. J Am Acad Dermatol 1989; 21:1165–1175.

89. Clark WH Jr, Elder DE, Van Horn M. The biologic forms of malignant melanoma. Hum Pathol 1986;17:443–450.

90. Sterling GB, Libow LF, Grossman ME. Pigmented nail streaks may indicate Laugier-Hunziker syndrome. Cutis 1988;42:325–26.

91. Lambert WC, Lambert MW, Mesa ML, Schneider LC, Fischman GJ, Abbey AH, et al. Melanoacanthoma and related disorders: simulants of acral-lentiginous (P-P-S-M) melanoma. Int J Dermatol 1987;26:508–510.

92. Clark WH Jr, Ainsworth AM, Bernardino EA, Yang CH, Mihm MC, Reed RJ. The developmental biology of primary human malignant melanoma. Semin Oncol 1975;2:83–103.

93. Breslow A. Thickness, cross-sectional areas and depth of invasion in the prognosis of cutaneous melanoma. Ann Surg 1970;172:902–908.

94. Kopf AW, Welkovich B, Frankel RE, Stoppelmann EJ, Bart RS, Rogers GS, et al. Thickness of malignant melanoma: global analysis of related factors. J Dermatol Surg Oncol 1987;13:345–390, 401–420.

95. Balch CM, Murad TM, Soong SJ, Ingalls AL, Halpern NB, Maddox WA. A multifactorial analysis of melanoma: prognostic histopathological features comparing Clark's and Breslow's staging methods. Ann Surg 1978;188:732–742.

96. Fletcher JR, White CR Jr, Fletcher WS. Improved survival rates of patients with acral lentiginous melanoma treated with hyperthermic isolation perfusion, wide excision and regional lymphadenectomy. Am J Surg 1986;151:594–598.

6

Cysts and Cystlike Lesions

—Frank A. Spinosa

The subject of bone tumors is complex and varied. The average practitioner, when faced with the challenge of diagnosis, must rely on an array of available tests. Diagnostic tools range from the inexpensive and easily performed radiograph to the ever-improving magnetic resonance imaging. Unfortunately, no single means of testing is sufficient in itself.

The simple office radiograph affords the practitioner a basic two-dimensional visualization of a suspected lesion and, in fact, is often the mechanism by which a tumor is discovered (as an incidental finding). The radiograph, however, cannot be used as a sole means of diagnosis since there is much overlap in the radiologic characteristics of bone tumors.

Tomography, the radiographic technique by which the x-ray source and film move synchronously in opposite directions, affords better depth perception of a lesion and improved visualization of its boundaries (1).

Radioisotopic skeletal imaging (bone scans) is a very sensitive but nonspecific test. Radioisotopes accumulate in areas of increased osteoblastic or vascular activity, producing a "hot spot" on the film's image (2). While this may be critical in locating a painful lesion (e.g., osteoid osteoma) in its early stages, this diagnostic tool cannot begin to classify a tumor or indicate whether it is benign or malignant unless metastases have occurred.

Computerized tomography (CT) is extremely helpful in imaging the size and boundaries of a lesion by using computerized reconstruction of axial tomography, giving an indication of a tumor's benign or malignant tendency. CT scans contrast soft or osseous tissue and thereby give further valuable information (3). While becoming more common, the CT scan is not accessible to all patients, is rather expensive, and exposes the patient to an appreciable amount of radiation.

Magnetic resonance imaging (MRI) eliminates exposure of the patient to radiation by utilizing a strong magnetic field to measure the activity of hydrogen atoms within body tissues (4). The tremendous size and cost of the units preclude its use by most smaller institutions. In addition, while the MRI provides unique clarity for soft tissue and bone marrow, its use for cortical bone lesions is limited.

The definitive way of making a bone-tumor diagnosis remains the biopsy and histologic analysis. It is by these means that a tumor is classified and categorized (5–7).

The classification of tumors is simplified by assigning a grading system to indicate the degree of pathology (8). Tumors may be graded on the basis of histology (9). Three grades are described by Jaffe (10). Grade I includes lesions with normal, mature cells, grade II exhibits some degree of atypical cells, and grade III indicates a malignancy with extensive atypical stromal cells.

The treatment of bone tumors often involves surgery. If a lesion can be totally excised without impairing a patient's function, this method may present a treatment with the least chance of recurrence. Often, though, curettage and bone graft is a more logical course.

To perform a curettage and bone graft, a rectangular window is made in the cortex overlying the lesion. The cortical "window" is carefully removed and saved for later use. The underlying lesion is thoroughly curetted and flushed with normal sterile saline and then packed with autogenous bone chips. Next, the area is covered with the cortical window, and overlying soft tissue is sutured to maintain its stability. Compression dressings and casting are used for an appropriate period of time (4, 6, 10).

A group of bone tumors which present problems in diagnosis are bone cysts and cystlike lesions. These include the relatively common

163

osteoid osteoma, fibroid dysplasia, enchondroma, unicameral bone cyst and nonossifying fibroma, the uncommon giant cell tumor, chondroblastoma, and chondromyxoid fibroma (6–7). This chapter will deal with these and other cystlike lesions which are distinguished by their clinical, radiologic, and microscopic characteristics (Table 6.1).

ANEURYSMAL BONE CYST

Aneurysmal bone cyst is so named because of its striking radiologic appearance rather than its histologic makeup (11). It exhibits a bulging (aneurysmal) cortex surrounding a cavity filled with sanguineous fluid (bone cyst) (Fig. 6.1) (12).

Malignant transformation does not occur, with rare exception. While it is unrelated to the solitary bone cyst histologically, a transformation of a solitary bone cyst into an aneurysmal bone cyst as a result of trauma was reported by Johnston and Fletcher in 1986 (13).

Clinical Presentation

Aneurysmal bone cyst is found in adolescents and young adults. It is rarely seen in a patient more than 20 years old. Females are more often affected than males (4). While the presenting patient often relates a history of local trauma which may exacerbate the lesion, this is not thought to be the etiology of the cyst (14).

Moderate swelling of increasing severity and local pain of several months duration are usually the presenting symptoms (6). The lesion can be rapidly progressive, expanding the cortex of bone within a 2-month period.

Etiology

The true pathogenesis of aneurysmal bone cysts is unknown, but one theory is that a venous occlusion causes an arteriovenous disparity that results in excessive arterial filling and inadequate venous drainage within an area of fibrous tissue (15). The fluid pushes against the lesion's borders causing expansion. The lesion may arise de novo or develop from a preexisting lesion (i.e., giant cell tumor, chondroblastoma, or fibrous dysplasia through secondary trauma).

Trauma alone is not thought to be a likely etiology in an aneurysmal bone cyst that originates within the interior of bone. However, it is possible that trauma may initiate a

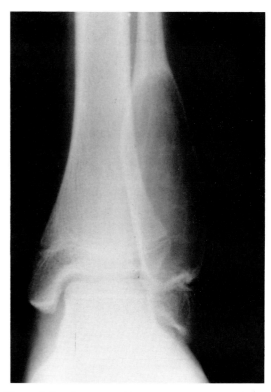

Figure 6.1. Aneurysmal bone cyst of the fibula before epiphyseal fusion.

soft-tissue lesion which erodes the outer surface of bone (16).

Site

The aneurysmal bone cyst usually affects the metaphysis of a long tubular bone, most often the femur. It is often seen in the vertebral column. The lesion is usually seen at the distal or proximal end of the shaft, and will only encroach upon the epiphyseal area after fusion of the growth center (9). When found in the foot, the calcaneus, metatarsals, and phalanges are common sites.

Radiologic Presentation

The radiographic appearance of the aneurysmal bone cyst is one of an eccentrically located lesion, up to 7 cm in length, that causes a bulging or ballooning of the cortex. The lesion is commonly described as having a "blown-out" appearance on x-ray (10).

Some trabeculation may be seen within the lesion in a honeycomb pattern. An elevated periosteum may also be seen on radiograph.

Codman's triangle may result from the periosteal elevation. The lesion is covered by a thin shell of bone. Its margin is usually well-circumscribed and sclerotic (17), although it may appear ill-defined on some radiographic views where the lesion lies closest to the thinned cortical border of bone.

Microscopic Examination

The aneurysmal bone cyst presents microscopically with a thin, osseous outer border surrounding blood-filled cavities with connective tissue septa. The outer shell may or may not have an endothelial lining. Multinuclear giant cells may be present. Normal blood vessels are not seen (10, 15).

Differential Diagnosis

Aneurysmal bone cyst is most often confused with giant cell tumor due to its radiographic appearance and the fact that giant cells are often seen histologically. Differentiation must be made on the basis of age and location of the lesions, since giant cell tumors are rarely seen in adolescent patients and do involve the epiphyseal region of bone (18, 19).

Other differential diagnoses include unicameral bone cyst, chondroblastoma, and fibrous dysplasia.

Treatment

Since aneurysmal bone cysts are benign, drainage, curettage, and packing with bone chips is the easiest and safest type of treatment. Healing may be complete in many cases even when some portions of the cyst wall are not completely removed. Total resection may be performed when it is a viable option. Recurrence has been reported in 10% of patients (10, 14).

Interestingly, the unroofing of the lesion reveals unclotted blood that is suggestive of vascular anomalies as an etiologic consideration.

UNICAMERAL BONE CYST

A unicameral bone cyst is a true fluid-filled cyst lined with a thin fibrous membrane. The fluid is straw-colored and the cavity is unicameral. The terms solitary bone cyst and unicameral bone cyst are used interchangeably (9, 14). Jaffe (10) divided the cysts into active and latent categories. The active bone cysts are found next to the epiphyseal growth plate and may continue to grow until epiphyseal fusion,

while latent bony cysts are found a distance from the epiphysis and are nearly always benign (20) (Fig. 6.2).

Clinical Presentation

Unicameral bone cysts are usually discovered in children and adolescents between the ages of 3 and 16 years, and seem to affect more males than females in a 2-to-1 predominance. The cysts are asymptomatic unless a pathologic fracture occurs (4, 6).

Needle biopsy will reveal yellow, straw-colored serous fluid surrounded by a thin layer of fibrous tissue. The fluid may be sanguineous if a pathologic fracture has occurred (21).

Laboratory studies including alkaline phosphatases are not characteristically abnormal.

Etiology

Various theories have been proposed as to the pathogenesis of unicameral bone cysts, including its formation during the stage of active bone growth or venous obstruction causing an obstruction of interstitial fluid drainage and subsequent cyst growth. Others suggest that a defect in the metaphysis causing osteolysis of bone by overactivity of osteoclasts without enough new bone replacement will cause the cyst (4, 9).

Site

Active unicameral bone cysts originate in the metaphysis adjacent to the epiphyseal plate and maintain growth potential. Latent cysts are almost always located in the diaphysis of long bones, most often the shafts of the proximal humerus and femur (9). It is normal

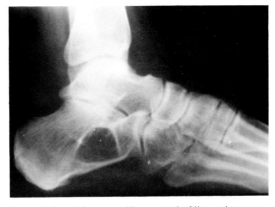

Figure 6.2.   Unicameral bone cyst of the calcaneus.

Table 6.1. Cystlike Lesions of Bone

Tissue of Origin or Differentiation	Tumor	Ages Affected	Clinical Presentation	Radiographic Presentation	Bone Sites Most Affected	Sex Ratio M:F	Benign/ Malignant
Fibrous connective tissue	Aneurysmal bone cyst	8–20	Local pain and swelling	Ballooning of cortex; "blown-out" appearance	Metaphysis of long bones, especially femur	1:1.5	Benign
	Unicameral bone cyst	3–16	Often asymptomatic unless pathologic fracture occurs	"Soap bubble" appearance; "fallen fragment" sign	Metaphysis of long bones, adjacent to epiphysis	2:1	Benign
	Giant cell tumor	20–35; rare below 15	Dull ache; local swelling	Poorly defined margins; usually no periostitis	Epiphysis of long bones, after fusion	1:1	Potentially malignant
	Pseudocysts	Adults over 40	Asymptomatic; pain is due to degenerative joint disease	Roundish radiolucency with sclerotic border	Femoral head or first metatarsal head	1:1	Benign
	Fibrous cortical defect	4 and over	Usually asymptomatic; regression is common	Multilocular; solitary or multiple lesions	Metaphysis of long bones near epiphyseal end	1.5:1	Benign
	Nonossifying fibroma	8–20	Often asymptomatic	Scalloped border; slight cortical bulge; multilocular	Metaphysis of long bones; does not invade epiphysis	1:1	Benign
	Fibrous dysplasia	5–20	Moderately painful; can be cosmetically deforming	Cortex bulged and thinned; borders not well-demarcated; no periosteal reaction; "shepherd's crook deformity" in femoral neck	Usually metaphyseal (less often epiphyseal) in long bones of leg and short bones of foot	1:3	Benign
Bone	Osteoid osteoma	10–25	Moderate to severe local pain, worse at night; symptoms relieved by aspirin	Radiolucent nidus surrounded by sclerotic density	Nidus usually seen in cortical bone, but also found in cancellous or subperiosteal bone	2:1	Benign
	Osteoblastoma	7–20	Local pain; local swelling may occur later	Eccentric expansile lytic lesions with thin cortical borders; spotty calcification may be seen within lesion	Vertebrae and small tubular bones of hands and feet; metaphyseal; may extend to diaphysis; never crosses epiphysis	2:1	Benign
Cartilage	Enchondroma	10–50	Occasionally mild pain and swelling; pathologic fractures are common	Oval radiolucency with ground-glass appearance; usually solitary	Metaphyseal in phalanges, metatarsals, and metacarpals; will extend to epiphysis after fusion	1:1	Benign

Table 6.1. Cystlike Lesions of Bone

Tissue of Origin or Differentiation	Tumor	Ages Affected	Clinical Presentation	Radiographic Presentation	Bone Sites Most Affected	Sex Ratio M:F	Benign/ Malignant
	Chondroblastoma	10–25	Mild pain and edema at adjacent joint; symptoms appear long after tumor development	Eccentrically located oval radiolucency; flecks of calcification noted within borders	Epiphyseal region of femur, tibia, humerus; also in calcaneus and talus	2:1	Benign
	Chondromyxoid fibroma	Under 30	Mild pain locally at tumor site	Ovoid lytic area; scalloped margins	Both long and flat bones; most often in tibia; usually metaphyseal, sometimes diaphyseal	1:1	Benign
Adipose	Intraosseous lipoma	Any age	Rarely symptomatic	Characteristically deep radiolucency; well-demarcated	Long bones of extremities; skull and ribs; usually metaphyseal, can be epiphyseal or diaphyseal	1:1	Benign
Mesenchyme	Intraosseous ganglion	25–50	Aching intermittent pain aggravated by activity	Solitary radiolucency with well-demarcated borders	Epiphyseal or metaphyseal, rarely diaphyseal; femur, tibia and calcaneus	1:1	Benign
Vascular	Hemangioma	5–45	Asymptomatic until pathologic fracture occurs	Multilocular expansile lytic lesions with vertical or honeycombed trabeculation	Metaphyseal: vertebrae, skull, pelvis	1:1.5	Benign
	Glomus tumor	35–60	Moderate to severe local pain	Nondescript central ovoid area of rarefaction	Distal phalanges of hands and feet	1:1	Benign
Reticuloendothelial	Eosinophilic granuloma	5–15	Often seen as an incidental finding; occasionally causes local pain and swelling	Irregular areas of radiolucency; periosteal reaction may be seen	Usually flat bones; sometimes long bones of extremities; metaphyseal or diaphyseal closer to midshaft	1:1	Benign
	Multiple myeloma	40–70	Severe aching bone pain	Multiple osteolytic lesions with "punched-out" appearance	Spine as well as flat bones	2:1	Malignant
Infectious process	Brodie's abscess	Any age	Chronic pain; inflammation, if present, is mild and localized	Small, lytic defect	Any bone	1:1	Not applicable

bone growth that displaces the latent cysts from epiphyseal cartilage. Unicameral bone cysts are also found in the tibia and fibula. They are rarely found in the foot, but of those lesions that have been most are seen in the calcaneus (10, 14).

Radiologic Presentation

The lesions are typically large radiolucent areas, oval in shape, but never erode through the cortex into soft tissue. They are usually centrally located within the bone and are bordered by a sclerotic margin. Although the cortex may show a slight bulge, periostitis is seen only following pathologic fractures. The oval, lucent presentation is often referred to as a "soap bubble" appearance.

The classic "fallen fragment sign" is seen when a fragment of bone at a superior periphery of the cyst breaks off, often secondary to trauma, and falls through the cyst's fluid by gravity to an inferior area of the lesion (6, 21).

Occasionally, the cyst will appear loculated with fine septa. They are usually 2–3 cm in size, but can grow to the entire length of a bone.

Microscopic Examination

The unicameral bone cyst is lined with fibrous tissue and filled with clear, amber fluid (4). Analysis of the fluid reveals components similar to serum. Some giant cells may be found. The lining consists of fibrous, fatty, and osseous tissues (6, 9, 20).

Differential Diagnosis

Enchondroma, giant cell tumor, and aneurysmal bone cysts are all included in the differential diagnosis of unicameral bone cysts due to their areas of radiolucency. None of the above-mentioned lesions, however, have the strikingly lucent appearance of the solitary bone cyst (10, 22).

Treatment

Little evidence exists that the cysts will resolve in time if left untreated.

Steroid injections into the cyst to cause resorption of the fluid may be helpful in a non-weight-bearing area, but the treatment of choice is drainage and curettage of the cyst with removal of the fibrous lining (22). Packing with autogenous bone will usually bring total healing with little chance of recurrence.

Resection of nonessential bones is also a consideration. In any case, the surgery is best performed after the lesion has grown away from the epiphyseal plate.

GIANT CELL TUMOR

Before the scientific literature designated specific benign bone tumors that presented with giant cells as aneurysmal, unicameral, chondroblastoma, and nonosteogenic fibroma, the lesions were considered to be variants of giant cell tumors (10, 23). Authors such as Jaffe and Lichtenstein began differentiating these so-called variants in the 1940s. Therefore, the true giant cell tumor is not a very common lesion. Approximately one-quarter of the lesions will recur and metastasis is a definite possibility (Fig. 6.3) (4, 6, 10).

Clinical Presentation

Giant cell tumors invariably occur in patients between the ages of 20 and 35 years. They are truly rare below age 15 and above age 50. The lesions do not often develop before the epiphyseal plate is closed (9–10, 14). Males and females are affected evenly in most studies.

Most patients present with a chief complaint of a dull ache occasionally associated with soft-tissue swelling. Sometimes the tumor is not detected until a pathologic fracture occurs, or it causes pain in a nearby joint (4, 6).

Etiology

The giant cell tumor arises from nonosteogenic connective tissue of bone marrow (14). Its pathogenesis has not been adequately determined although trauma has been implicated.

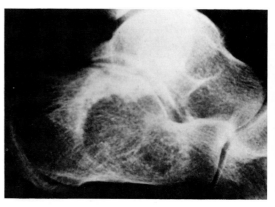

Figure 6.3. Giant cell tumor of the calcaneus.

Site

The giant cell tumor is quite commonly found at the end of a long tubular bone, often involving the epiphyseal end and the adjacent metaphysis (9). While these tumors are most often found in the distal portions of the tibia, femur, and fibula, the os calcis is the most common location in the foot. They have been reported in metatarsals and phalanges, always beginning at the epiphyseal end (10). It is important to note that the tumor is able to extend into the epiphysis from its adjacent metaphyseal origin only after epiphyseal fusion. An open epiphyseal plate, rare in the typically older patient with giant cell tumor, prevents extension of the lesion (6).

Radiologic Presentation

Radiographic appearance of giant cell tumor exhibits a more or less well-demarcated area of radiolucency with minimal trabeculation (6, 24). The tumor presents initially as an eccentrically placed lesion that will grow to encompass the entire width of a bone and eventually weaken the cortex (9). Periosteal reactions and cortical erosions can occur and may herald a malignant transformation.

It is obvious that there is no typical radiographic appearance of a giant cell tumor. Multiple tumors are rarely encountered. The solitary lesion is often round and may exhibit a "soap bubble" appearance (4, 6). Although its margins are well-circumscribed, it usually lacks a sclerotic border.

Microscopic Examination

The tissue of giant cell tumor is a stroma of multinuclear giant cells with moderately strong vascular supply. Giant cells are often found in histologic specimens of bone tumors other than an actual giant cell tumor (10, 14). Some lesions of bone that demonstrate giant cells are aneurysmal bone cyst, solitary bone cyst, fibrous dysplasia, osteoblastoma, and chondroblastoma (17).

Therefore, the appearance of giant cells in a lesion is not sufficient evidence for making a diagnosis. Frequent mitoses are seen in those lesions which are potentially malignant (9).

Differential Diagnosis

The differential diagnosis of giant cell tumor will obviously include all lesions which exhibit giant cells (e.g., aneurysmal bone cyst, unicameral bone cyst, nonosteogenic fibroma, and chondroblastoma) (9).

The lesion must be differentiated from the brown tumors of hyperparathyroidism that, on gross appearance, can mimic giant cell tumor since both have soft reddish-brown features (14). Laboratory studies such as serum calcium and alkaline phosphatase will help in differentiating the two lesions (6).

A solitary enchondroma may have a similar radiographic appearance but will not involve the end of a bone.

Treatment

Curettage and bone grafting of the lesion appears to be the best treatment, as is resection of the lesion in a nonessential area such as the proximal end of the fibula (10). Unfortunately, the recurrence rate is great, and since there is a 10% possibility of malignant change, total removal is imperative (6). Failure of initial therapy may result in the need to amputate, and even then, one must employ the use of diagnostic tests such as radioisotope bone scan to detect possible metastases.

PSEUDOCYSTS

Cystic lesions found in association with osteoarthritis are described as pseudocysts or subchondral bone cysts. They are multiple and multilocular (25). Pseudocysts are reported as accompanying findings of degenerative joint disease and are not symptomatic of themselves (Fig. 6.4).

Clinical Presentation

Pseudocysts will appear in areas of osteoarthritis, bony sclerosis, and joint space narrowing (25). The pain experienced by a patient will be due to degenerative joint disease changes and its accompanying capsulitis and bursitis. The pseudocyst will be discovered as an incidental roentgen finding.

Etiology

Pseudocysts appear to arise from the degeneration of fibrocartilage secondary to trauma (26). Landell (27) suggests that the trauma of degenerative joint disease causes defects in cartilage and subsequent cyst formation in subchondral bone.

Site

Pseudocysts are found most often at the femoral head in patients with degenerative joint

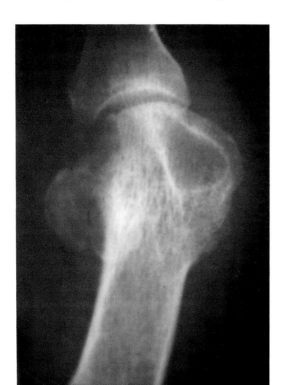

Figure 6.4.   Pseudocyst of the first metatarsal head.

disease and at the first metatarsal head in patients with hallux abducto valgus deformity (26, 28). While the literature is replete with references to subchondral bone cysts of the femur, Lemont and Smith (26) in 1982 were the first to describe the lesions at the first metatarsal head.

Radiologic Presentation

Pseudocysts are commonly seen in radiographs of bunion deformities as roundish radiolucencies of the first metatarsal head. They usually have distinct sclerotic borders, and erosions seem to occur in such atrophic conditions as rheumatoid arthritis (25).

Microscopic Examination

Pseudocysts consist of a thick fibrous border of sclerotic bone surrounding gelatinous fluid of cartilaginous, osseous, and adipose cells (25–26).

Differential Diagnosis

Pseudocysts are characteristic in their small size, radiographic location, and gross presence of a thick, clear, yellow fluid in their centers

(29). Differential diagnoses should include enchondromas and solitary bone cysts.

Treatment

Treatment of the pseudocyst per se is unnecessary except in the adjunctive treatment of an osteoarthritic joint. The lesion itself will not recur if resected, but the underlying osteoarthritis may produce other pseudocysts.

FIBROUS CORTICAL DEFECT

Fibrous cortical defect is a rather common osteolytic lesion of fibrous tissue found in children. It is estimated that up to 40% of all children will develop at least one lesion in their childhood. The lesion is most often asymptomatic and undergoes spontaneous regression as the child grows older (4, 6, 10). Edeiken and Hodes (4) postulate that "bone islands" seen as incidental findings in adults may be remnants of regressed fibrous cortical defects. The lesions that do not regress form a nonossifying fibroma (Fig. 6.5).

Clinical Presentation

Fibrous cortical defect is most frequently found in children between the ages of 4 and 8 years. Males with this condition predominate over females in approximately a 1.5-to-1 ratio (30–31). Pain is rarely reported, and regression usually takes place within 2 years of discovery (4).

Etiology

It has been suggested by Jaffe (10) and Lichtenstein (14) that the periosteum of bone produces fibrous tissue which erodes the adjacent cortical bone, causing fibrous cortical defects.

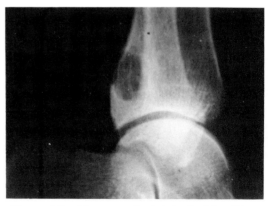

Figure 6.5.   Fibrous cortical defect of the tibia.

Site

Fibrous cortical defect is commonly found in the metaphysis of a long tubular bone, near the epiphyseal plate (30). The most frequent locations are the distal femur and the proximal fibula or tibia (6). The lesions occasionally occur in the diaphysis of long bones, but rarely in the epiphysis.

Radiologic Presentation

Fibrous cortical defect will appear on x-ray as a roundish or oval radiolucency approximately 2 cm in diameter. The lesion's border is well-defined and mildly sclerotic (6, 30). The lesions may be solitary or multiple in number. They are located eccentrically in bone and often cause thinning of the overlying cortex. The lesion will appear multilocular or lobulated.

Microscopic Examination

Histologic study of fibrous cortical defect reveals only nonspecific fibrous and osteoid tissue. Diagnosis must be aided by the clinical and radiographic presentations.

Differential Diagnosis

Fibrous cortical defect may be confused with its later sequela, nonossifying fibroma, or with the benign lesions of chondromyxoid fibroma and giant cell tumor (4, 31).

Treatment

Treatment is unnecessary, unless the lesion causes pain in a rare instance, or unless it develops into nonossifying fibroma with potential for pathologic fracture. If needed, treatment is excision or curettage and bone grafting (32).

NONOSSIFYING FIBROMA

Nonossifying fibroma, also known as nonosteogenic fibroma, was formerly thought to be a variant of giant cell tumor. It is a fibrous bone tumor which is benign in nature. It is the result of the continued development of a fibrous cortical defect (Fig. 6.6) (6).

Clinical Presentation

Nonossifying fibroma occurs in older children and young adults between the ages of 8 and 20 years (10). Most lesions are seen as incidental findings, as is true of fibrous cortical defect (14). The lesion is not frequently pain-

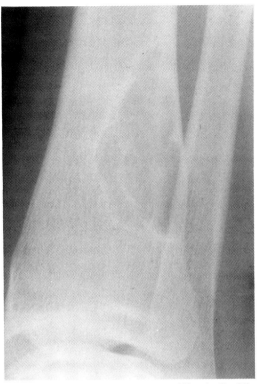

Figure 6.6. Nonossifying fibroma of the shaft of the tibia.

ful, although it is more symptomatic than fibrous cortical defect. Malignant transformation has not been reported (9).

Etiology

Hatcher (31) suggests local failures of ossification as a possible cause of nonossifying fibroma, while Jaffe (10) implicates aberrant development of periosteum. In any case, the lesions are developmental defects rather than primary bone tumors (9).

Site

Nonossifying fibroma begins in the end of a long tubular bone. The most common host is the femur; however, the lesion is found in all long bones of the lower extremity (4, 6). The lesion does not invade the epiphysis but rather originates a short distance away in the metaphysis (30).

Radiologic Presentation

Nonossifying fibroma appears as an oval osteolytic multilocular area about 4 cm in diameter. The cortex bulges slightly, and a dense sclerotic scalloped border is seen. The lesions are not frequently multiple in number (14). No periostitis is seen.

Microscopic Examination

Spindle-shaped cells of connective tissue make up the basic histologic presentation of nonossifying fibroma. Hemosiderin deposits may also be found (14).

Differential Diagnosis

The differential diagnosis of nonossifying fibroma is similar to that of fibrous cortical defect in that it includes chondromyxoid fibroma and giant cell tumor.

Treatment

Surgery should only be performed if pain is present or if a pathologic fracture occurs. Healing of a fracture often results in eradication of the lesion. Curettage with autogenous bone chip packing or block resection of the affected area are the treatments of choice.

FIBROUS DYSPLASIA

Fibrous dysplasia is a benign lesion characterized by the presence of fibrous and osseous tissue in focal areas of otherwise normal bone. The tumor varies in shape and size; however, the danger of malignant transformation is very slight (10, 33).

Fibrous dysplasia sometimes presents with such clinical features as hyperthyroidism, precocious puberty, and abnormal yellowish-brown skin pigmentation. These cases are labeled Albright's syndrome (10).

The widely differing shapes seen in radiographs are due to the uneven replacement of normal bone with fibrous tissue (Fig. 6.7) (4, 34).

Clinical Presentation

Fibrous dysplasia may be noticed in patients as early as 5 years old. It is rare for the lesions to be first discovered in adulthood, since fibrous dysplasia is usually quiescent by that time (9, 14). It is not unusual for the lesions to be discovered when a pathologic fracture occurs.

Jaffe (10) grouped fibrous dysplasia into four categories, including monostotic (involving one bone), monomelic (involving one extremity), polystotic (involving multiple bones), and polystotic associated with Albright's syndrome (9, 33). The most common type is monostotic.

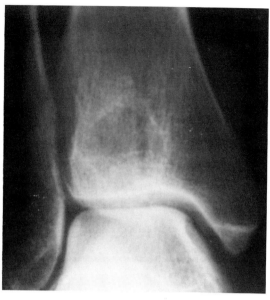

Figure 6.7. Fibrous dysplasia of the tibia.

The lesions are sometimes moderately painful, depending upon which bone is involved and may be cosmetically deforming (10). Females are more often affected than males, in a ratio of almost 3 to 1 (10).

Etiology

Fibrous dysplasia, along with other tumors of fibrous tissue origin, is considered to be a developmental defect of osseous mesenchyme tissue (9, 14). There is no familial tendency noted and no evidence that the tumor has a basis in endocrine dysfunction (10).

Site

The lesions of fibrous dysplasia characteristically occur near the ends of long tubular bones, the proximal femur being the most common site when the involvement is monostotic (9). Polystotic involvement often affects several bones of the lower limb, including the femur, fibula, tibia, and foot (10, 34). Foot involvement has been reported in the metatarsals, phalanges, and tarsal bones (33, 35).

The lesions usually are seen in the metaphyseal area, although epiphyseal involvement has been reported (33, 36).

Radiologic Presentation

Radiographic interpretation of fibrous dysplasia may be somewhat difficult because the lesions do not have well-demarcated borders common to benign bone tumors (9). Periosteal reaction is not usually observed, and the cortex may appear bulged but thinned (9).

A characteristic of the roentgen appearance of fibrous dysplasia in the femur is a lateral deviation in the neck area called "shepherd's crook deformity," more commonly seen in the polystotic form (9, 34). Widening of the bone occurs, and the lesion appears multilocular.

The radiographic presentation may vary from an irregularly lucent area to one of a ground-glass appearance.

Microscopic Examination

The connective tissue cells of fibrous dysplasia are rich in alkaline phosphatase (14).

Differential Diagnosis

The café-au-lait type of skin pigmentation occasionally seen in fibrous dysplasia sometimes causes an investigator to consider an association with von Recklinghausen's neurofibromatosis. Since neurofibromatosis has a recognized genetic tendency, the two diseases are not considered linked (10).

Unicameral bone cyst, enchondroma, Paget's disease, giant cell tumor, and aneurysmal bone cyst must all be included in the differential diagnosis of fibrous dysplasia due to its varying radiographic appearance (34). Diagnosis must be made by biopsy.

Treatment

The interruption of the deforming ability of fibrous dysplasia is only accomplished by its total resection (32). Excision or curettage and bone grafting are indicated in children. The adult lesion does not often continue to grow or deform its host bone, and therefore need not be treated (9, 34). If a large lesion is excised from the femur, the deficit created may require an inlay strut.

The abnormal skin pigmentation has not been successfully treated. Disfigurements caused by bony abnormalities are alleviated by proper resection of the lesion (10).

OSTEOID OSTEOMA

Osteoid osteoma is a small, benign bone tumor, first described by Jaffe (10) in 1935. It is characterized by local pain that is worse at night but relieved by salicylates. Osteoid osteoma is not a rare tumor and accounts for up to 10% of benign tumors (37). It does not undergo malignant transformation (Fig. 6.8) (4, 14, 38).

Clinical Presentation

Osteoid osteoma is approximately twice as common in males as in females. The lesion is often seen in older children and young adults, typically aged 10–25 years. It is rare to find it in patients over age 35 (9, 39).

Patients diagnosed as having osteoid osteoma often present with moderate to severe local pain which is worse during inactivity. Consequently, most pain is reported at night. Symptoms are never systemic, but the pain usually increases in severity. It is well-known that aspirin provides quick, short-term relief and that it is used as a tool in the diagnosis of the lesion (40). On the average, patients will present approximately 6 months to 2 years following the onset of symptoms.

The pain produced by the lesion often precedes its appearance on radiograph. Immobilization does not seem to relieve pain, and conversely, the pain of osteoid osteoma may cause the patient to guard the limb which, over a period of time, will cause disuse muscle atrophy (41). Local heat and edema may sometimes be seen in subperiosteal osteoid osteoma.

Etiology

The etiology of osteoid osteoma is undetermined. Trauma has been ruled out as a possible etiology, although an inflammatory origin or a healing and reparative process is sometimes considered (42, 43).

Site

The nidus may develop in cortical, cancellous, or subperiosteal bone. Although they can be found in almost any bone, approximately

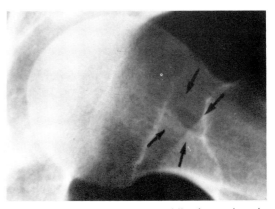

Figure 6.8.   Osteoid osteoma of the femoral neck. *Arrows* indicate radiolucent defect of osteoid osteoma.

50% of these tumors are found in the tibia and femur. Many cases have been reported in the small bones of the hands and feet, and cases have been reported in the talus and calcaneus. When found in the femoral neck, the osteoid osteoma will cause less sclerosis, and osteoporosis of the femoral head and neck commonly results (6, 9, 10, 14).

Radiologic Presentation

Osteoid osteoma is most often 1 cm or less in size. Radiographically, the osteoid osteoma appears as a small radiolucency, the nidus, surrounded by a sclerotic area of cortical thickening. The nidus is usually round or oval. It is initially uncalcified. If the nidus later calcifies, it will appear radiopaque with a lucent halo surrounding it within the outer zone of sclerosis. This outer sclerotic margin is an area of reactive bone formation (4, 6, 44).

The most common area in which the lesion's nidus is found is in cortical bone. The greatest radiographic changes are seen in cortical osteoid osteoma. When found in cancellous bone, less surrounding osteosclerotic change will be seen about the nidus, but may occur at some distance from it. The lesion is least often seen subperiosteally, appearing as a soft-tissue mass adjacent to bone. These subperiosteal lesions affect nearby joints, causing synovitis. The nidus may or may not be centrally located within the sclerotic zone, and this must be considered when surgical excision is attempted (4, 6, 9).

Microscopic Examination

The nidus is comprised of interconnecting trabeculae of osseous tissue in an area of vascular connective tissue. This area is the osteoid osteoma proper. Many unmyelinated nerve fibers are found about the blood vessels within the nidus, and it is thought that this is the source of the tremendous pain produced by osteoid osteomas. The surrounding zone of sclerosis is comprised of reactive perifocal bone (6, 10).

Differential Diagnosis

The roentgenographic appearance of osteoid osteoma is often classic in appearance, but tomography and radionuclide bone scans aid in locating the tumor. The appearance of the nidus of osteoid osteoma can mimic the bony sequestrum of osteomyelitis.

The differential diagnosis must also include sclerosing osteomyelitis of Garré, especially when the nidus is not visible. In this case, the clinical presentation must be closely examined.

Osteogenic sarcoma is also considered in the radiographic differential, while osteoblastoma will appear histologically similar (4, 14, 45). It should be remembered that most benign tumors are painless, with the exception of osteoid osteoma, chondroblastoma, and chondromyxoid fibroma.

Treatment

When left untreated, the lesion will cause pain indefinitely. Even after many years duration, the nidus almost never shows signs of involution or regression. Dramatic relief is usually obtained following complete surgical excision of the lesion. Curettage is the treatment of choice, but if the nidus is not completely removed, recurrence is the rule. Intraoperative radiographs are helpful during curettage. The surrounding sclerotic bone will recede after the nidus is removed (10, 46, 47).

OSTEOBLASTOMA

Osteoblastomas are vascular, fibroplastic, osseous-forming lesions that are always benign (9). They are actively growing tumors that are similar to a large osteoid osteoma (Fig. 6.9).

Clinical Presentation

Osteoblastoma is most common in older children and young adults, with most cases being reported in patients between ages 7 and 20 (14, 48). Males are more frequently affected than females (6). The patient often complains of pain and, in time, local swelling will occur.

Etiology

The etiology of osteoblastoma is unknown. As in osteoid osteoma, however, an inflammatory origin and rapid osseous healing may be factors in its pathogenesis (4, 49).

Site

The vertebrae are most often affected by osteoblastoma, followed by small tubular bones of the hands and feet (49). The tumors are located in the metaphysis and occasionally extend to the diaphysis. The open epiphyseal plate is never crossed (4, 10).

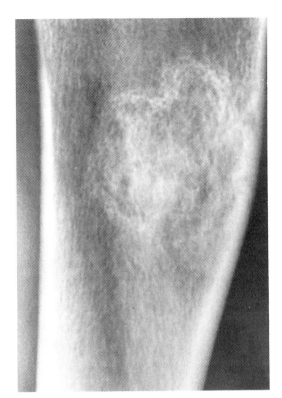

Figure 6.9. Osteoblastoma of the femur. (From Edeiken J, Hodes PJ. Roentgen diagnosis of diseases of bone. 2nd ed. Baltimore: Williams & Wilkins, 1973:866.)

Radiologic Presentation

Radiographically, one notes expansile, often eccentric lytic lesions with thin cortical borders (6). Spotty calcification may be noted within the tumor, which ranges in size from 2 to 12 cm (6, 48). Pathologic fracture may be the reason for the radiographic finding of osteoblastoma.

Microscopic Examination

The presence of osteoblasts and giant cells in a vascular connective tissue stroma are characteristic of osteoblastoma (4, 6).

Differential Diagnosis

The increased osteoclastic activity of osteoblastoma often causes it to be confused with giant cell tumor (9). In addition, it is histologically similar to osteoid osteoma (6). Its lack of periosteal new bone formation differentiates the lesion from osteogenic sarcoma.

Treatment

Resection and/or curettage of the lesion is usually sufficient for a cure as there is little fear of malignant transformation. Recurrence is rare.

ENCHONDROMA

Enchondroma is a fairly common benign tumor, usually solitary, which often affects one of the phalanges. The lesion is a cartilaginous growth that develops in the interior of bone (14). The systemic presentation of multiple enchondromatosis, involving several bones, is known as Ollier's disease, while enchondromas seen with hemangiomatosis is called Maffucci's syndrome (10, 50). The lesion is known to undergo malignant change into chondrosarcoma infrequently in long bones and very rarely in short, tubular bones (Fig. 6.10) (10, 50).

Clinical Presentation

Enchondroma appears to have no predilection for either sex. It seems to affect patients between the ages of 10 and 50 years (10, 14). Patients will present with locally mild pain and swelling due to distention of the affected bone or after pathologic fracture occurs (10, 14).

Etiology

Enchondromas arise from aberrant cartilage cells from the adjacent epiphysis or may have a primary etiology from connective tissue of the bone marrow (9).

Site

The bones most commonly affected are the phalanges, metatarsals, and metacarpals, but

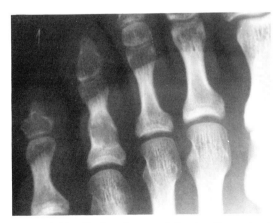

Figure 6.10. Enchondroma of the fourth proximal phalanx.

enchondromas are also seen in larger bones of the limb such as the tibia, femur, or humerus. The tumor begins in the metaphysis of bone but only extends into the epiphyseal region if the growth plate is closed. An enchondroma may grow large enough to involve a large portion of the shaft (10).

Radiologic Presentation

Enchondroma appears as an oval radiolucency with radiopaque foci of calcification within its borders, giving it a ground-glass appearance that is characteristic of these lesions. A fine radiopaque line separates the lesion from normal bone (4, 51).

Microscopic Examination

The hyaline cartilaginous cells of enchondroma exhibit a small, single nucleus in contrast to other normal cartilage cells (50). In older lesions, progressive calcification and grouping of cells will occur (9).

Differential Diagnosis

The radiographic appearance of enchondroma will be similar to that of fibrous dysplasia, unicameral bone cyst, or aneurysmal bone cyst because of its lucent, expansile features (10, 51). Giant cell and chondroblastoma must also be considered (51).

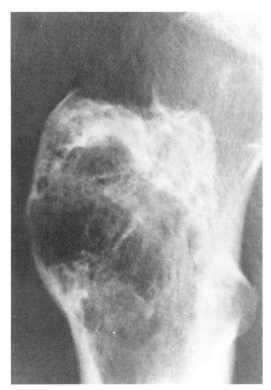

Figure 6.11. Chondroblastoma of the greater trochanter. (From Edeiken J, Hodes PJ. Roentgen diagnosis of diseases of bone. 2nd ed. Baltimore: Williams & Wilkins, 1973:884.)

Treatment

Only those lesions which present with clinical symptoms should be considered for treatment. The treatment of choice for these benign lesions is, by far, curettage and filling of the defect with autogenous bone chips. Healing is uneventful.

CHONDROBLASTOMA

Chondroblastoma is a primary benign tumor of bone which develops from cartilaginous cells. It occurs most often in teenage boys but is rather uncommon (14). The tumor appears to destroy the epiphyseal cartilage of a bone (9). Chondroblastoma is recognized by its tendency for focal calcification within its borders. It is sometimes known as Codman's tumor, for the investigator who originally labeled it a giant cell tumor variant (Fig. 6.11) (4, 10).

Clinical Presentation

Chondroblastoma affects males twice as often as females and is most commonly seen in patients between the ages of 10 and 25

years (52–53). The presenting symptoms are rather mild, and the patient is frequently not seen until months or years after the development of the lesion (54). The clinical symptoms appear in an adjacent joint where pain and edema may be present, and the examining physician should, therefore, rule out meniscal pathology (53).

Etiology

The chondroblastoma seems to result from the presence of excessive calcium in the cell membranes of chondroblasts that subsequently causes the necrosis, chondrification, and calcification of the cellular material (14, 53).

Site

Chondroblastoma is often found in the ends of the femur and tibia and in the proximal end of the humerus (10). It has also been reported in the talus and calcaneus (52). The lesion is most commonly seen in the epiphysis, although it may involve an adjacent portion of the metaphysis (10, 54).

Radiologic Presentation

The lesion of chondroblastoma appears roundish or oval in shape on radiograph, measuring from 3–5 cm in diameter (54) and eccentrically located in the epiphyseal region. It appears somewhat radiolucent with flecks of calcification within its borders. Some cortical bulging may be noted.

Microscopic Examination

Chondroblasts and components of hyaline cartilage are seen in the histologic examination of chondroblastoma. Large polyhedral cells and giant cells may also be present (14).

Differential Diagnosis

Chondroblastoma may appear similar to giant cell tumor on x-ray, especially since it favors the ends of tubular bones. It must be remembered, however, that the giant cell patient is often between the ages of 20 and 40, with closed epiphyseal plates. The chondroblastoma will form in the epiphysis before fusion and may later cross into the metaphysis (6, 9, 14).

Other considerations for differential diagnosis are chondromyxoid fibroma, because of its cartilaginous tissue, and enchondroma, because radiographs show foci of calcification within the tumor (4).

Treatment

Radiation therapy was sometimes used on chondroblastomas in the 1940s and 1950s, with the unhappy result of producing some transformations of the lesions into chondrosarcomas (54). Curettage and bone grafting is adequate therapy since recurrence is rare (53).

CHONDROMYXOID FIBROMA

Chondromyxoid fibroma is a benign bone tumor which originates from cartilage-forming connective tissue. This is a rare tumor that is not invasive and is difficult to differentiate from other tumors derived from cartilage-forming tissue (Fig. 6.12) (4, 6, 55, 56).

Clinical Presentation

This tumor is seen in patients under 30 years of age and seems to affect males and fe-

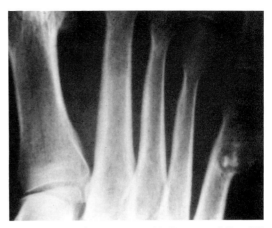

Figure 6.12. Chondromyxoid fibroma of the fifth metatarsal.

males equally. Mild pain experienced locally at the tumor site is the most likely presentation (4, 55). Pathologic fractures are not common (55, 56).

Etiology

Pathogenesis of chondromyxoid fibroma is not proven. The lesion may be a manifestation of cartilage dysplasia since the cartilage forming connective tissue from which it is derived is different from that of enchondroma or chondroblastoma (56).

Site

The lesion is found in both long and flat bones, but most often in the tibia (55). It has been reported in the calcaneus, metatarsals, and phalanges (56). It favors the metaphyseal region of bone and, to a lesser extent, the diaphysis.

Radiologic Presentation

The tumor appears as an ovoid lytic area, not seen in the epiphyseal region unless plate fusion has occurred (55). It averages 3 cm in diameter and may cause the cortex to expand and thin (6). Calcifications may be present within the lesion, and its margins may appear scalloped (4, 6, 55).

Microscopic Examination

The lesion will exhibit chondroid and fibrous tissue histologically. The large size of the cartilage cells causes the lesion to resemble a malignant chondrosarcoma (4, 9, 10).

Differential Diagnosis

The differential diagnosis of chondromyxoid fibroma must include unicameral bone cyst, giant cell tumor, aneurysmal bone cyst, and nonossifying fibroma when examined radiographically since it is a benign, expansile radiolucency (14). A chondrosarcoma will appear similar histologically (6).

Treatment

Since the lesion is absolutely benign, surgical excision or curettage can be approached without trepidation. Recurrence, however, is reported more often in curettage and bone grafting than in block resection (10).

INTRAOSSEOUS LIPOMA

An intraosseous lipoma is a benign tumor composed of adipose tissue. It rarely presents as a primary bone lesion, the incidence of which is 1/1000 bone tumors (57). More often, the lipoma per se is seen as a soft-tissue lesion or a capsular lipoma of the knee joint (10). It is quite unusual for an intraosseous lipoma to undergo malignant degeneration (Fig. 6.13).

Clinical Presentation

The lesion is rarely symptomatic and is often an incidental finding on x-ray. There appears to be no distinct age or sex predilection (10, 58). If symptoms are present, they usually consist of mild pain and swelling locally.

Etiology

The etiology of intraosseous lipoma may be some type of bony infarct or traumatic fatty degeneration secondary to fracture causing a walling off of adipose tissue (58). Many authors, however, believe that the lesion is a true benign primary bone tumor.

Site

The intraosseous lipoma can occur in the long bones of the extremities, or the skull and ribs (6). The bones of the lower extremity are more frequently affected. While the lesions may be found in the epiphysis or diaphysis, the majority of the lesions have been discovered in the metaphyseal region (58).

Radiologic Presentation

The radiographic presentation is one of an expansile lesion with a well-demarcated but thinned cortex (6). Sclerotic borders are infrequently noted. The presentation of the lesion on x-ray and, especially, computerized tomographic scans is one of a characteristically deep radiolucency due to the adipose content of the lesion (58). Larger lesions appear lobulated.

Microscopic Examination

Histologic diagnosis is difficult due to the fact that the marrow normally yields adipose cells. The characteristic appearance of intraosseous lipoma, however, is of very large fat cells interspersed with irregular bone (59).

Differential Diagnosis

A diagnosis of intraosseous lipoma cannot be made without tissue biopsy due to the extensive differential diagnoses (32). Included in the differentials are pseudocysts, aneurysmal bone cysts, giant cell tumors, fibrous dysplasia, and unicameral bone cysts (58).

Treatment

There is no reported recurrence of intraosseous lipoma following treatment by curettage and bone grafting or excision. Pathologic fractures are rarely reported, and the lesion is never malignant, indicating that treatment may be deferred if the patient is asymptomatic (57–59). It must be noted that statistics are small due to the rare nature of the lesion.

INTRAOSSEOUS GANGLION

Intraosseous ganglion is an extremely rare lesion of bone. Some authors consider them to be synonymous with synovial bone cysts (60). There is, however, no evidence that these lesions originate from the cartilaginous defects seen in osteoarthritis (Fig. 6.14) (61).

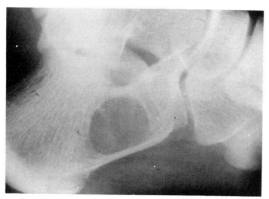

Figure 6.13. Intraosseous lipoma of the calcaneus.

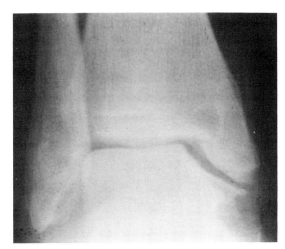

Figure 6.14.   Intraosseous ganglion of the tibia.

Microscopic Examination

The lesions contain myxoid fibrous tissue and fibroblasts similar to that found in pseudocysts or soft-tissue ganglia (60). The mucoid centers are yellowish in color and gelatinous in consistency.

Differential Diagnosis

Intraosseous ganglia appear radiologically similar to such solitary lesions as enchondroma, unicameral bone cyst, and giant cell tumors. They are differentiated from pseudocysts by their larger size and solitary nature (60). In addition, joint surfaces are usually normal in intraosseous ganglion.

Brodie's abscess of osteomyelitis must be ruled out due to the radiolucent cystic appearance (63).

Treatment

Treatment, as is usual with benign bone tumors, is curettage and bone chip grafting. Treatment is often unnecessary unless the lesion is large, is in a weight-bearing area, or undergoes pathologic fracture.

OSSEOUS HEMANGIOMA

Hemangioma of bone is quite a rare entity. While hemangiomas are common lesions in soft tissue and vertebrae, their presence in the axial skeleton is not often seen (65). Even more rare are multiple lesions of hemangiomas of bone, which are called cystic angiomatosis (Fig. 6.15).

Clinical Presentation

The lesions range in size from 2 mm to 7 cm (6). The average is 1–2 cm in diameter (62). There is no apparent sex predilection, but it is more often observed in young or middle-aged adults (62). Pain, if present, is aching and intermittent and is aggravated by activity (61). Swelling is rarely seen. Laboratory values are normal and do not assist in the diagnosis (63).

Etiology

The pathogenesis of these lesions is unknown. Trauma is a usual suspect, as seen in the pseudocysts of degenerative joint disease. Hicks (64) suggested that synovial differentiation of connective tissue was a possible cause.

Site

Intraosseous ganglia occur most often in the epiphyseal or metaphyseal regions of long bones. They are rare in the diaphysis (62). The most common location for the lesions are the femur and tibia near the articulating surfaces. The lesion has been reported in the os calcis and the medial malleolus of the tibia (60).

Radiologic Presentation

The intraosseous ganglion presents as a radiolucency with clearly demarcated sclerotic borders. The lesions are round or oval and are uni- or multilocular. They are usually solitary. There is usually no periostitis or bulging of the cortex (63).

Clinical Presentation

Osseous hemangiomas are found in a wide range of patient ages, from infancy to adulthood (4, 6, 9). The lesions may remain asymptomatic and unnoticed until trauma causes a pathologic fracture, usually during adolescence.

The lesions are rarely malignant; however, Lichtenstein (14) has reported a case of hemangioma of the os calcis that underwent malignant transformation years following radiation therapy. There appears to be a slight predilection for females over males (10).

Etiology

The etiology of hemangioma of bone remains unknown. Jaffe (10) proposed that most asymptomatic osseous hemangiomas may actually be clusters of varicosities.

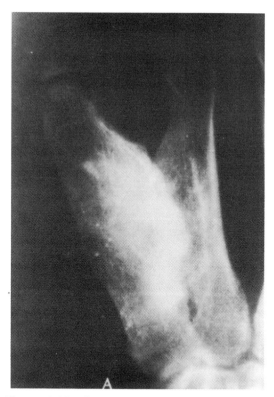

Figure 6.15. Osseous hemangioma of the fifth metacarpal. (From Greenfield GB. Radiology of bone diseases. 2nd ed. Philadelphia: Lippincott, 1975:479.)

Site

Hemangiomas of bone are found in the vertebrae, skull, pelvis, and, least often, in the hands and feet. They are most often seen in the metaphyseal area of bone but can appear at one end of the diaphysis (4, 14).

Radiologic Presentation

The lesion appears as expansile osteolytic areas with thin sclerotic margins. It widely varies in size from 2 mm to 3 cm (4, 6). Larger hemangiomas may appear multilocular, and periosteal reaction may be seen. A pattern of vertical or honeycombed trabeculation is sometimes seen as a result of stress on the host bone (4, 9, 14).

Microscopic Examination

Osseous hemangiomas are cavernous with numerous thin-walled vascular channels (4). These channels are seen in clusters with connective tissue septa interspersed.

Differential Diagnosis

Due to their expansile potential, osseous hemangiomas must be differentiated from such lesions as aneurysmal bone cysts. Lichtenstein (14) reports a case of hemangioma in a calcaneus that was diagnosed radiographically as a giant cell tumor before the lesion was surgically excised and a pathology report obtained.

Treatment

Hemangiomas of bone respond well to excision, with little or no recurrence. However, unless the lesion is large or subject to pathologic fracture, treatment may not be necessary (32).

INTRAOSSEOUS GLOMUS TUMOR

A glomus tumor of bone is an arteriovenous anastomosis intertwined with nerve fibers. Its appearance in bone is rare.

Clinical Presentation

The lesion is usually no larger than 0.5 cm in diameter. It has no predilection for either sex or age but is more often seen in middle-aged to older adults. The lesion is painful due to the unmyelinated nerve fibers wrapped around it.

Etiology

A glomus may exist as a normal finding in the medullary canals of bone, especially in the distal phalanges of the hands and feet (10). It is possible that pressure at the ends of these bones will cause some erosion of the bone and irritation of the glomus.

Site

Although rarely seen, intraosseous glomus tumors are found in the distal phalanges of the hands and feet more often than other areas.

Radiologic Presentation

The radiographic appearance of glomus tumor of bone is a nondescript central ovoid area of rarefaction (6, 14). A diagnosis cannot be made merely by x-ray presentation.

Microscopic Examination

On histologic inspection, the glomus tumor is seen as a characteristic anastomosis of arteries and veins within unmyelinated neural filaments (66).

Differential Diagnosis

When seen in the small bones of the hands and feet, intraosseous glomus tumors will resemble enchondromas or intraosseous ganglions and lipomas (6).

Treatment

Thorough excision or curettage will result in complete healing with no recurrence since these lesions are always small in size and benign in nature.

EOSINOPHILIC GRANULOMA

Intraosseous eosinophilic granuloma is a lesion of focal necrosis within a bone, probably of bacterial or viral origin. It is usually solitary but can be found as multiple lesions. Its features are similar to those of histiocytosis X, and it is considered to be an expression of one of the lipid storage diseases (Fig. 6.16) (66, 67).

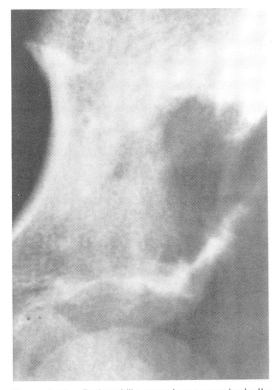

Figure 6.16. Eosinophilic granuloma superior to the acetabulum. (From Edeiken J, Hodes PJ. Roentgen diagnosis of diseases of bone. 2nd ed. Baltimore: Williams & Wilkins, 1973:334.)

Clinical Presentation

Eosinophilic granuloma is seen most often in patients between the ages of 5 and 15 years. There is no predilection for either sex, and the lesions are sometimes discovered as incidental findings on radiograph (14). More often, the patient will present with pain and mild swelling at the area of bone involvement.

Etiology

Lichtenstein (14) has suggested that eosinophilic granuloma may be a result of Letterer-Siwe disease, but other authors propose a bacterial or viral etiology (9).

Site

Eosinophilic granuloma is most frequently found in the flat bones, especially the pelvis, but long bones of the upper and lower extremities have also been implicated (67). The lesion is seen in the metaphysis and diaphysis of bone, closer to the midshaft than the ends. It rarely crosses the open epiphyseal plate (9).

Radiologic Presentation

Eosinophilic granuloma of bone will present radiographically with confluent areas of osseous destruction causing irregular areas of radiolucency within bone, not unlike osteomyelitis. Periosteal reaction is not uncommon. Some sclerosis will be seen about the lesion and some trabeculation within it (6, 14).

Microscopic Examination

Histiocytes and reticuloendothelial cells are seen in histologic preparations of eosinophilic granuloma, but the diagnostic feature is the great number of eosinophils clustered within the lesion. Giant cells may be present (66).

Differential Diagnosis

Due to the fact that the lesion is seen in the midshaft of long bones, and is accompanied by periosteal reaction, the differential diagnosis must include osteomyelitis and Ewing's sarcoma (4, 67).

Treatment

Excision or curettage is acceptable treatment for eosinophilic granuloma, but spontaneous healing is most often seen (9).

MULTIPLE MYELOMA

Multiple myeloma is the most common malignant bone tumor. It arises from the bone marrow cells and will present with diffuse skeletal involvement. The lesions are not osteoblastic, but rather, are destructive (Fig. 6.17) (14, 66).

Clinical Presentation

Multiple myeloma will typically affect patients between the ages of 40 and 70 years and is rare in children (4, 14). Males are affected twice as often as females. The patient with multiple myeloma will present with severe aching bone pain, most commonly back pain. Pathologic fracture and anemia are often the presenting symptoms (6, 9, 68).

Etiology

It is thought that multiple myeloma may be caused by a chronic irritation and inflammation of the bone marrow causing plasma cell inflammatory reaction (66). A subsequent anaplastic proliferation occurs, and multiple foci of bone are seen (68).

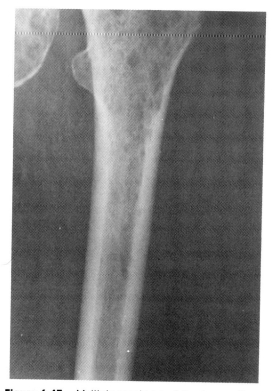

Figure 6.17. Multiple myeloma of the femur. (From Edeiken J, Hodes PJ. Roentgen diagnosis of diseases of bone. 2nd ed. Baltimore: Williams & Wilkins, 1973:1038.)

Site

Multiple myeloma involves the spine as well as flat bones of the ribs, pelvis, and skull due to its red marrow origin (68). Ultimately, every bone may come to be involved (14).

Radiologic Presentation

The lesions of multiple myeloma will appear on x-ray as multiple osteolytic lesions with a "punched-out" appearance. These lesions may become confluent to extend throughout the entire bone. Periosteal reaction is not seen (6, 14).

Microscopic Examination

Immature groups of plasma cells are seen microscopically, some with mitotic activity. Some giant cells may also be present (66).

Differential Diagnosis

The diagnosis of multiple myeloma is best accomplished by bone marrow biopsy. Differentiation from other neoplasms are rarely needed since the disease presents such a characteristic clinical and radiographic picture.

Treatment

No successful treatment is available for multiple myeloma, as it is always fatal. Death is often the result of renal failure caused by the production of nephrotoxic Bence Jones protein (66, 68).

BRODIE'S ABSCESS OF OSTEOMYELITIS

Brodie's abscess, while not a true cyst or tumor, will give a radiographic appearance similar to bone cysts such as unicameral or osteoid osteoma. It is a chronic abscess of bone which remains in a relatively quiescent state (Fig. 6.18) (66).

Clinical Presentation

Patients with Brodie's abscess complain of chronic persisting pain, with no other systemic manifestations (69). If present, inflammation will be mild and localized.

Etiology

The etiology of Brodie's abscess is the same for any type of osteomyelitis, in that an organism invades the bone by a hematogenous route, direct extension, or contiguous inoculation (70, 71).

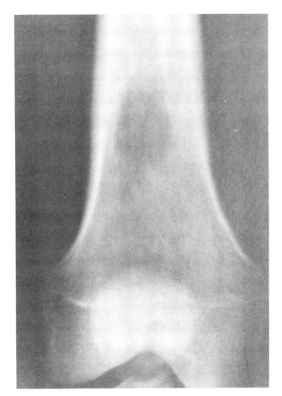

Figure 6.18. Brodie's abscess of the femur. (From Rogers LF. Bone tumors and related conditions. Juhl JH, Crummy AB, eds. Essentials of radiologic imaging. 5th ed. Philadelphia: Lippincott, 1987:186.)

Site

Brodie's abscess is often located centrally in the metaphysis of bone. Any bone may be involved.

Radiologic Presentation

Radiographically, Brodie's abscess will appear as a small, lytic, bony defect within a dense zone of the metaphyseal region of bone. It is a radiolucent lesion with only minimal sclerotic margins (4, 69).

Microscopic Examination

Histologic study will reveal the organism infecting the host bone. Gram stains and all necessary cultures should be utilized (70).

Differential Diagnosis

Definitive diagnosis is only made through biopsy and culture. Aerobic, anaerobic, fungal, and acid-fast cultures should all be utilized. Tuberculosis of bone, seen in some children and young adults with positive tu-

berculin tests, may be detected by the acid-fast culture (70).

Brodie's abscess can be differentiated radiographically from osteoid osteoma since it has no nidus (6).

Treatment

The goal of treatment of Brodie's abscess is to eradicate the lesion by curettage and evacuation. The entire infected bone must be removed and appropriate antibiotics maintained until all signs of inflammation have resolved (69).

REFERENCES

1. Schlefman BS. Radiology. In: McGlamry ED, ed. Fundamentals of foot surgery. 1st ed. Baltimore: Williams & Wilkins, 1987:136–173.
2. Mettles FA, Guiberteau MJ. Essentials of nuclear medicine imaging. 1st ed. New York: Grune & Stratton, 1983:214–244.
3. Rogers LF. Bone tumors and related conditions. In: Juhl JH, Crummy AB, eds. Essentials of radiologic imaging. 5th ed. Philadelphia: Lippincott, 1987:131–177.
4. Edeiken J, Hodes PJ. Roentgen diagnosis of diseases of bone. 2nd ed. Baltimore: Williams & Wilkins, 1973.
5. Berlin SJ. A laboratory review of 67,000 foot tumors and lesions. J Am Podiatr Assoc 1984; 74:341–347.
6. Greenfield GB. Radiology of bone diseases. 2nd ed. Philadelphia: Lippincott, 1975.
7. Bernstein AL, Jacobs AM, Oloff LM, Gilula L. Cyst and cystlike lesions of the foot. J Foot Surg 1985;24:3–17.
8. Coley BL. Neoplasms of bone. 2nd ed. New York: Paul B. Hoeber, 1960.
9. Gilmer WS Jr, Higley GB Jr, Kilgore WE. Atlas of bone tumors. St. Louis: Mosby, 1963.
10. Jaffe HL. Tumors and tumorous conditions of the bones and joints. Philadelphia: Lea and Febiger, 1968.
11. Kaplan RK, Pupp GR, Feldman AC. Aneurysmal bone cysts with emphasis on roentgenologic diagnosis. J Foot Surg 1981;20:204–209.
12. Erseven A, Garti A, Weigl K. Aneurysmal bone cyst of the first metatarsal bone mimicking malignant tumor. Clin Orthop 1983;181:171–174.
13. Johnston CE, Fletcher RR. Traumatic transformation of unicameral bone cyst into aneurysmal bone cyst. Pediatr Orthop 1986;9: 1441–1446.
14. Lichtenstein L. Bone tumors. 5th ed. St. Louis: Mosby, 1977.
15. Dahlin DC, McLeod RA. Aneurysmal bone cyst and other nonneoplastic conditions. Skeletal Radiol 1982;8:243–250.
16. McNamara G, Beheshti F, Saunders TG, Globo SM. Aneurysmal bone cyst of a metatarsal. J Am Podiatr Assoc 1982;72:356–359.

17. Katz JB. Aneurysmal bone cyst of the phalanx. J Am Podiatr Assoc 1980;70:356–357.
18. Diercks RL, Sauter AJ, Mallens WM. Aneurysmal bone cyst in association with fibrous dysplasia: a case report. J Bone Joint Surg (Br) 1986;68:144–146.
19. Michota RS, Perdiue RL, McGee TP. Aneurysmal bone cyst/lipoma of toe. J Am Podiatr Assoc 1978;68:725–731.
20. Epstein J, Wertheimer SJ. Unicameral bone cyst of the calcaneus. J Am Podiatr Assoc 1984;74:76–79.
21. Gordon SL, Denton JR, McCann PD, Parisien MV. Unicameral bone cyst of the talus. Clin Orthop 1987;215:201–205.
22. Frankel SL, Chioros PG, Sidlow CJ. Steroid injection of a unicameral bone cyst of the calcaneus: literature review and two case reports. J Foot Surg 1988;27:60–65.
23. Jaffe HL, Lichtenstein L, Portis RB. Giant cell tumor of bone; its pathologic appearance, grading, supposed variants and treatment. Arch Pathol 1940;30:993.
24. Wold LE, Swee RG. Giant cell tumor of the small bones of the hands and feet. Semin Diagn Pathol 1984;1:173–184.
25. Weissman SD. Radiology of the foot. 1st ed. Baltimore: Williams & Wilkins, 1983:223.
26. Lemont H, Smith JS. Subchondral bone cysts of the head of the first metatarsal. J Am Podiatr Assoc 1982;72:233–236.
27. Landell JW. The bone cysts of osteoarthritis. J Bone Joint Surg 1953;45:643.
28. Rhaney KR, Lamb DW. The cysts of osteoarthritis of the hip: a radiological and pathological study. J Bone Joint Surg (Br) 1955;37:663.
29. Levine B, Kanat IO. Subchondral bone cysts, osteochondritis dissecans, and Legg-Calvé-Perthes disease: a correlation and proposal of their possible common etiology and pathogenesis. J Foot Surg 1988;27:75–79.
30. Sontag LW, Pyle SI. The appearance and nature of cystlike areas in the distal femoral metaphysis of children. Am J Roentgenol Radium Ther Nucl Med 1941;46:185–191.
31. Hatcher CH. The pathogenesis of localized fibrous lesions in the metaphysis of long bones. Ann Surg 1945;122:1016–1020.
32. Lewis MM. Bone tumor surgery. 1st ed. Philadelphia: Lippincott, 1988:1.1–2.6.
33. Duncan GS. Monostotic fibrous dysplasia of the foot. J Foot Surg 1987;26:301–303.
34. Perlman MD, Schor AD, Gold ML. Fibrous dysplasia: a case report and literature review. J Foot Surg 1987;26:317–321.
35. Gibson MJ, Middlemiss CM. Fibrous dysplasia of bone. Br J Radiol 1971;44:1–4.
36. Nixon AW, Lurdin VR. Epiphyseal involvement in polyostotic fibrous dysplasia: a report on two cases. Radiology 1973;106:167–170.
37. Perdiue RL, Olin FH. Osteoid osteoma of talus. J Am Podiatr Assoc 1980;70:353–355.
38. Meissner PJ Jr, Mauro G. Osteoid osteoma: a literature review and case report. J Foot Surg 1981;20:25–27.
39. Kahn MD, Tiano FJ, Lillie RC. Osteoid osteoma of the great toe. J Foot Surg 1983;22:325–328.
40. Spinosa FA, Freundlich WA, Roy PP. Osteoid osteoma of the hallux. J Foot Surg 1985;24:370–372.
41. Estersohn HS, Day JC. Osteoid osteoma. J Am Podiatr Assoc 1981;71:568–571.
42. Patterson BT, Peters VJ. Osteoid osteoma of the fourth metatarsal. J Am Podiatr Assoc 1981;71:328–330.
43. Alkalay I, Grunberg B, Daniel M. Osteoid osteoma in an ossicle of the big toe. J Foot Surg 1987;26:246–248.
44. Short LA, Mattana GW, Benton VG. Osteoid osteoma in the medial malleolus. J Foot Surg 1988;27:264–267.
45. Hamilos DT, Cervetti RG. Osteoid osteoma of the hallux. J Foot Surg 1987;26:397–399.
46. Potter WA, Epstein EP. Osteoid osteoma of the os calcis. J Am Podiatr Assoc 1972;62:435–437.
47. Goranson K, Johnson RP. Osteoid osteoma of the os calcis. Orthop Rev 1986;15:98–102.
48. Francis DR. A rare case of digital benign osteoblastoma. J Am Podiatr Assoc 1980;70:358–360.
49. Segal P, Hoeffel JC, Abadou H, Dehoux E, Adnet JJ, Herbinet P. Osteoblastoma of the first metatarsal bone. J Radiol 1987;68:533–535.
50. Perlman MD, Gold ML, Schor AD. Enchondroma: a case report and literature review. J Foot Surg 1988;27:556–560.
51. Yale I, Conway DH, Carrel JM, et al. Enchondroma. J Am Podiatr Assoc 1976;66:631–637.
52. Katz JB, Hunt DW. Chondroblastoma of the calcaneus: a case report. J Am Podiatr Assoc 1975;65:184–187.
53. Bloem JL, Mulder JD. Chondroblastoma: a clinical and radiological study of 104 cases. Skeletal Radiol 1985;14:1–9.
54. Jaffe HL, Lichtenstein L. Benign chondroblastoma of bone. Am J Pathol 1942;18:969.
55. Van Horn JR, Lemmens JA. Chondromyxoid fibroma of the foot: a report of a missed diagnosis. Acta Orthop Scand 1986;57:375–377.
56. Alchermes SL, Rusnack T, Alchermes LA. Chondromyxoid fibroma. J Am Podiatr Assoc 1984;74:363–367.
57. Dahlin D. Bone tumors. 3rd ed. Springfield: Charles C Thomas, 1978:149.
58. Leeson MC, Kay D, Smith BS. Intraosseous lipoma. Clin Orthop 1983;181:186–190.
59. Lauf E, Mullen BR, Ragsdale BD, Kanat IO. Intraosseous lipoma of distal fibula. J Am Podiatr Assoc 1984;74:434–439.
60. Kenan S, Graham S, Lewis M, Yabut SM. Intraosseous ganglion in the first metacarpal bone. J Hand Surg (Am) 1987;12:471–473.
61. Rubenstein SA, Bardfeld LA. Ganglia (synovial cysts) of bone. J Foot Surg 1988;27:71–74.
62. Menendez LR, Chandler DR, Moore TM, Schwinn CP. Diaphyseal intraosseous ganglion. Clin Orthop 1988;227:310–312.
63. Newland Z, Moore RM. Intraosseous ganglion of the ankle. J Foot Surg 1986;25:241–246.
64. Hicks JD. Synovial cysts in bone. Aust NZ J Surg 1956;26:138–143.
65. Brailsford JF. Ossifying haematomata and other single lesions mistaken for sarcomata. Br J Radiol 1948;21:157.

66. Robbins SL. Pathology. 3rd ed. Philadelphia: Saunders, 1967:326–372.
67. Lichtenstein L. Histiocytosis X (eosinophilic granuloma of bone, Letterer-Siwe disease, and Schüller-Christian disease): further observations of pathological and clinical importance. J Bone Joint Surg (Am) 1964;46:76.
68. Bayrd ED, Heck FJ. Multiple myeloma. J Am Med Assoc 1947;133:147.
69. Rigault P. Infectious and traumatic disorders. In: Maroteaux P. Bone diseases of children. 1st ed. Philadelphia: Lippincott, 1979:331–345.
70. Buchanan RE, Gibbons NE, eds. Bergey's manual of determinative bacteriology. 8th ed. Baltimore: Williams & Wilkins, 1974:599–861.
71. Ingerman M, Abrutyn E. Osteomyelitis: a conceptual approach. J Am Podiatr Med Assoc 1986;76:487–492.

Suggested Readings

Jaffe N. Bone tumors in children, vol II. 1st ed. Littleton: PSG Publishing Co, 1979.
Madiefsky L, Wasiak GA. Outpatient surgery of a unicameral bone cyst of the calcaneus. J Foot Surg 1986;25:73–77.
Stroh JW, Butler JD. Osteoid osteoma: case presentation and discussion. J Am Podiatr Assoc 1974;64:713–717.
Toth SP. Bone cyst, osteoid osteoma: a case report. J Am Podiatr Assoc 1970;60:404–406.
Weinstein F. Roentgenology of the foot. 1st ed. St. Louis: Warren H Green, 1974.
West A, Polito MA. Aneurysmal bone cyst of the foot. J Am Podiatr Assoc 1981;71:446–449.
Zohn DA, Mennell JM. Musculoskeletal pain: diagnosis and physical treatment. 1st ed. Boston: Little, Brown & Co, 1976.

Cartilaginous and Osseous Neoplasms

—German C. Steiner

CARTILAGINOUS TUMORS OF THE FOOT

Cartilaginous tumors of bone are the most common neoplasms of the skeletal system. However, the frequency of these tumors in the foot is relatively rare. In the series reported in two major textbooks of bone pathology (Dahlin and Unni (1) and Schajowicz (2)) the incidence of cartilaginous tumors in the foot varies from 2.4% to 5.7%, respectively. Although infrequent, all major types of cartilaginous neoplasms are present in the foot. The majority of the lesions are benign and, in the series of Dahlin and Unni (1) and Schajowicz (2), only 22 and 9.5%, respectively, were malignant.

Subungual exostosis is discussed in the group of cartilaginous tumors. Although Schajowicz (2) thinks it is an osteochondroma, we think it is a separate entity and describe it as such here.

Enchondroma (Chondroma)

Enchondroma is the second most common benign cartilaginous tumor of the skeletal system, after osteochondroma. It occurs between the second and sixth decades of life (1, 2). Most tumors are found in the short tubular bones of the hand and, less frequently, the bones of the foot. Thirty-eight out of 454 chondromas in the series of Schajowicz (2) occurred in the foot (approximately 8%). In our experience, enchondroma is the most common tumor of the foot; this is also the experience of Dahlin and Unni (1) and Schajowicz (2). The phalanges are the most common sites, followed by the metatarsal and tarsal bones (2).

Clinically, the lesions manifest by swelling or intermittent pain, which often is due to a pathologic fracture following injury. Radiologically, enchondromas consist of a radiolucency of the medullary cavity with varying degrees of expansion of the bone and thinning and scalloping of the overlying cortex, with occasional reactive marginal sclerosis (3, 4). In the phalanges and metatarsals, the lesions involve the midshaft of the bone and, when the epiphyseal plate is closed, they often extend to the articular end of the bone. Pathologic fractures are common. Punctate radiodensities are a frequent and important diagnostic feature that favors enchondroma (3) (Figs. 7.1 and 7.2). If the tumor in the foot is radiolucent without calcification, other possibilities should be considered (e.g., giant cell tumor, aneurysmal bone cyst, simple bone cyst, or reparative giant cell granuloma (3–5)). Destruction of the cortex and soft-tissue extension of the tumor raises the possibility of malignancy.

Histologically, the cartilaginous tissue is poorly to moderately cellular with abundant intercellular matrix, disposed in a lobulated pattern (Fig. 7.3). Focal calcification of the matrix is variable, and reactive ossification around the lobules can be observed. The presence of cell pleomorphism in enchondroma of small bones of the hands and feet is a relatively common finding and does not indicate malignancy, because these lesions behave in a benign fashion (2). Malignant transformation of a solitary enchondroma is rare.

Curettage is the treatment of choice and most lesions are cured, although occasional recurrence occurs. In enchondromas involving the distal phalanges, phalangectomy may be indicated.

Periosteal Chondroma

Periosteal chondroma is a benign cartilaginous tumor arising from the periosteal surface of the bone (4, 6). In the foot, the lesions are located in the phalanges and occur usually in young people. Radiologically, there is a juxtacortical soft-tissue mass associated with erosion and scalloping of the underlying cortex (4, 6). Patchy calcification of the tumor may be present (Fig. 7.4). Histologically, it is similar to enchondroma.

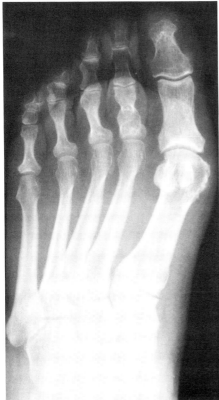 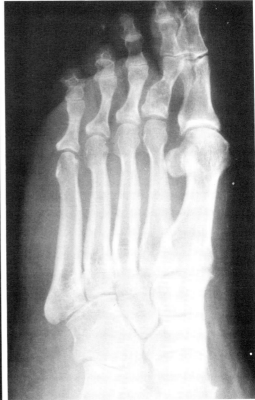

Figure 7.1. Enchondroma. Forty-nine-year-old female with lesion in proximal phalanx of second toe. There is expansion of the bone, with thinning of the cortex and patchy calcification within the lesion.

Enchondromatosis

Enchondromatosis is a nonhereditary abnormality of cartilage growth, characterized by the presence of multiple enchondromas mainly in the hands. It is manifested usually in early childhood with often unilateral involvement of the skeleton, particularly a limb (Fig. 7.5). The bones of the foot are less frequently involved than the hands (7). Malignant transformation to chondrosarcoma in the foot may occur (7).

Solitary Osteochondroma

Osteochondroma (osteocartilaginous exostosis) is the most frequent tumor of bone and accounts for 40–46% of benign tumors in any major reported series (1, 2). It tends to occur in the second decade of life; most patients are under 20 years of age. Most osteochondromas originate from the metaphysis of the distal end of the femur and proximal ends of the tibia and humerus. They arise less frequently from the distal tibia and fibula. Any bone preformed in cartilage can give rise to an osteochondroma.

The bones of the foot are rarely involved and account for approximately 1–5% of osteochondromas in three major reported series (1, 2, 8). In this site, the lesions may occur in older patients.

The most common sites of osteochondromas in the foot are the metatarsals and tarsal bones, followed by the phalanges (1, 2, 8–12). Of the tarsal bones, the calcaneus is the most frequent site. Schajowicz (2) reported 10 lesions in that bone.

Osteochondromas of the foot manifest clinically by the presence of a painless mass noted on palpation, sometimes increasing in size over several years. More often, the mass is painful, and the symptoms increase with the progression of time. Ambulation and long periods of standing tend to aggravate the symptoms. Occasionally, the tumor is found incidentally during a routine radiographic examination of the foot (Fuselier et al. (9), case 2).

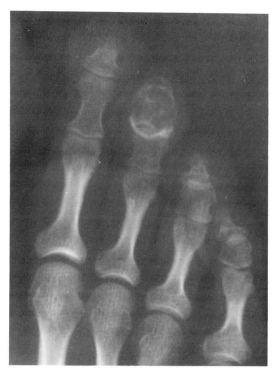

Figure 7.2. This enchondroma of the distal phalanx of the third toe has produced expansion of the bone with marginal sclerosis. The tumor was treated by distal phalangectomy. Patient was a 33-year-old female.

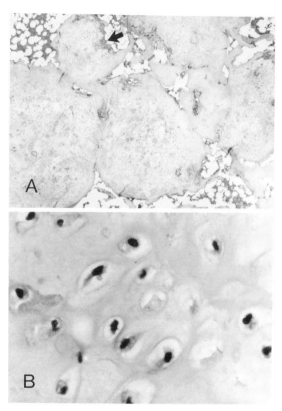

Figure 7.3. **A,** enchondroma. Low-power photomicrograph showing a lobulated pattern of poorly cellular cartilage. There is focal calcification and ossification of the matrix (*arrow*). (Original magnification, X42) **B,** high-power view of enchondroma. The chondrocytes are of uniform size and lie within lacunae in the matrix. (Original magnification, X480)

Rarely, a bursa can develop over the osteochondroma (bursa exostotica), and the patient may experience acute pain and swelling (4).

Clinical examination reveals the presence of a hard, deeply fixed mass in the foot. In large lesions, the mass may be multilobulated, and the overlying skin tight and stretched over the mass.

RADIOLOGY

There is an exostotic mass arising from the cortical surface of the bones. The lesion can be sessile or pedunculated and extend into the soft tissues (Fig. 7.6). In tumors arising from the metatarsals, the exostoses may project into the interosseous space and produce erosion of the adjacent metatarsal (9, 12).

At the site of origin of the osteochondroma, the cortex of the host bone is interrupted and continues into the stalk or base of the exostosis (3, 4, 13). In order to demonstrate this relationship, proper x-ray views or computerized axial tomography (CAT) may be necessary. The cartilage cap overlying the exostosis is not

calcified, and it is not visible on the radiograph. Radiodensities may be seen in the stalk of the lesion, and they represent islands of calcified cartilage that have become incorporated into the bone (4). If multiple calcifications are seen scattered throughout the cartilage cap and away from the stalk, the possibility of malignant transformation to chondrosarcoma should be strongly considered (14).

PATHOLOGY

Grossly, osteochondromas have a smooth or lobulated surface and are partially covered with a cartilaginous cap which varies in thickness according to the patient's age and the growth activity (4). The cap usually measures several millimeters in thickness (Fig. 7.7). In older patients, it becomes thinned, or is replaced by fibrous tissue. Histologic examina-

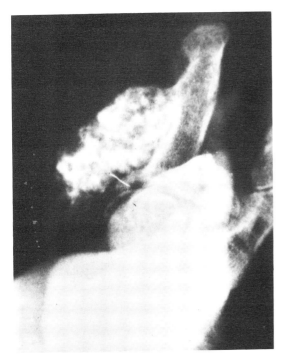

Figure 7.4. Periosteal chondroma arising from the phalanx of the great toe, showing marked calcification. The patient was a 61-year-old male.

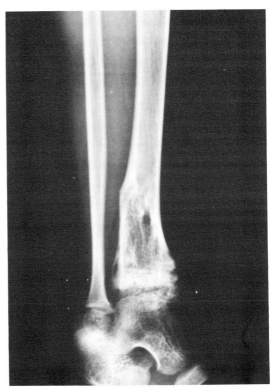

Figure 7.5. Enchondromatosis of the distal tibia. The epiphyseal growth plate of the tibia was involved by the process, leading to growth disturbance. There was also involvement of the femur of the same limb. Patient is a 6-year-old boy.

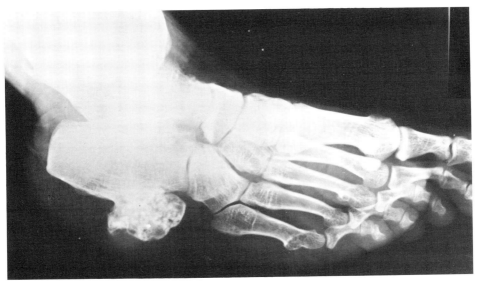

Figure 7.6. Osteochondroma arising from the calcaneus in a 24-year-old male. The radiograph demonstrates interruption of the cortex at the base of the lesion and continuity of the bone of the calcaneus into the osteochondroma. The stalk of the lesion shows patchy calcification.

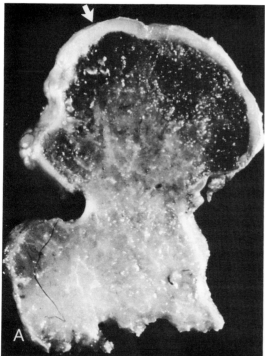
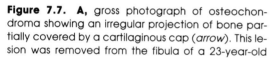
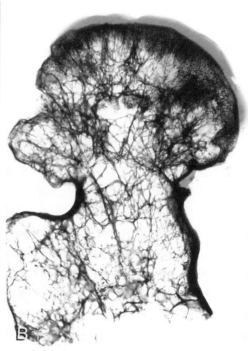

Figure 7.7. A, gross photograph of osteochondroma showing an irregular projection of bone partially covered by a cartilaginous cap (*arrow*). This lesion was removed from the fibula of a 23-year-old male. **B,** radiograph of osteochondroma illustrated in *A*. The cartilaginous cap covering the lesion on top is not calcified.

tion of the cap reveals hyaline cartilage composed of cartilage cells of uniform size. In the deeper part, the cells are aligned in columns resembling the epiphyseal growth plate. Active endochondral ossification is usually seen at the chondro-osseous junction (Fig. 7.8). Underlying the cartilage is the cancellous bone of the stalk of the exostosis.

TREATMENT

The treatment for osteochondroma is surgical excision, and the majority of patients are cured without recurrence. Most osteocartilaginous exostoses are benign, and malignant transformation is rare, probably less than 1% (1, 2). The presence of a thick cartilaginous cap in an adult showing extension into the adjacent soft tissue, associated radiologically with dispersed calcification, is an indication of malignant transformation to chondrosarcoma (14). These malignant tumors are well-differentiated and may show subtle histologic abnormalities.

The origin of osteochondroma is not known, but Virchow's theory of displacement of cartilage from the growth plate followed by subperiosteal growth is probably the best explanation, as discussed by Schajowicz (2).

Hereditary Multiple Exostosis (Multiple Osteochondromatosis)

This is an inherited condition, autosomal dominant, that manifests during childhood by the presence of multiple bumps and protuberances, particularly around the knee, ankle, shoulder, and wrist (Figs. 7.9 and 7.10). The risk of malignant transformation is greater than in solitary osteochondroma and ranges around 10% (1, 2).

Bizarre Parosteal Osteochondromatous Proliferation (BPOP)

This is a disorder that should be differentiated from osteochondroma (15, 16). In the foot, it involves the phalanges and metatarsals. Contrary to osteochondroma, in which the stalk merges with the cortical and medullary bone at the site of origin, in BPOP, the lesion arises directly from the cortex. Histologically, there is cartilaginous and osseous prolifera-

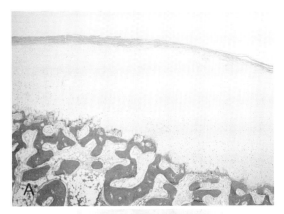

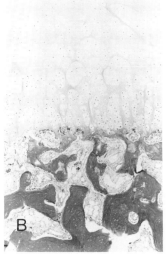

Figure 7.8. A, low-power photomicrograph of osteochondroma showing the cartilaginous cap overlying cancellous bone. (Original magnification, X75) **B,** mid-power view of the cartilage-osseous junction demonstrating enchondral ossification. (Original magnification, X130)

tion, but it is disorganized when compared with osteochondroma (15, 16).

Dysplasia Epiphysialis Hemimelica (Trevor's Disease)

This is a developmental disorder of childhood, characterized by asymmetric cartilaginous overgrowth of one or several epiphyses of a limb. It is common in the ankle and foot and affects one side of the extremity (17–19). Clinically, the lesions of the foot manifest by pain, deformity, and restricted motion. Equinus deformity of the ankle may occur. The radiographic features demonstrate irregular radiopacities projecting from the distal epiphysis of the tibia and fibula, talus, calcaneus, navicular, or cuneiform bones (Fig. 7.11).

Pathologically, the lesion consists of hyaline cartilage with a central area of cancellous bone and active endochondral ossification. The cartilaginous surface resembles osteochondroma, which explains why this lesion has been called epiphyseal osteochondroma (17).

This disorder may be familial (19). It is benign and surgical resection is usually curative, but multiple recurrences can occur (17).

Subungual Exostoses

Subungual exostoses is a benign proliferation of bone arising from the distal phalanges, particularly of the toes, and less frequently of the fingers (1, 20, 21). It occurs in the second and third decades of life. The great toe is, by far, the most frequent site, but the other toes are also affected. The patients complain of pain and swelling that is usually present for several weeks but sometimes for up to 10 years (20, 21). On physical examination, there is a firm mass palpable in the distal region of the toe, sometimes under the nailbed. There may be swelling and ulceration of the overlying skin and subungual region. Radiologically, there is an exostotic growth of bone arising from the distal portion of the phalanx, usually on the dorsal and medial aspect (20, 21). There is no periosteal reaction and no destruction of the distal phalanx to suggest a malignant process (Figs. 7.12 and 7.13).

Histologically, the exostosis consists of trabeculae of lamellar bone covered distally with a cap of fibrocartilaginous tissue with endochondral ossification (Fig. 7.14).

Subungual exostosis should be differentiated from osteochondroma, which is a common benign neoplasm, by the following features: it arises from the distal tuft of the phalanx and not the metaphysis as the osteochondroma; it is formed by a cap of fibrocartilage, and it is not a neoplasm but rather a reactive process and, therefore, does not undergo malignant transformation. Patients with subungual exostosis do not have associated osteochondromatosis (21).

The clinical presentation of subungual exostosis can confuse the initial examiner as to the nature of the lesion. The involvement of the nailbed with ulceration may raise the possibilities of chronic paronychia, pyogenic granuloma, subungual melanoma, or carcinoma. An initial biopsy may show active cellular cartilaginous proliferation that can be mistaken for a chondrosarcoma (21).

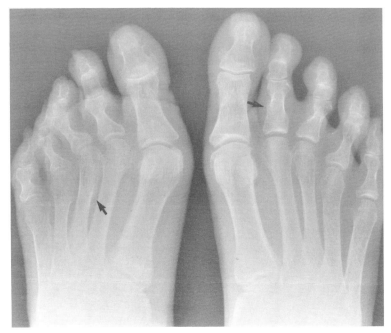

Figure 7.9. Osteochondromatosis. There are multiple small exostotic lesions in both feet involving the phalanges and a metatarsal (*arrows*). Patient is a 57-year-old female.

It is probable that trauma and infection play a role in the pathogenesis of this condition. Treatment should include resection of the bony stalk, including the covering fibrocartilaginous cap; this will avoid recurrence. It is recommended, if possible, to wait until the lesion matures to solid bone before removal (20).

Chondroblastoma

Chondroblastoma is a relatively rare, benign tumor arising, most often, in the epiphysis of long bones, in relation to the epiphyseal growth plate. It favors the second decade of life. The most frequent sites are both epiphyses of the femur, and the proximal epiphysis of the tibia and the humerus (1, 2, 8). The tarsal bones are the next most common sites for chondroblastoma (slightly over 7% in a review article) (8). The talus is more frequently involved than the calcaneus (22). The navicular bone, metatarsals, and phalanges are rare locations.

The clinical manifestations are pain, insidious in onset and sometimes of considerable duration, suggesting that the lesion grows slowly. Local swelling may be noted.

Radiologically, there is evidence of radiolucency of the affected bone. The lesion can be well-circumscribed and discrete or large, and associated with patchy calcification. Marginal

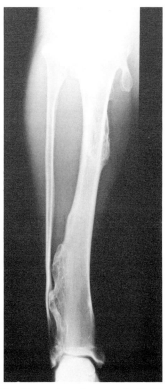

Figure 7.10. Osteochondromatosis. Multiple osteochondromas are seen involving the tibia. There is compression of the distal fibula by one of the lesions. Patient is a 24-year-old female.

Figure 7.11. Dysplasia epiphysialis hemimelica. **A,** **B,** there are radiodense masses in the ankle adjacent to the talus (arrow). The patient is a 3-year-old boy who had a "bump" in the foot since early infancy. There has been increasing pain and decreased motion of the ankle.

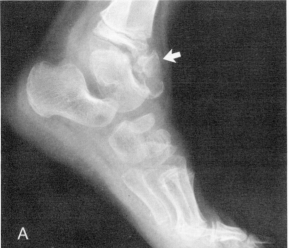

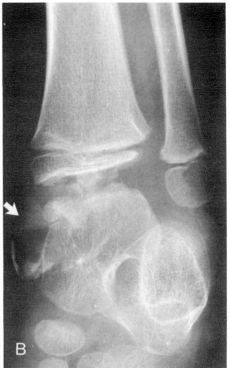

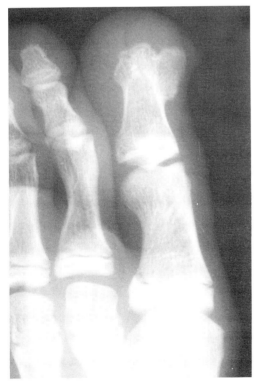

Figure 7.12. Subungual exostosis in a 14-year-old boy. Radiograph of lesion arising from the distal phalanx of the great toe. The patient injured his great toe 6 months before, and since then had swelling and tenderness, and pain while playing sports.

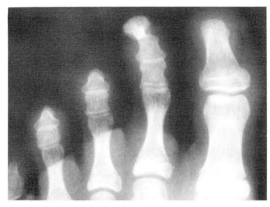

Figure 7.13. Lesion arising from the distal phalanx, second toe, in an 11-year-old girl.

sclerosis around the lesion is often observed (Fig. 7.15). The talus may be deformed by the tumor, with partial collapse of the upper surface.

The histologic features characteristic of chondroblastoma are the presence of large polygonal cells with scanty cytoplasm and prominent nuclei with occasional indentations. The cells are disposed in dense aggregates with sparse intercellular matrix. Multinucleated giant cells are frequently present and calcification of the matrix around the individual cells ("chicken-wire pattern") or in focal areas of the tumor is often noted (Fig. 7.16).

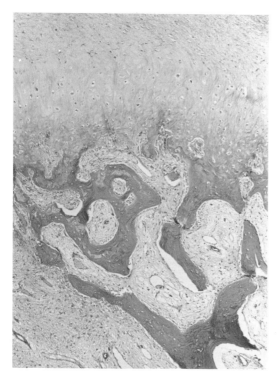

Figure 7.14. Photomicrograph of subungual exostosis. The trabecular bone is covered by fibrocartilage that merges with the overlying connective tissue. This lesion resembles osteochondroma. There is focal ossification at the chondro-osseous junction. (Original magnification, ✕180)

Foci of cartilaginous differentiation may be seen. Reactive ossification is also noticed in the tumor, and it may be extensive enough so that the lesion can be mistaken for osteoblastoma. If numerous giant cells are observed, a diagnosis of giant cell tumor may be erroneously considered. Secondary cystic changes have been described in chondroblastoma in up to 17% of cases (2). Cystic chondroblastomas have been documented in the foot (23, 24). The treatment for this benign tumor is curettage, and most lesions are cured. There are, however, a small number of cases that may recur, and a few can follow a locally aggressive course with soft-tissue infiltration (22). In a recent report, a chondroblastoma of the talus invaded the adjacent calcaneus (25).

Malignant transformation is very rare. Most chondroblastomas of the foot are solitary lesions. However, rare reports of multifocal tumors have been documented. One patient had tumors in the tibia and calcaneus (26), and an-

other had chondroblastomas in the left talus and right tarsal navicular (22).

Chondromyxoid Fibroma

This is a rare benign tumor of bone that is most common in the second and third decades of life. It is more frequent in the lower extremities, particularly in the tibia (one-third of all cases), foot, femur, and fibula. In a review of 340 chondromyxoid fibromas from the literature, 64 cases (18.8%) involved the foot (8). The calcaneus and metatarsals are affected with approximately equal frequency; the talus and phalanges are rare sites (1, 2, 8).

The clinical symptoms are nonspecific and characterized by progressive pain and swelling that can be present for several years. If there is expansion of the bones such as the calcaneus, a palpable mass may be noted.

Radiologically, there is radiolucency of the bone, often with a multilobulated and bubbly appearance. The periphery of the lesion is sclerotic and scalloped and expansion of the bone is a frequent finding (27) (Figs. 7.17 and 7.18). Calcification of the tumor is very rare, compared with chondroblastoma. Differential diagnosis in the calcaneus should include simple bone cyst, which is a lesion more frequent than chondromyxoid fibroma, but tends to occur in the anterior region of the bone and lacks the scalloped sclerotic appearance of chondromyxoid fibroma.

Histologically, the tumor consists of an ill-defined lobulated pattern of stellate cells separated by abundant pale-stained matrix. Lacunar spaces are seen around some cells indicating cartilaginous differentiation. There is increased cellularity at the periphery, where giant cells are usually identified (Fig. 7.19). In resected specimens, the tumor is seen expanding the bone and growing in a nodular fashion, surrounded by reactive sclerotic bone.

Curettage is the treatment of choice. Recurrence occurs in approximately 15–20% of cases (1, 2, 8). It is usually due to incomplete removal because the tumor grows in a lobular pattern into the bone, and, therefore, a thorough curettage is difficult to carry out (8).

Some chondromyxoid fibromas of the foot may be locally aggressive and extend into the soft tissues (8, 28). In one case studied by the author, the tumor was primary in the metatarsal bone, recurred despite a ray resection, and, finally, invaded the adjacent bone and

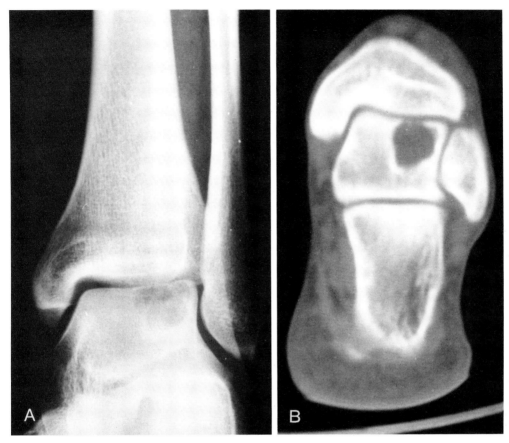

Figure 7.15. Chondroblastoma. **A,** osteolytic lesion in the talus with some degree of marginal sclerosis. **B,** the lesion is clearly seen in the CAT scan. No calcification is noted. Patient is a 27-year-old male.

soft tissues, requiring a partial resection of the foot.

Chondrosarcoma

Excluding multiple myeloma, chondrosarcoma is the second most common primary neoplasm of the skeletal system, after osteosarcoma. It affects males more frequently than females and occurs in adults and older people, usually between 30 and 75 years (1). The most frequent sites of chondrosarcoma are the femur, pelvis, humerus, scapula, ribs, and tibia. The foot is rarely a site for chondrosarcoma. In the Mayo Clinic series (1), 9 out of 634 chondrosarcomas originated in the foot (1.4%). The tarsal bones, particularly the calcaneus, are the most common sites, followed by the phalanges and metatarsals (1, 2, 29–36). Most chondrosarcomas of the foot bones are primary, although secondary chondrosarcomas arising in patients with solitary

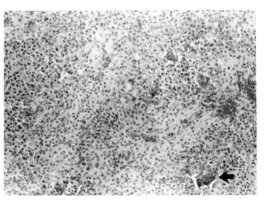

Figure 7.16. Photomicrograph of chondroblastoma showing dense aggregates of polygonal cells with focal calcification around individual cells (*arrow*). (Original magnification, X160)

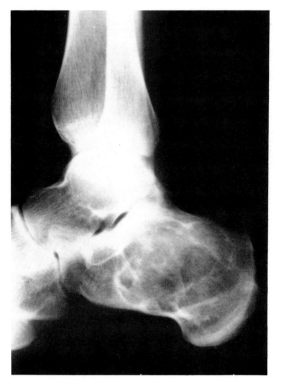

Figure 7.17. Chondromyxoid fibroma. The lesion in the calcaneus is large and osteolytic with sclerotic scalloped margins. Twenty-nine-year-old female with pain for the last 3 years.

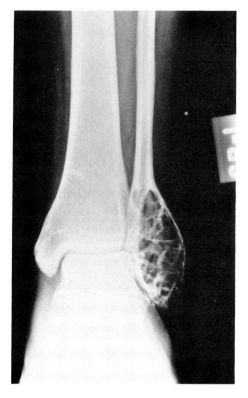

Figure 7.18. This tumor is located in the distal fibula and the cortex is expanded and thin. There is prominent trabeculation within the lesion. The patient is a 42-year-old female.

osteochondromas (31), hereditary multiple exostosis (32), and enchondromatosis do occur (1, 7).

The patients complain of increasing pain and swelling, or progressive enlargement of a toe, that lasts from several months to up to 10 years. In some tumors, there is minimal or complete absence of pain and, although this is uncommon, it has also been noted in chondrosarcomas involving other parts of the skeleton (31).

Radiologically, the affected bone shows central expansion and destruction of the medullary cavity associated with thinning and destruction of the cortex. In most cases, the tumor has extended into the soft tissues, and, in some reports, this was quite prominent (33, 35) (Fig. 7.20). Patchy or punctate calcification of the tumor is a common radiographic finding, and it has been found in approximately two-thirds of the cases (36). The presence of cortical destruction and soft-tissue extension in a cartilaginous tumor is a radiologic sign of local aggressiveness and is essential for the di-

agnosis of chondrosarcoma, as opposed to enchondroma.

In chondrosarcomas arising in osteochondromas, the radiologic appearance is most helpful for the diagnosis: the presence of patchy calcification dispersed throughout a large cartilage cap and away from the stalk of the osteochondroma (14) (Fig. 7.21).

Grossly, the tumors can measure up to 12 cm and consist of whitish cartilaginous tissue with areas of gritty calcification (36) (Fig. 7.21 B). In some cases, the tumor may be gelatinous with a mxyoid appearance. Evidence of lobulation is sometimes more obvious in the component of the tumor that is invading soft tissue. Histologically, chondrosarcoma of the foot does not differ from chondrosarcoma of other sites and consists of moderately to highly cellular cartilaginous tissue showing varying degrees of cell pleomorphism and nuclear atypia (Fig. 7.22). The tumor grows in a lobulated fashion and areas of degeneration and necrosis are noted. Mito-

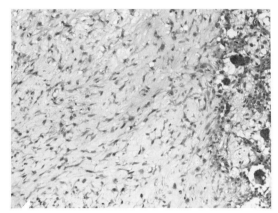

Figure 7.19. Photomicrograph of chondromyxoid fibroma. The tumor cells are stellate in shape and are separated by abundant matrix. At the periphery of the myxoid lobules there are multinucleated giant cells. (Original magnification, X260)

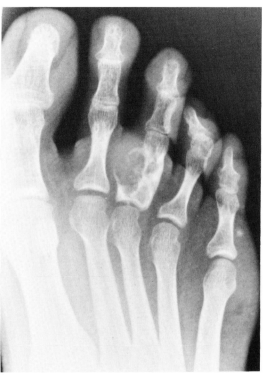

Figure 7.20. Chondrosarcoma. Radiograph shows osteolytic lesion in proximal phalanx of third toe, with expansion and destruction of the medial cortex and focal soft-tissue extension. The patient was a 28-year-old male with swelling of the toe for 6 months.

ses are rare. Patchy calcification of the matrix is seen to a variable degree, and reactive ossification around the tumor lobules can be recognized. These latter findings correlate with the patchy densities seen radiographically.

Most chondrosarcomas of the foot are of low grade (grade 1) or moderate grade (grade 2) of malignancy (36). In some grade 1 chondrosarcomas, the histologic differentiation from chondromas may be a difficult problem, because it is well-known that enchondromas of tubular bones of the feet may show cellular pleomorphism and yet still be benign (2). In these cases, tumor infiltration of the bone marrow is an indication of malignancy, together with invasion of the cortex and soft tissues.

The treatment for chondrosarcomas of the foot depends on the size and location of the tumor and includes amputation of the digit, ray resection, and partial, or complete, amputation of the foot, if necessary (36). An adequate resection from the onset will avoid the development of local recurrence and the possibilities of distant metastases. Two out of 12 patients reported by Dahlin and Salvador (36) with chondrosarcomas of the foot developed pulmonary metastases.

Cartilaginous tumors can occur in the soft tissues of the foot, and they are usually benign. They may be quite cellular histologically and can recur following excision, but they behave in a benign fashion and do not metasta-

size (37). Therefore, these benign soft-tissue chondromas of the foot should be recognized as distinct entities and different from the tumors arising in the bone.

Most chondrosarcomas of the foot are of the ordinary or conventional histologic type. The foot is rarely involved with other infrequent types of chondrosarcomas, such as myxoid chondrosarcoma (38) and mesenchymal chondrosarcoma (39).

OSSEOUS TUMORS OF THE FOOT

Osseous tumors are the second most common neoplasms of the skeletal system after cartilaginous neoplasms. The incidence of these lesions in the foot is rare for the most part: they account for 1.4 and 5.6% of the osseous tumors in Dahlin and Unni (1) and Schajowicz's (2) series, respectively. Benign osseous tumors are more frequent than malignant ones.

Figure 7.21. Chondrosarcoma arising at the site of an osteochondroma of the calcaneus that was removed 10 years previously. Patient is a 30-year-old female. **A,** there is patchy calcification scattered throughout the soft tissue, consistent with chondrosarcoma (14). **B,** amputation specimen. There are white nodular areas of cartilage involving the soft tissues (*arrow*).

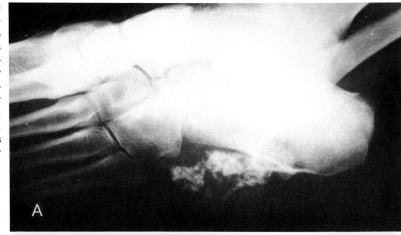

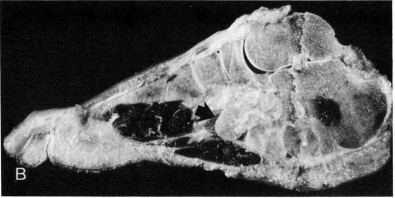

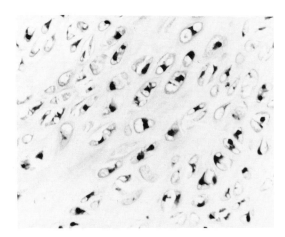

Figure 7.22. Photomicrograph of chondrosarcoma, showing moderate to marked degree of cellularity. There is evidence of cellular pleomorphism and nuclear hyperchromasia. (Original magnification, X320)

Osteoid Osteoma

Osteoid osteoma is a relatively rare, benign, bone-forming lesion which usually measures less than 1 cm in diameter. It occurs more frequently in males and has a predilection for young people, particularly in the second decade of life. The femur, especially the proximal end, and the tibia account for at least 50% of all cases (1, 2).

The frequency of osteoid osteoma in the foot varies from 4.0 to 15.4% (1, 2, 40, 41). It is the second most common benign tumor of the foot after chondromas (1, 2). The talus is by far the most common site and many reports have been published of this tumor in that location, as mentioned by Capanna et al. (40). In that article, the authors reviewed their experience and found 68 cases of osteoid osteoma and osteoblastoma in the foot. Of the 68 cases, 40 were located in the talus and 33 were osteoid osteomas (40). The calcaneus, other tarsal bones, metatarsals, and phalanges are less frequent sites for this lesion (42, 43).

The typical symptom of osteoid osteoma of the foot is pain that is often continuous and increases by weight bearing and walking. The pain often awakens the patient at night. It is promptly relieved within 20–30 minutes by taking aspirin. This pain pattern and its relief by salicylates is typical of most osteoid osteomas (41). It may be present for a few months up to a few years before diagnoses (40, 42). There are, however, occasional cases of painless osteoid osteomas (44).

Some lesions in the foot are accompanied by limping, muscle atrophy, and decreased range of motion of the joint adjacent to the affected bone (42). Some patients note the presence of local swelling of the foot or ankle and even redness and warmth of the soft tissues (40). If the tumors are juxtaarticular, the symptoms may mimic an inflammatory arthritis as a result of associated synovial reaction (40). There is usually tenderness of the nidus on touch, and pressure on it causes pain.

RADIOGRAPHIC FEATURES

The lesion consists of a small radiolucent nidus that measures a few millimeters in diameter, and it is located in the subperiosteal region or within the cancellous bone. Involvement of the cortical bone by osteoid osteoma of the foot is less frequent than in the femur and tibia (42).

In the talus, most osteoid osteomas are subperiosteal and are often located in the neck near the ankle joint (40) (Figs. 7.23 and 7.24). Central calcification of the nidus is frequently seen, and reactive marginal sclerosis, when present, is usually mild and not prominent. This latter feature differentiates subperiosteal and cancellous osteoid osteomas from cortical osteoid osteomas, which show marked marginal sclerosis (42). If the lesions are adjacent to joints, there is evidence of degenerative arthritis, and this may create diagnostic difficulties (42).

Not all osteoid osteomas are recognized initially by routine x-rays (42, 45), and we have seen cases in which plain radiographs showed minimal or no abnormalities at all (Fig. 7.25). Three out of 10 osteoid osteomas of the foot reported by Shereff et al. (42) had normal routine x-rays, and the lesions were detected on tomograms. If a patient has typical symptoms of osteoid osteoma and the plain radiographs are normal, computed tomography should be performed; this is probably the best technique to localize the nidus. Radionuclide scan can also be helpful. In some cases, it may take several months before the nidus is identified by routine x-rays. Magnetic resonance imaging is a

new modality being used recently for the detection of osteoid osteoma (46) (Fig. 7.25C).

PATHOLOGY

If the lesion is removed intact, the nidus is rounded and measures a few millimeters or 1 cm maximum in diameter. It is usually reddish, and gritty and distinct from the surrounding bone; less frequently, it is whitish and heavily calcified.

Histologically, it consists of a delicate trabecular pattern of woven bone separated by a fibrovascular stroma, with abundant osteoblastic activity (Fig. 7.26). There is a variable amount of osteoid matrix in the nidus. The density of the nidus seen radiologically is a reflection of the degree of mineralization of the lesion.

TREATMENT

The treatment for osteoid osteoma is surgical excision either by curettage or en block resection. This usually effects a cure.

Recurrence of symptoms is usually due to failure to remove the nidus, and rarely due to

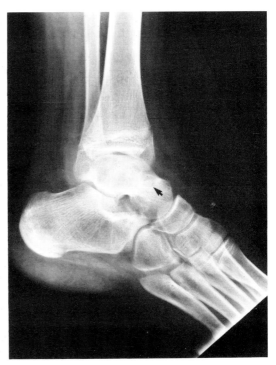

Figure 7.23. Osteoid osteoma arising from the neck of the talus in an 11-year-old girl (*arrow*). The nidus is radiodense and there is little marginal sclerosis. The patient had ankle pain relieved by aspirin. She had antalgic gait and there was decreased dorsiflexion of the ankle.

Figure 7.24. Lesion arising in the posterior talus in a 34-year-old female. **A,** plain radiograph (*arrow*). **B,** CAT scan. The lesion is lytic with focal calcification.

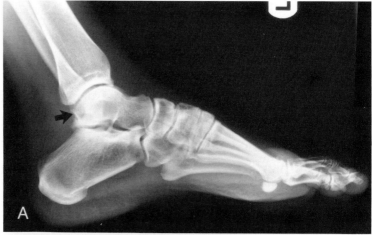

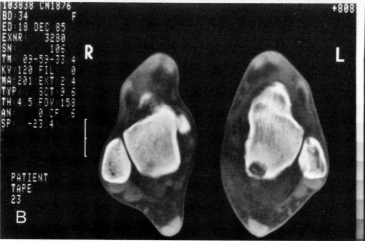

incomplete removal (41). There are cases in which the patient's symptoms disappeared despite the fact that the pathologist failed to find the nidus (47). One of the biggest problems encountered by the surgeon is the intraoperative localization of the nidus. In a recent article, Ayala et al. (48) recommend giving the patient preoperative tetracycline. At the time of surgery, the tissue removed can be examined immediately under an ultraviolet lamp; the lesional tissue shows a strong fluorescence, but the reactive and normal bone do not (48). We found this technique useful in most but not all of our cases that received tetracycline.

Osteoblastoma

Osteoblastoma is an infrequent benign bone-forming neoplasm closely related to osteoid osteoma, but of larger size.

It has a predilection for young people, particularly in the second decade of life. It occurs most commonly in the spine and long bones. The frequency in the foot varies from 1.5 to 9.6% (1, 2, 8). The talus is the most common site (8, 40, 49). The symptom of osteoblastoma is pain that is usually milder than in osteoid osteoma, does not increase at night, and has a limited response to aspirin (40, 41). Ankle swelling, redness and warmth, decreased range of motion, and limping may be other accompanying symptoms.

Radiographic features consist of a radiolucent defect measuring at least 1.5 cm in diameter, associated with mild surrounding reactive bone (Fig. 7.27). The lesion may look like a large osteoid osteoma, including the presence of central calcification. Osteoblastomas of the talus involve the body or neck and may be subperiosteal (40). The tumor often expands

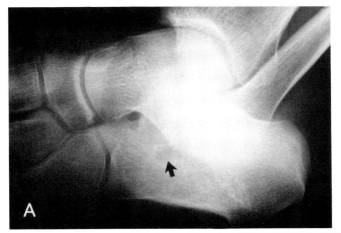

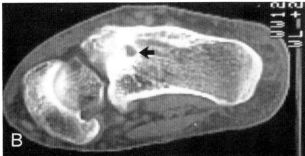

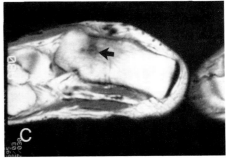

Figure 7.25. Osteoid osteoma of the calcaneus. **A,** the lesion is hardly recognizable in the routine x-ray (*arrow*). **B,** computed tomograph demonstrates the nidus better than does the plain film (*arrow*). **C,** magnetic resonance imaging shows an area of low-intensity signal in the nidus (*arrow*). Proton density.

the bone. Histologically, it resembles osteoid osteoma, although the lesion can be more cellular and vascular with a prominent trabecular pattern (Fig. 7.28).

Osteoblastoma is closely related to osteoid osteoma, but because of its larger size and different behavior it is considered a separate en-

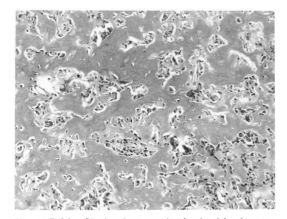

Figure 7.26. Photomicrograph of osteoid osteoma. There are irregular trabeculae of immature bone separated by a stroma composed of mature osteoblasts. (Original magnification, X220)

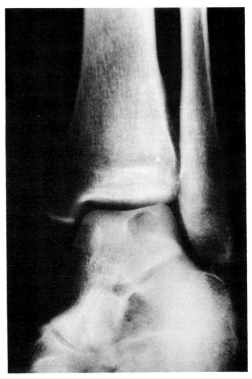

Figure 7.27. Osteoblastoma. There is a radiolucent lesion in the talus with marginal sclerosis.

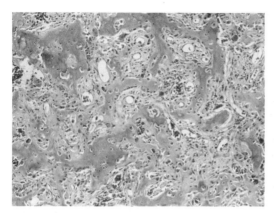

Figure 7.28. Osteoblastoma. The trabeculae of immature bone are separated by abundant vascular stroma with prominent osteoblastic proliferation. (Original magnification, X220)

tity. It is more aggressive than osteoid osteoma, tends to recur more frequently, and there are a few cases of malignant transformation (41). In one case, reported by the author, the tumor was locally aggressive in the foot and involved at least two bones (50) (Fig. 7.29).

Osteosarcoma

Osteosarcoma is the most common primary malignant tumor of bone excluding myeloma. It has a predilection for the second decade of life, and more than 50% of the patients are males. The metaphyseal region of the long bones around the knee is the most common localization (1, 2). The distal metaphyses of the tibia and fibula are infrequent sites.

The foot is a rare site for osteosarcoma. From a total of 2,843 osteosarcomas reported in several papers (1, 2, 8, 52–54), 22 tumors occurred in the foot (0.7%), 13 lesions were located in the tarsal bones, and 9 in the metatarsals. The calcaneus is probably the most frequent site. The phalanges are exceedingly rare sites; to our knowledge there is only one case reported in the literature (55). The age incidence of osteosarcoma of the foot is often older than that of osteosarcoma of long bones.

The clinical symptoms are nonspecific, and the patients complain of swelling of the affected part of the foot, associated with pain of a few weeks to a few months' duration. On physical examination, a mass is frequently palpated in the affected bone. Radiologically, there is usually destruction of the involved bone with increased density and extension beyond the cortex into the soft tissues. The de-

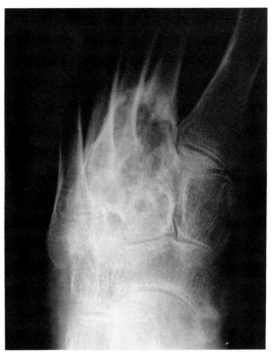

Figure 7.29. Aggressive osteoblastoma. There is a large destructive lesion involving the second metatarsal, second cuneiform, and possibly other bones. Patient was a 22-year-old male with pain for 3½ years.

gree of radiodensity may be prominent. In two calcaneal osteosarcomas seen by the author, the bone was extensively sclerotic (Figs. 7.30 and 7.31).

Histologically, the tumor resembles osteosarcoma of long bones. It is composed of pleomorphic cells with hyperchromatic nuclei and frequent mitoses and shows varying amounts of neoplastic bone (Fig. 7.32). In the lesions with radiologic evidence of sclerosis, there is a marked degree of tumor bone which is heavily mineralized. In this instance, the malignant cells lose their anaplastic features as they become entrapped in the sclerotic bone, and the tumor may be erroneously diagnosed as osteoblastoma or osteoid osteoma. In a recent report of a sclerosing osteosarcoma of toe phalanx, the initial biopsy material was mistaken for an osteoid osteoma (55).

The treatment for osteosarcoma of the foot is below-the-knee amputation if the tumor arises in the tarsal bones. If it originates in the metatarsal bones, a Syme's amputation should be considered instead of a below-knee amputation (51). CAT and magnetic resonance imag-

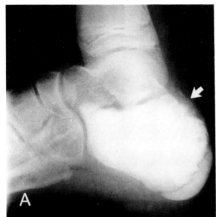
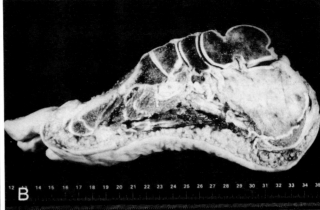

Figure 7.30. Sclerotic osteosarcoma in a 14-year-old male, who complained of swelling and dull pain of the heel of 3 weeks' duration. **A,** the tumor produced a marked radiodensity of most of the calcaneus. There is focal cortical destruction posteriorly (*arrow*). **B,** amputation specimen shows involvement of the entire calcaneus except for the posterior epiphysis. (Courtesy of Dr. Leonard Kahn, Long Island Jewish Hospital, Long Island, NY.)

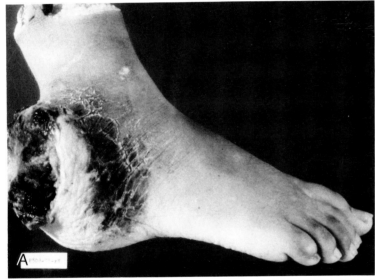

Figure 7.31. Osteosarcoma of calcaneus in a 16-year-old female. **A,** unusual soft-tissue infiltration with extensive ulceration of the skin. Amputated specimen. **B,** radiograph demonstrates increased density of the calcaneus with tumor extension into the soft tissues posteriorly. The joints were not involved. (Courtesy of Dr. Juan J. Segura, Costa Rica.)

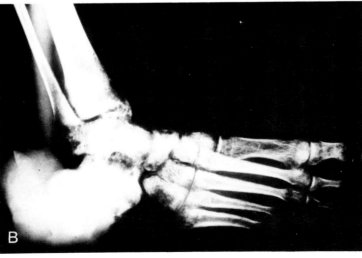

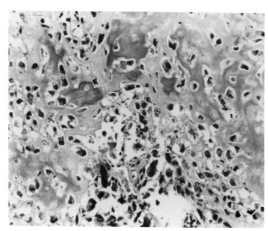

Figure 7.32. Photomicrograph of osteosarcoma. There are pleomorphic malignant cells with large nuclei, separated by tumor osteoid and bone. (Original magnification, X320)

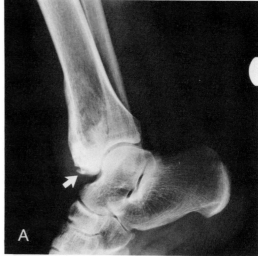

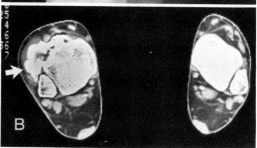

Figure 7.33. Parosteal osteosarcoma arising from the anterior cortex of the distal tibia. **A,** there is increased density and thickness anteriorly (*arrow*). **B,** computed tomograph showing the parosteal origin of the tumor with soft-tissue extent (*arrow*). The medullary cavity of the tibia is spared. The patient is a 38-year-old female with a slow-growing ankle mass for 3 years.

ing are very helpful in outlining the degree of tumor extent in the metatarsal lesions prior to surgery (51).

Due to the rarity of foot osteosarcoma, there is little experience on the prognosis and survival rate. Some authors suggest that it has a somewhat better long-term prognosis than does osteosarcoma of long bones, although there is a high propensity for pulmonary metastasis. All six patients with osteosarcoma of metatarsal bones collected by Sneppen et al. (56) died of their tumor. One osteosarcoma of a tarsal bone seen by the author died of pulmonary metastases in 2½ years.

Parosteal Osteosarcoma

The osteosarcoma described previously is the conventional type arising from the medullary cavity of the bone; it is high-grade malignant and metastasizes frequently. Parosteal osteosarcoma is a less-frequent tumor arising from the surface of the bone; it is low-grade malignant and has a better prognosis than the conventional medullary osteosarcoma. Most parosteal osteosarcomas favor the posterior region of the distal femur. They rarely involve the distal tibia (57, 58) (Fig. 7.33). In a collected series of 164 cases, four lesions originated in the foot (2, 57–59). Two tumors arose in the metatarsals, a third in the calcaneus, and the fourth in the tarsal bones (2, 57–59). There is another case report of a parosteal osteosarcoma arising in a metatarsal bone (60). In a case studied by the

writer, the patient developed progressive enlargement of the foot of 6 years' duration, thought to be myositis ossificans (Fig. 7.34).

Histologically, the tumors are low-grade malignant and composed of well-differentiated spindle cells admixed with organized lamellar bone (Fig. 7.35). They involve the surface of the cortex and infiltrate into the adjacent soft tissues. The medullary cavity of the bone is spared in most cases.

Treatment is partial resection of the foot or amputation. Prognosis is better than in conventional osteosarcoma. However, in one calcaneal (case 11) (59) and one tarsal (case 15) (58) tumor, the patients died of metastatic disease.

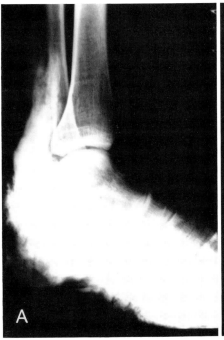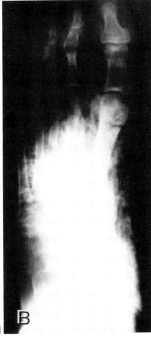

Figure 7.34. A, B, parosteal osteosarcoma. A 28-year-old male with extensive radiodensity involving the soft tissues of the sole of the foot and ankle. The patient died of pulmonary metastasis 2 years after amputation. This case was previously reported (case 15) (58).

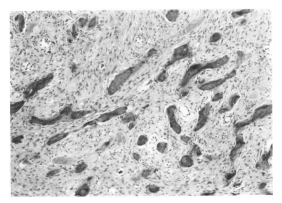

Figure 7.35. Photomicrograph of parosteal osteosarcoma. It consists of well-differentiated spindle cells separated by thin trabecular bone. (Original magnification, X180)

·ACKNOWLEDGMENT

The author would like to thank Ms. Hilda Castro for typing the manuscript.

REFERENCES

1. Dahlin D, Unni K. Bone tumors. General aspect and data on 8,542 cases. 4th ed. Springfield, IL: Charles C Thomas, 1986.
2. Schajowicz F. Tumors and tumor-like lesions of bone and joints. New York: Springer-Verlag, 1981.
3. Norman A. Tumor and tumor-like lesions of the bones of the foot. Semin Roentgenol 1970; 5:407–418.
4. Steiner GC. Benign cartilage tumors. In: Taveras JM, Ferrucci JT, eds. Radiology—diagnosis—imaging—intervention, vol 5. Philadelphia: Lippincott, 1986.
5. Lorenzo J, Dorfman HD. Giant cell reparative granulomas of short bones of the hands and feet. Am J Surg Pathol 1980;4:551–563.
6. Freiberg TA, Hembree JL, Laine W. Periosteal chondroma: a review of the literature and case report. J Foot Surg 1986;25:54–57.
7. Campbell CJ. Tumors of the foot. In: Jahss MH, ed. Disorders of the foot, vol 1. Philadelphia: Saunders, 1982.
8. Huvos AG. Bone tumors. Diagnosis, treatment and prognosis. Philadelphia: Saunders, 1979.
9. Fuselier CO, Binning T, Kushner D, Kirchwehm WW, Rice JRD, Hetherington V, Kahl RL, Hanley DC, West A, Gray J, Berkey SF, Merritt HN, Scherer DC, Ways GA. Solitary osteochondroma of the foot: an in-depth study with case reports. J Foot Surg 1984;23:3–24.
10. Rosen JS. Solitary osteochondroma of the metatarsal. J Am Podiatr Assoc 1983;73:261–262.
11. Greenberg D, Lenet MD, Sherman M. A large osteochondroma of the third toe. J Am Podiatr Assoc 1983;73:208–211.
12. Chioros PG, Frankel SL, Sidlow CJ. Unusual osteochondroma of the foot and ankle. J Foot Surg 1987;26:407–411.
13. Renton P, Stripp WJ. The radiology and radiography of the foot. In: Klenerman L, ed. The foot and its disorders. Blackwell Scientific Publications, 1982.
14. Norman A, Sissons HA. Radiographic hallmarks

of peripheral chondrosarcomas. Radiology 1984;151:589–596.

15. Nora FE, Dahlin DC, Beabout JW. Bizarre parosteal osteochondromatous proliferations of the hands and feet. Am J Surg Pathol 1983; 7:245–250.

16. deLange EE, Pope TL, Fechner RE, Keats TE. Case report 428. Skeletal Radiol 1987;16: 481–483.

17. Kettelkamp DB, Campbell CJ, Bonfiglio M. Dysplasia epiphysealis hemimelica. A report of fifteen cases and a review of the literature. J Bone Joint Surg 1966;48:746–766.

18. Fasting OJ, Bjerkreim I. Dysplasia epiphysealis hemimelica. Acta Orthop Scand 1976;47: 217–225.

19. Hensinger RN, Cowell HR, Ramsey PL, Leopold RG. Familial dysplasia epiphysealis hemimelica, associated with chondromas and osteochondromas. J Bone Joint Surg (Am) 1974; 56:1513–1516.

20. Miller-Breslow A, Dorfman HD. Dupuytren's (subungual) exostosis. Am J Surg Pathol 1988; 12:368–378.

21. Landon GC, Johnson KA, Dahlin DC. Subungual exostosis. J Bone Joint Surg (Am) 1979;61:256–259.

22. Dahlin DC, Ivins JC. Benign chondroblastoma. A study of 125 cases. Cancer 1972;30: 401–413.

23. Barbera C, Pinotti N, Klein MJ, Lewis MM. An unusual case of cystic chondroblastoma of the calcaneus: a case report. Bull Hosp Joint Dis Orthop Inst 1988;48:88–92.

24. Steiner GC, Kantor EB. Ultrastructure of aneurysmal bone cyst. Cancer 1977;40: 2967–2978.

25. Ohno T, Kadoya H, Park P, Yamanashi M, Wakayama K, Ihtsubo K, et al. Case report 382. Skeletal Radiol 1986;15:478–483.

26. Roberts PF, Taylor JG. Multifocal benign chondroblastoma: report of a case. Hum Pathol 1980;11:296–298.

27. Tang J, Gold RH, Mirra JM. Case report 454. Skeletal Radiol 1987;16:675–678.

28. Van Horn JR, Lemmens JAM. Chondromyxoid fibroma of the foot. Report of a missed diagnosis. Acta Orthop Scand 1986;57:375–377.

29. Joseph R, Stones GF, Klein DE, Cavuoto JW. Chondrosarcoma of the foot; diagnosis and treatment. J Am Podiatr Med Assoc 1987; 77:223–227.

30. Wu KK. Chondrosarcoma of the foot. J Foot Surg 1987;26:449–455.

31. Lewis MM, Marcove RC, Bullough PG. Chondrosarcoma of the foot. A case report and review of the literature. Cancer 1975;36:586–589.

32. Wicks IP, Fleming A. Chondrosarcoma of the calcaneum and massive soft tissue calcification in a patient with hereditary and acquired connective tissue diseases. Ann Rheum Dis 1987; 46:346–348.

33. DeBenedetti MJ, Waugh TR, Evanski PM, Jordon I, Kruger M. Chondrosarcoma of the talus. A case report. Clin Orthop 1978;136: 234–237.

34. Wu KK, Guise ER. Chondrosarcoma of the foot; a report of three new cases plus a review of the medical literature. Orthopaedics 1978;1: 380–383.

35. Pachter RM, Albert M. Chondrosarcoma of the foot skeleton. J Bone Joint Surg (Am) 1964; 46:601–607.

36. Dahlin DC, Salvador AH. Chondrosarcomas of bones of the hands and feet—a study of 30 cases. Cancer 1974;34:755–760.

37. Dahlin DC, Salvador AH. Cartilaginous tumors of the soft tissues of the hand and feet. Mayo Clin Proc 1974;49:721–726.

38. Steiner GC, Greenspan A, Jahss M, Norman A. Myxoid chondrosarcoma of the os calcis. A case report. Foot Ankle 1984;5:84–91.

39. Nakashima Y, Unni KK, Shives TC, Swee RG, Dahlin DC. Mesenchymal chondrosarcoma of bone and soft tissue. A review of 111 cases. Cancer 1986;57:2444–2453.

40. Capanna R, Van Horn JR, Ayala A, Picci P, Bettelli G. Osteoid osteoma and osteoblastoma of the talus. Skeletal Radiol 1986;15:360–364.

41. Norman A. Benign osteoblastic tumors. In: Taveras MJ, Ferrucci JT, eds. Radiology—diagnosis—imaging—intervention, vol 5. Philadelphia: Lippincott, 1986.

42. Shereff MJ, Cullivan WT, Johnson KA. Osteoid osteoma of the foot. J Bone Joint Surg (Am) 1983;65:638–641.

43. Hamilos DT, Cervetti RG. Osteoid osteoma of the hallux. J Foot Surg 1987;26:397–399.

44. Wiss DA, Reid BS. Painless osteoid osteoma of the finger. Report of three cases. J Hand Surg 1983;8:914–917.

45. Stapor DJ, Jacobs RL. Osteoid osteoma of the talus. A case study. Bull Hosp Joint Dis Orthop Inst 1987;47:273–277.

46. Yearger BA, Schiebler ML, Wertheim SB, Schmidt RG, Torg JS, Perosio PM, et al. MR imaging of osteoid osteoma of the talus. Case report. J Comput Assist Tomogr 1987;11: 916–917.

47. Sim FH, Dahlin DC, Beabout JW. Osteoid osteoma; diagnostic problems. J Bone Joint Surg (Am) 1975;57:154–159.

48. Ayala AG, Murray JA, Erling MA, Raymond AK. Osteoid osteoma: intraoperative tetracycline-fluorescence demonstration of the nidus. J Bone Joint Surg (Am) 1986;68:747–751.

49. Giannestras NJ, Diamond JR. Benign osteoblastoma of the talus. A review of the literature and report of a case. J Bone Joint Surg (Am) 1958;40:469–478.

50. Steiner GC. Ultrastructure of osteoblastoma. Cancer 1977;39:2127–2136.

51. Wu KK. Tumor review: osteogenic sarcoma of the foot. J Foot Surg 1987;26:269–271.

52. Ohno T, Abe M, Tateishi A, Kako K, Miki H, Sekine K, et al. Osteogenic sarcoma. A study of 130 cases. J Bone Joint Surg (Am) 1975; 57:397–404.

53. Uribe-Botero G, Russell WO, Sutow WW, Martin RG. Primary osteosarcoma of bone. A clinicopathologic investigation of 243 cases, with necropsy studies in 54. Am J Clin Pathol 1977; 67:427–435.

54. Weinfeld MS, Dudley HR Jr. Osteogenic sarcoma. A follow up study of the ninety-four cases observed at the Massachusetts General Hosp

from 1920–1960. J Bone Joint Surg (Am) 1962; 44:269–276.

55. Mirra JM, Kameda N, Rosen G, Eckardt J. Primary osteosarcoma of toe phalanx: first documented case. Review of osteosarcoma of short tubular bones. Am J Surg Pathol 1988;12: 300–307.

56. Sneppen O, Dissing I, Heerfordt J, Schiodt T. Osteosarcoma of the metatarsal bones. Review of the literature and report of a case. Acta Orthop Scand 1978;49:220–223.

57. Unni KK, Dahlin DC, Beabout JW, Ivins JC. Parosteal osteogenic sarcoma. Cancer 1976; 37:2466–2475.

58. Ahuja SC, Villacin AB, Smith J, Bullough PG, Huvos AG, Marcove RC. Juxtacortical (parosteal) osteogenic sarcoma. Histological grading and prognosis. J Bone Joint Surg (Am) 1977; 59:632–647.

59. Lorentzon R, Larsson SE, Boquist L. Parosteal (juxtacortical) osteosarcoma. A clinical and histopathological study of 11 cases and a review of the literature. J Bone Joint Surg (Br) 1980; 62:86–92.

60. Kliman MD, Fornasier VL, Hastings DE. Parosteal osteosarcoma of the fourth metatarsal bone. Foot Ankle 1982;3:50–52.

8

Summary

—Carol Cambas

Neoplasms of the foot and leg are increasingly encountered in podiatric practice. Since the publication of Dr. Steven Berlin's *Soft Somatic Tumors of the Foot: Diagnosis and Surgical Management* (1976), there has been no single current reference of this nature to assist doctors in the differential diagnosis and treatment of this disease. This text helps to fill that gap.

Contributors to this volume were asked to summarize recent findings in their specialties and advise clinicians of their expertise relevant to treating neoplasms and clarifying correct procedures (diagnostic and therapeutic).

"Current Etiologic Theories of Neoplasia" summarizes current thinking on the possible causes of this disease. The main theme of the entire volume is that cancer is a multifactorial event. There is no single cause, but there may be, and usually are, multiple factors that can produce neoplastic tumors, transform benign ones into malignant forms, and make the treatable disease untreatable. Podiatrists and medical doctors must be aware of all the potential factors that may be involved. Dr. McCarthy succinctly reviews scientific advances in our understanding of the role of genetics, cell reproduction, viruses, the immune system, and the interaction among them in healthy individuals, as well as what may go wrong to produce neoplasms. Environmental factors, such as stress and nutrition, are also discussed, as are their possible etiologic roles.

"Epidemiology of Neoplasms of the Foot" provides information on world-wide incidence rates, frequency of different tissue type tumors, and the percentage of benign versus malignant conditions. Dr. Shore systematically analyzes and summarizes descriptive data on the epidemiology of neoplasms that are not currently available in the clinical literature in any single source (most are case series).

The remainder of the chapter focuses on malignant neoplasms: bone, soft tissue, melanoma, and nonmelanotic skin cancer. He points out that data on the epidemiology of foot neoplasms are sparse and that a need for current data exists. There is also a relatively untapped area for future investigation in documenting epidemiologic and clinical aspects of foot malignancies associated with AIDS. He concludes by pointing out that podiatry needs "alert clinicians" to detect new clues on the etiology or other characteristics of neoplasms and that these individuals may have valuable insights for medical sciences.

The psychology of cancer is an extremely important issue. The extraordinary stress that always accompanies such a diagnosis can produce terror in a patient. It can also lead to lapses of judgment on the part of the doctor and the patient.

In "The Psychologic Aspects of Cancer," Dr. Applebaum discusses psychologic ramifications in the doctor and the patient, as well as the interaction between them. Too frequently, doctors forget that such diagnoses are often equivocal. They have been trained to be decisive, and it is either difficult or impossible for them to get beyond the dictates of their training and the emotional need to conform to it.

Prognosis is even more difficult. Predictions are mainly statistical probabilities; the future cannot be predicted by medical science.

Healing comes through wildly diverse means. While scientific advances in learning to recognize, diagnose, and treat diseases have been remarkable, there is still a great deal we do not know in medicine.

Dr. Applebaum discusses the history of the idea of a mind-body split in Western culture and medicine, including Freud's struggle with it. Scientific attitudes can, and do, change for a variety of reasons. In the last 25 years, the mind-body split paradigm has been largely replaced by the idea of holistic medicine.

Previously, psychosomatic medicine was mostly anecdotal. However, as knowledge increases and technology advances, new fields are being created. Psychoneuroimmunology deals with the effect of mental attitudes on the body's resistance to disease by way of the "mind," brain, and immune system. There is now hard evidence of the effect on the body of emotional states (e.g., on blood pressure). Distress and loneliness are related to reduced levels of γ-interferon.

His research supports the hypothesis that there is a cancer-disposing and maintaining state of mind. Inhibited aggression may be a causal factor.

A backlash against the holistic view is now developing. [The term holistic medicine has been usurped by a host of medical "quacks" to cover a broad range of nonprofessional, unproven techniques and treatments, utilizing anecdotal statements to support their work. Holistic medicine that refers to treating the whole patient (brain, body, disease) is a different issue, one that should be supported—Eds.] Some doctors say patients are coming to them demanding expertise in which they were trained and are proficient, not a good bedside manner.

Perhaps the most critical aspect of treating patients with neoplasms is being able to differentiate benign from malignant conditions. Dr. Cole's chapter reviews current knowledge of the cellular basis of neoplasia, but most of this section deals with correct procedures in obtaining a complete history and performing an exhaustive physical examination. It outlines the data a good history should contain and explains the potential clinical significance of each. There is also an extensive delineation of the correct sequence of steps to perform in a physical examination, what specific things to look for, and what their potential clinical significance might be. Podiatrists are physicians, and they must be aware that what they see on the lower extremity may be a clue to disease elsewhere in the body. They must then refer the patient to the correct medical doctor.

Dr. Cole also discusses the importance of biopsy and of selecting a pathologist. Technologic advances of the past few decades introduced more sophisticated equipment for use in biopsy procedures that also has made more accurate diagnosis, treatment, and prognosis possible.

The remainder of this book consists of chapters written by podiatrists and medical doctors with expertise in treating various neoplasms of the foot and leg. Each distinguished contributor discusses his or her experience and expertise with specific diagnostic measures and follow-up procedures, differential diagnosis, treatment, and prognosis with specific types of soft-tissue and osseous neoplasms. There is a separate, complete chapter on vascular, muscular, tenosynovial, nervous, fibrous, adipose, and cutaneous neoplasms. The chapter on osseous neoplasms has been included to complete the volume.

Index

Page numbers in *italics* denote figures; those followed by "t" denote tables.

Acanthoma, clear cell, 151
Acanthosis nigricans, 150
Achilles tendon
    normal, *81*
    thickening due to seronegative spondyloarthropathy,
        86–87
Acoustic neuroma, 104
Acquired immune deficiency syndrome, Kaposi's sarcoma
    in, 55–59, 154
Adenocarcinoma, digital papillary, 154
Adenolipomatosis, 144
Adenoma, digital papillary, 151
Adenovirus, 6
Adipose tissue tumors, 143–148
    adiposis dolorosa, 147
    angiomyolipoma, 147
    lipofibromatous hamartoma, 147–148
    lipoma, 143–145
    lipoma arborescens, 147
    liposarcoma, 145–147
    nevus lipomatosus superficialis, 147
    piezogenic papules, 147
Adiposis dolorosa, 147
Adult T cell leukemia/lymphoma, 8
Albright's syndrome, 172
Aneurysmal bone cyst, 164–165, *168*
    clinical presentation of, 164
    differential diagnosis of, 164
    etiology of, 164
    histology of, 164
    radiologic appearance of, 164
    site of, 164
    treatment of, 164
Angioendotheliomatosis, malignant, 153–154
Angiography
    of fibrous tumors, 123–124
    of tenosynovial neoplasia, 81–83
    of vascular tumors, 46–47
Angiokeratoma circumscriptum, 151
Angioleiomyoma, 65–67, 151
    age and sex distribution of, 65–66
    clinical features of, 66
    diagnostic procedures for, 66
    differential diagnosis of, 66
    etiology of, 65
    histology of, 66
    locations of, 65
    origin of, 65
    prevalence of, 65
    recurrence of, 66–67

size of, 66
    treatment of, 66
Angiolipoma, 144
Angiomyolipoma, 147
Angiosarcoma, 53–55
    on angiography, 46
    of bone, 55
        clinical features of, 55
        diagnosis of, 55
        prognosis of, 55
        treatment of, 55
    cutaneous, without lymphedema, 54
    of deep soft tissue, 54
    grading of, 53
    incidence of, 53
    locations of, 53
    lymphedema and, 54
    metastases of, 53
    postirradiation, 54
    prognosis of, 53
Antioncogenes, 5
Antoni types A and B tissue, 107, *107*, 111
Arsenical keratoses, 151–152, *152*

Basal cell carcinoma, 153
    epidemiology of, 29
    etiology of, 29
Bednar's tumors, 135
Biopsy procedures, 43–44
    electron microscopy, 44
    handling of specimens, 43
    incisional vs. excisional biopsy, 43
    special stains, 43–44
Bizarre parosteal osteochondromatous proliferation, 190
Blue nevus, 156–157
Blue rubber bleb nevus, 49–50
"Bone islands," 170
Bone lesions, 163–183
    aneurysmal bone cyst, 164–165, *168*
    angiosarcoma, 55
    bizarre parosteal osteochondromatous proliferation, 190
    Brodie's abscess, 182–183, *183*
    chondroblastoma, *176*, 176–177, 192–194, *195*
    chondromyxoid fibroma, *177*, 177–178, 194–195,
        196–197
    chondrosarcoma, 25, 195–197, *197–198*
    curettage and bone grafting for, 163
    cystlike, 166t–167t
    diagnosis of, 163
        computed tomography, 163

Bone Lesions—*continued*
  magnetic resonance imaging, 163
  radiography, 163
  scintigraphy, 163
  tomography, 163
  dysplasia epiphysialis hemimelica, 191, *193*
  enchondroma, *175*, 175–176, 186, *187–188*
  enchondromatosis, 186, *189*
  eosinophilic granuloma, 181, *181*
  epidemiology of, 24–25
  etiology of, 25
  fibrous cortical defect, *170*, 170–171
  fibrous dysplasia, *172*, 172–173
  giant cell tumor, *168*, 168–169
  grading of, 163
  hereditary multiple exostosis, 190, *192*
  intraosseous ganglion, 178–179, *179*
  intraosseous glomus tumor, 180–181
  intraosseous lipoma, 178, *178*
  leiomyosarcoma, 68–69
  metastatic, 26
  multiple myeloma, 181–182, *182*
  nonossifying fibroma, *171*, 171–172
  osseous hemangioma, 179–180, *180*
  osteoblastoma, 174–175, *175*, 200–202, *201–202*
  osteochondroma, 187–190, *189–191*
  osteoid osteoma, *173*, 173–174, 198–200, *199–201*
  osteosarcoma, 202–204, *203–204*
  parosteal osteosarcoma, 204, *204–205*
  periosteal chondroma, 186, *189*
  pseudocysts, 169–170, *170*
  subungual exostoses, 191–192, *193–194*
  unicameral bone cyst, 165–168, *168*
Bowen's disease, 152, *152*
Branham's test, 45
Brodie's abscess, 182–183, *183*
  clinical presentation of, 182
  differential diagnosis of, 183
  etiology of, 182
  histology of, 183
  radiologic appearance of, 183
  site of, 183
  treatment of, 183
Burkitt's lymphoma, 11
Bursa exostotica, 188

Cachexia, 17
Café-au-lait spots, 104
Cancer
  cellular basis of, 40
  diagnosis of, 40–44
  principal features of, 40
  variable biologic behavior of, 40
Carotenoids, 18
Cartilaginous tumors, 186–197
  bizarre parosteal osteochondromatous proliferation, 190
  chondroblastoma, *176*, 176–177, 192–194, *195*
  chondromyxoid fibroma, *177*, 177–178, 194–195,
    196–197
  chondrosarcoma, 195–197, *197–198*
  dysplasia epiphysialis hemimelica, 191, *193*
  enchondroma, *175*, 175–176, 186, *187–188*
  enchondromatosis, 187, *189*
  hereditary multiple exostosis, 190, *192*
  incidence of, 186
  osteochondroma, 187–190, *189–191*
  periosteal chondroma, 186, *189*
  subungual exostosis, 191–192, *193–194*

Cell cycle, 6
  definition of, 6
  effect of oncogenes on, 2
  G_o state of, 6
  phases of, 6
  of tumors, 6
Cherry angioma, 48
Chondroblastoma, *176*, 176–177, 192–194, *195*
  age distribution of, 192
  clinical presentation of, 176, 192
  cystic, 194
  differential diagnosis of, 177
  etiology of, 176
  histology of, 177, 193–194, *195*
  malignant transformation of, 194
  radiologic appearance of, 177, 192–193
  site of, 176–177, 192
  treatment of, 177, 194
Chondroma, periosteal, 186, *189*
Chondromatosis, synovial, 87–88
Chondrosarcoma, 195–197, *197–198*
  age and sex distribution of, 195
  clinical features of, 196
  epidemiology of, 25
  grading of, 197
  histology of, 196, *198*
  pathology of, 196, *198*
  radiologic appearance of, 196
  sites of, 195
  treatment of, 197
Codman's tumor. *See* Chondroblastoma
Colony stimulating factors, 3–4
  clinical applications of, 4
  cloned types of, 3–4
  function of, 3
  role in leukemia pathogenesis, 4
Communication, 33–34
Computed tomography
  of fibrous tumors, 124
  of liposarcoma, 147
  of neural tumors, 111
  of tenosynovial neoplasia, 83
  of vascular tumors, 47
Condyloma acuminata, 16–17
Contrast arthrography, of tenosynovial neoplasia, 83
Cutaneous tumors, 149–159
  basal cell carcinoma, 29, 153
  epidemiology of, 24, 25t, 27–29
  melanocytic, 156–159
    benign, 156–157
    melanoma, 157–159, *158–159*
    premalignant, 157
  nonmelanocytic, 149–156
    benign dermal, 151
    benign epidermal, 149–150, *149–150*
    Kaposi's sarcoma, 55–59, 154–156, *155*
    lymphoma, 156
    malignant dermal, 153–154
    malignant epidermal, 152–153, *153*
    metastatic disease, 156
    premalignant, 151–152, *152–153*
  squamous cell carcinoma, 29, 152–153, *153*
Cysts
  bone, 166t–167t
  cutaneous, 150
  tenosynovial, 86
Cytomegalovirus, 58
  Kaposi's sarcoma and, 58

in renal transplant recipients, 58

Dercum's disease, 147
Dermatofibroma, 151
Dermatofibrosarcoma protuberans, 135
    clinical features of, 135
    diagnosis of, 135
    differential diagnosis of, 133, 135
    histology of, 135
    sites of, 135
    treatment of, 135
DNA tumor viruses, 8–13
    Epstein-Barr virus, 11–12, *12*
    human papilloma virus, 9–11, *10*
    in humans vs. animals, 8–9
    mechanism of neoplastic transformation by, 9
Dupuytren's contracture, 129
Dysplasia epiphysialis hemimelica, 191, *193*

Eccrine poroma, 149–150
    malignant, 154
Elastofibroma, 126
    age and sex distribution of, 126
    clinical features of, 126
    etiology of, 126
    treatment of, 126
Electron microscopy, 44
Elephantiasis neuromatosa, 104
Empathic responses, 34
Enchondroma, *175*, 175–176, 186, *187–188*
    age distribution of, 186
    clinical presentation of, 175, 186
    differential diagnosis of, 176
    etiology of, 175
    histology of, 176, 186, *188*
    in Maffucci's syndrome, 175
    in Ollier's disease, 175
    radiologic appearance of, 176, 186
    sites of, 175–176, 186
    treatment of, 176, 186
Enchondromatosis, 187, *189*
Enthesopathy, 80, *83*
Eosinophilic granuloma, 181, *181*
Epidemiology, 24–30
    of bone tumors, 24–26
        chondrosarcoma, 25
        metastatic, 26
        osteosarcoma, 25
        Paget's sarcoma, 25
    incidence rates, 24
    of malignant melanoma, 27–29
    of nonmelanotic skin cancer, 29
        basal cell carcinoma, 29
        squamous cell carcinoma, 29
    of soft tissue neoplasms, 26–27
        fibrosarcoma, 26–27
        Kaposi's sarcoma, 26
        rhabdomyosarcoma, 27
        synovial sarcoma, 27
    type of tissue affected, 24, 25t
Epidermal growth factor, 2, 3
    as progression factor, 3
    receptor for, 3
Epidermolysis bullosa dystrophica, 152, *153*
Epithelioid sarcoma, 154
Epstein-Barr virus, 11–12, *12*
    activation in immunosuppressed persons, 11
    in Burkitt's lymphoma, 11–12, *12*

in nasopharyneal carcinoma, 12
silent infection with, 11

Factor VIII-related antigen, 45
    in Kaposi's sarcoma, 58
Fasciitis, 125
    nodular, 125
        clinical features of, 125
        epidemiology of, 125
        etiology of, 125
        histology of, 125
        treatment of, 125
    proliferative, 125
        clinical features of, 125
        epidemiology of, 125
        histology of, 125
        treatment of, 125
Fiber, dietary, 19
Fibroblastoma, giant cell, 128
    clinical features of, 128
    histology of, 128
    sites of, 128
    treatment of, 128
Fibrolipoma, 144
Fibroma, 125
    calcifying aponeurotic, 128
        clinical features of, 128
        developmental phases of, 128
        histology of, 128
        recurrence of, 128
    chondromyxoid, *177*, 177–178, 194–195, *196–197*
        age distribution of, 194
        clinical presentation of, 177, 194
        differential diagnosis of, 178, 194
        etiology of, 177
        histology of, 177, 194, *197*
        radiologic appearance of, 177, 194
        site of, 177, 194
        treatment of, 178, 194
    nonossifying, *171*, 171–172
        clinical presentation of, 171
        differential diagnosis of, 172
        etiology of, 171
        histology of, 172
        radiologic appearance of, 171–172
        site of, 171
        treatment of, 172
    peritendinous, 88
    of tendon sheath, 126
        clinical features of, 126
        epidemiology of, 126
        etiology of, 126
        histology of, 126
        treatment of, 126
Fibromatosis, 128–130
    classification of, 128
    definition of, 128
    infantile digital, 127
        histology of, 127
        prognosis of, 127
        recurrence of, 127
    juvenile hyalin, 127–128
        clinical features of, 127
        histology of, 127–128
        treatment of, 128
    palmar, 129
    plantar, *129*, 129–130
        age distribution of, 129–130

Fibromatosis—*continued*
   etiology of, 130
   histology of, 130
   incidence of, 129
   other fibromatoses with, 130
   treatment of, 130
Fibrosarcoma, 130–132
   adult, 131–132
     age and sex distribution of, 131
     clinical features of, 131
     etiology of, 132
     histology of, 131
     low- vs. high-grade, 131
     prognosis of, 131
     sites of, 131
     treatment of, 131–132
   congenital and infantile, 132
     clinical features of, 132
     histology of, 132
     treatment of, 132
   epidemiology of, 26–27
   etiology of, 27
   histology of, 130
Fibrous cortical defect, *170*, 170–171
   in children, 170
   clinical presentation of, 170
   differential diagnosis of, 171
   etiology of, 170
   histology of, 171
   radiologic appearance of, 171
   site of, 171
   treatment of, 171
Fibrous dysplasia, *172*, 172–173
   in Albright's syndrome, 172
   clinical presentation of, 172
   differential diagnosis of, 173
   etiology of, 172
   histology of, 173
   radiologic appearance of, 172–173
   site of, 172
   treatment of, 173
Fibrous histiocytoma, 132–137
   cutaneous, 132
   differential diagnosis of, 132–133
   histology of, 132
   juvenile xanthogranuloma, 133–134
   malignant, 135–137
     angiomatoid type, 137
     classification of, 135
     differential diagnosis of, 133
     giant cell type, 136–137
     inflammatory type, 137
     myxoid type, 136
     storiform-pleomorphic type, 135–136
   of subcutaneous and deep tissues, 132
   treatment of, 133
Fibrous tumors, 120–137
   benign, 120, 125–126
     elastofibroma, 126
     fibroma, 125
     fibroma of tendon sheath, 126
     keloid, 126
     nodular fasciitis, 125
     proliferative fasciitis, 125
     proliferative myositis, 125
   classification of, 120–123
   diagnostic procedures for, 123–124
     angiography, 123–124

     computed tomography, 124
     magnetic resonance imaging, 124
     radiography, 123
     scintigraphy, 123
     ultrasonography, 124
     xeroradiography, 123
   fibrohistiocytic, 132–137
     atypical fibroxanthoma, 134
     Bednar's tumors, 135
     benign fibrous histiocytoma, 132–133, *133*
     dermatofibrosarcoma protuberans, 135
     juvenile xanthogranuloma, 133–134
     malignant fibrous histiocytoma, 135–137
     reticulohistiocytoma, 134
     xanthoma, 134–135
   fibromatosis, 128–130
     palmar, 129
     plantar, *129*, 129–130
   incidence of, 120
   of infancy and childhood, 126–128
     calcifying aponeurotic fibroma, 128
     categories of, 126
     fibrous hamartoma of infancy, 127
     giant cell fibroblastoma, 128
     infantile digital fibromatosis, 127
     infantile myofibromatosis, 127
     juvenile hyalin fibromatosis, 127–128
   knuckle pads, 130
   malignant, 120, 130–137
     adult fibrosarcoma, 131–132
     congenital and infantile fibrosarcoma, 132
Fibroxanthoma, atypical, 134
Fine-needle aspiration cytology, 84–86, *85*
   contraindication to, 84
   definition of, 84
   handling of specimens for, 84–86
   indications for, 84
   limitations of, 86
   procedure for, 84, *85*

Ganglion, 86
   intraosseous, 178–179, *179*
     clinical presentation of, 179
     differential diagnosis of, 179
     etiology of, 179
     histology of, 179
     radiologic appearance of, 179
     site of, 179
     treatment of, 179
Germinal center hyperplasia, 14
Giant cell fibroblastoma, 128
Giant cell lipoma, 144–145
Giant cell tumor
   of bone, *168*, 168–169
     clinical presentation of, 168
     differential diagnosis of, 169
     etiology of, 168
     histology of, 169
     radiologic appearance of, 169
     site of, 169
     treatment of, 169
   malignant, 90
   of tendon sheath, 88–90, 90t, 151
     etiology of, 88
     histology, 88–89
     large-joint vs. digital-type, 89–90, 90t
Glomangiosarcoma, 52
Glomus tumor, 51, 151

clinical features of, 51
diagnostic tests for, 51
  Hildreth's ischemia test, 51
  Love's pin test, 51
differential diagnosis of, 51
intraosseous, 180–181
  clinical presentation of, 180
  differential diagnosis of, 181
  etiology of, 180
  histology of, 180
  radiologic appearance of, 180
  site of, 180
  treatment of, 181
location of, 51
metastatic potential of, 51
pain of, 51
roentgenography of, 51
treatment of, 51
Granular cell tumor, 75–76
age and sex distribution of, 75
clinical features of, 75
diagnostic procedures for, 76
differential diagnosis of, 76
histology of, 75–76
malignant vs. benign, 75
origin of, 75
synonyms for, 75
treatment of, 76
Granuloma
eosinophilic, 181, *181*
  clinical presentation of, 181
  differential diagnosis of, 181
  etiology of, 181
  histology of, 181
  radiologic appearance of, 181
  site of, 181
  treatment of, 181
pyogenic, 48, *49*, 151
  appearance of, 48
  blood supply of, 48
  etiology of, 48
  location of, 48
  size of, 48
  treatment of, 48
Granulomatous synovitis, 88
Growth factors, 3

Hamartoma
fibrous, of infancy, 127
  epidemiology of, 127
  histology of, 127
  prognosis of, 127
  sites of, 127
lipofibromatous, 147–148
Hemangioendothelioma
malignant, on angiography, 46
Masson's intravascular, 55
Hemangiomas, 47–51
capillary, 47–48
  cherry angioma, 48
  juvenile hemangioma, 48
  pyogenic granuloma, 48, *49*
cavernous, 48–50
  appearance of, 48
  blue rubber bleb nevus, 49–50
  Klippel-Trenaunay syndrome, 50
  Maffucci's syndrome, 50
  nevus flammeus, 50

verrucous hemangioma, 49
classification of, 47
of deep tissue, 50–51
etiology of, 47
Kasabach-Merritt syndrome due to, 47
of muscle, 50–51
of nerve, 51
osseous, 179–180, *180*
  clinical presentation of, 179
  differential diagnosis of, 180
  etiology of, 179
  histology of, 180
  radiologic appearance of, 180
  site of, 180
  treatment of, 180
phleboliths in, 46, 47
synovial, 50, 88
Hemangiopericytoma, 52–53
on angiography, 46
clinical course of, 52
clinical features of, 52
definition of, 52
diagnosis of, 52
histology of, 52
locations of, 52
malignancy of, 52
metastases of, 52
recurrence of, 52
treatment of, 52–53
Hepatitis B virus, 12–13
in hepatocellular carcinoma, 12
structure of, 12
Hereditary multiple exostosis, 190, *192*
Hildreth's ischemia test, 51
Histoid leproma, *149*
History taking, 40–42
Host defense mechanisms, 16
Human immunodeficiency virus infection, 1
Human papilloma virus, 9–11, *10*
classification of, 9
cofactors in malignant transformation of, 11
genetic structure of, 9
involucrin expression and, 10
mechanism of infection with, 10
types found in various disorders, 9–10
Human T cell leukemia viruses, 8
Hutchinson's melanotic freckle, 29
Hyperkeratosis, punctate, 149, *150*
Hypersensitivity, delayed, *14*, 14–15

Immunohistochemistry, to diagnose vascular tumors, 45–46
Immunologic basis for malignancy, 15–16
Immunosuppressed persons, Kaposi's sarcoma in, 56–58, 154
Incidence rates. See also Epidemiology
definition of, 24
Infectious mononucleosis, 11
Interferon, 16–17
antitumor effects of, 16
classes of, 16
clinical use of, 17
function of, 16
for Kaposi's sarcoma, 58–59
natural and recombinant forms of, 17
for premalignant lesions, 16–17
production costs for, 17
routes of administration for, 17
tumor regression due to, 16

Interferon—*continued*
  types I and II, 16
Involucrin, 10

Kager's triangle, 80, 81
Kaposi's sarcoma, 55–59, *57*, 154–156, *155*
  African, 56
  in AIDS patients, 26, 154
  on angiography, 46
  cells of origin of, 55
  classic, 55–56
  classification of, 154
  clinical course of, 155
  clinical features of, 154
  diagnosis of, 58
  diseases associated with, 55
  epidemic, 56–57
  epidemiology of, 26, 154
  etiology of, 58, 154
  histopathology of, 155
  in immunosuppressed persons, 58, 154
  incidence of, 154
  lymphedema and, 154–155
  sites of, 154
  treatment of, 58–59, 155–156
  types of, 55
Kasabach-Merritt syndrome, 47, 151
Keloid, 126
  clinical features of, 126
  epidemiology of, 126
  histology of, 126
  treatment of, 126
Keratoacanthoma, 150, *150*
Keratoses
  arsenical, 151–152, *152*
  scar, 152
  stucco, 149, *149*
Klippel-Trenaunay syndrome, 50
Knuckle pads, 130
  age and sex distribution of, 130
  definition of, 130
  on foot, 130
  histology of, 130

Ledderhose's disease, *129*, 129–130
  age distribution of, 129–130
  etiology of, 130
  histology of, 130
  incidence of, 129
  other fibromatoses with, 130
  treatment of, 130
Leg ulcers, lymphangiosarcoma and, 54
Leiomyoma, 64–67
  appearance of, 64
  deep, 65
    age and sex distribution of, 65
    clinical features of, 65
    differential diagnosis of, 65
    histology of, 65
    locations of, 65
  definition of, 64
  locations of, 64
  multiple cutaneous, 64–65
    age and sex distribution of, 64
    clinical features of, 64
    histology of, 64–65
    inheritance pattern of, 64
  pain of, 64

solitary cutaneous, 65
  age and sex distribution of, 65
  clinical features of, 65
  differential diagnosis of, 65
  etiology of, 65
  histology of, 65
  locations of, 65
  origin of, 65
vascular, 65–67
  age and sex distribution of, 65–66
  clinical features of, 66
  diagnostic procedures for, 66
  differential diagnosis of, 66
  etiology of, 65
  histology of, 66
  locations of, 65
  origin of, 65
  prevalence of, 65
  recurrence of, 66–67
  size of, 66
  treatment of, 66–67
Leiomyosarcoma, 67–69
  clinical features of, 68
  cutaneous and subcutaneous, 67
    age and sex distribution of, 67
    clinical features of, 67
    differential diagnosis of, 67
    histology of, 67
    location of, 67
    size of, 67
  osseous, 68–69
    clinical features of, 68
    diagnostic procedures for, 68–69
    mitotic activity in, 69
    prognosis of, 69
    treatment of, 69
  prognosis of, 69
  treatment of, 69
  of vascular origin, 67–68
    clinical features of, 68
    differential diagnosis of, 68
    histology of, 68
    venous vs. arterial, 67–68
Lentigo simplex, 156
Leopard syndrome, 156
Leu-7 antibody, 112
Leukemia, cutaneous, 156
Lipoblastoma, 144
Lipoma, 143–145, 151
  age distribution of, 143
  angiolipoma, 144
  clinical features of, 143
  fibrolipoma, 144
  growth of, 143
  histology of, 144
  infiltrating vs. noninfiltrating, 144
  intraosseous, 178, *178*
    clinical presentation of, 178
    differential diagnosis of, 178
    etiology of, 178
    histology of, 178
    incidence of, 178
    radiologic appearance of, 178
    site of, 178
    treatment of, 178
  lipoblastoma, 144
  peritendinous, 88
  pleomorphic, 144–145

sites of, 143
solitary, 144–145
spindle-cell, 144
treatment of, 145
Lipoma arborescens, 147
Lipomatosis, 145
familial multiple, 145
multiple symmetric, 145
Liposarcoma, 145–147
on angiography, 147
clinical features of, 146
on computed tomography, 147
diagnosis of, 146–147
incidence of, 145
metastasis of, 146
myxoid, 146
pleomorphic, 146
round cell, 146
sclerosing, 146
sex distribution of, 145
sites of, 146
treatment of, 146
well-differentiated, 146
Lisch nodules, 104
Love's pin test, 51
Lymphangiosarcoma, 54
Lymphatic drainage, 43
Lymphokines, 15
Lymphoma, cutaneous, 156

Macrobiotic diets, 17
Macrophages, activated, 15
Madelung's disease, 144
Maffucci's syndrome, 50, 151, 175
Magnetic resonance imaging, 44
of fibrous tumors, 124
of tenosynovial neoplasia, 83–84, 84t
of vascular tumors, 47
Malignant melanoma, 157–159, 158–159
acral lentiginous, 157–158, 158
Breslow's thickness of, 159
Clark's levels of invasion of, 159
clinical features of, 157
epidemiology of, 27–28, 157
etiology of, 28–29
of foot, 28
histopathology of, 158–159, 159
incidence of, 157
interferon for, 16
lentigo maligna, 158
management of, 159
mortality from, 157
nodular, 158
pathologic types of, 157
prognosis of, 28
serum phenylalanine and tyrosine levels in, 19
staging of, 159
subungual, 158
superficial spreading, 158
verrucous, 157, 158
Masson's intravascular hemangioendothelioma, 55
Melanocytes, 101
Metastases
of angiosarcoma, 53
of bone tumors, 26
cutaneous, 156
of glomus tumors, 51
of hemangiopericytoma, 52

of liposarcoma, 146
of malignant schwannoma, 99, 117
of myositis ossificans, 76
Milroy's disease, 155
Molecular hybridization, 2
Moles, 156
Molluscum fibrosum, 104
Morton's neuroma
clinical manifestations of, 103, 103
sex distribution of, 98
site of, 98
surgery for, 114
Multiple myeloma, 181–182, 182
clinical presentation of, 182
differential diagnosis of, 182
etiology of, 182
histology of, 182
radiologic appearance of, 182
site of, 182
treatment of, 182
Murine sarcoma viruses, 3
Muscle, 63
development of, 63
smooth, 63
striated, 63
structure of, 63
Muscular neoplasms, 63–77
angioleiomyoma, 65–67
hemangioma, 51
leiomyoma, 64–65
leiomyosarcoma, 67–69
myoblastoma, 75–76
myositis ossificans, 76–77
origin of, 64
primary vs. secondary, 64
rhabdomyoma, 69–70
rhabdomyosarcoma, 70–75
of smooth muscle, 64
of striated muscle, 64
Myelin-associated glycoprotein, 112
Myoblastoma, 75–76
age and sex distribution of, 75
clinical features of, 75
diagnostic procedures for, 76
differential diagnosis of, 76
histology of, 75–76
malignant vs. benign, 75
origin of, 75
synonyms for, 75
treatment of, 76
Myofibromatosis, infantile, 127
clinical course of, 127
etiology of, 127
histology of, 127
multicentric vs. solitary, 127
nomenclature of, 127
spontaneous remission of, 127
Myositis, proliferative, 125
clinical features of, 125
epidemiology of, 125
etiology of, 125
histology of, 125
treatment of, 125
Myositis ossificans, 76–77
clinical features of, 77
definition of, 76
diagnostic procedures for, 77
differential diagnosis of, 77

Myositis ossificans—*continued*
    dystrophic, 76
    etiology of, 77
    histology of, 77
    lab findings in, 77
    metastatic, 76
    prognosis of, 77
    treatment of, 77
    variants of, 76–77
Myxolipoma, 144
Myxoma of nerve sheath
    histopathology of, 106
    site of, 98

Nerve, hemangioma of, 51
Neural tumors, 97–118
    age distribution of, 97–98
    classification of, 99–101
    clinical manifestations of, 102–105
    diagnostic methods for, 110–113
    differential diagnosis of, 109–110
    histopathology of, 105–108
    incidence of, 97
    pathogenesis of, 101–102
    prognosis of, 115–118
    sex distribution of, 98
    sites of, 98–99
    treatment of, 113–115
Neuroblastoma
    age distribution of, 98
    clinical manifestations of, 103
    diagnosis of, 111
    prognosis of, 116
    sex distribution of, 98
    site of, 98–99
Neurofibroma, 151
    diagnosis of, 111
    differential diagnosis of, 109, 110t
        cutaneous, 109
        of peripheral nerve, 109
        plexiform, 109
    histopathology of, 106, *106*
    malignant transformation of, 97
    pathogenesis of, 101
    prognosis of, 116
    sex distribution of, 98
    sites of, 99
Neurofibromatosis, *121*, 151
    age distribution of, 98
    café-au-lait spots in, 104
    chromosomal abnormality in, 101
    clinical manifestations of, 100–101, 103–105, *104–105*
    CNS effects of, 104
    cutaneous effects of, 104
    differential diagnosis of, 109–110, 110t, *111*
    incidence of, 97
    malignant schwannoma and, 97
    malignant tumors in, 105, 114, 118
    osseous effects of, 104–105
    prognosis of, 117–118
    sites of, 99, *100*
    treatment of, 113
Neurofibrosarcoma, 154
    histopathology of, 108
    prognosis of, 118
    sites of, 99
    treatment of, 115
Neuroma
    acoustic, 104
    age distribution of, 98
    clinical manifestations of, 103, *103*
    histopathology of, 108
    Morton's. See Morton's neuroma
    prognosis of, 115–116
    sites of, 98–99
    treatment of, 114
Neurothekeoma
    clinical manifestations of, 103
    differential diagnosis of, 110
    histopathology of, 106
    sex distribution of, 98
Nevus
    blue, 156–157
    blue rubber bleb, 49–50
    common melanocytic, 156
    compound, 156
    congenital melanocytic, 157
    dysplastic, 29, 157
    intradermal, 156
    junctional, 156
    melanotic risk of, 28–29
    spitz, 157
    strawberry, 48
Nevus flammeus, 50
    osteohypertrophic, 50
Nevus lipomatosus superficialis, 147
Nutrition, role in tumorigenesis, 17–19
    dietary fiber, 19
    phenylalanine and tyrosine, 19
    vitamin A, 18–19
    vitamin C, 18
    vitamin E, 18

Ollier's disease, 175
Oncogenes, 1–6
    activation of, 4–5
        by chromosomal translocations, 4–5
        by gene overexpression, 5
        by point mutations, 4
    cellular, 2
    growth factors and, 3–4
    historical recognition of, 1–2
    in human tumors, 1
    number of, 1
    precursors of, 1
    products of, 2
        DNA-binding proteins, 2
        GTP-binding (*ras*) proteins, 2–3
        protein kinases, 2–3
    proto-oncogenes, 2
    viral, 6–13. See also Viral oncogenesis
        definition of, 1
Oncosuppressor genes, 5
Os tibiale externum syndrome, 87
Osgood-Schlatter disease, 87
Osteoblastoma, 174–175, *175*, 200–202, *201–202*
    age distribution of, 200
    aggressive, 202, *202*
    clinical presentation of, 174, 200
    differential diagnosis of, 175
    etiology of, 174
    histology of, 175, 200, *202*
    radiologic appearance of, 175, 200
    site of, 174, 200
    treatment of, 175
Osteochondritis dissecans, 87

etiology of, 87
radiographic evaluation of, 87
sites of, 87
Osteochondroma, 187–190, *189–191*
age distribution of, 187
cliical features of, 187–188
incidence of, 187
pathology of, 189–190, *190*
radiologic appearance of, 188
sites of, 187
treatment of, 190
Osteochondromatosis, multiple, 190, *192*
Osteoid osteoma, *173*, 173–174, 198–200, *199–201*
age and sex distribution of, 198
clinical presentation of, 173, 198–199
differential diagnosis of, 174
etiology of, 173
histology of, 174, 199, *201*
incidence of, 198
pathology of, 199
radiologic appearance of, 174, 199
site of, 173–174, 198
treatment of, 174, 199–200
Osteosarcoma, 202–204, *203–204*
age and sex distribution of, 202
clinical presentation of, 202
epidemiology of, 25
histology of, 202, *204*
parosteal, 204, *204–205*
histology of, 204, *205*
prognosis of, 204
sites of, 204
treatment of, 204
prognosis of, 204
sites of, 202
treatment of, 202–204

Paget's sarcoma, 25
Periosteal chondroma, 186, *189*
Peritendinitis, 80
definition of, 80
on ultrasound, 80, *82*
Perivascular cuffing, *14*, 14–15
Peutz-Jehgers syndrome, 156
Phleboliths, 46–47
in hemangiomas, 46, 47
plain film appearance of, 46
Physical examination, 42–43
auscultation, 43
inspection, 42
lymph drainage, 43
measurements, 43
palpation, 42–43
Piezogenic papules, 147
Pigmented villonodular synovitis, 88, *89–90*
histology of, 88
localized vs. diffuse, 88
radiographic signs of, 88
sites of, 88
symptoms of, 88
Platelet-derived growth factor, 3
Port-wine stain, 50
Proliferating angioendotheliomatosis, 53
malignant, 53
reactive, 53
Proto-oncogenes, 2
activation of, 4–5
by chromosomal translocations, 4–5

by gene overexpression, 5
by point mutations, 4
definition of, 1
mechanisms of effects on cell proliferation, 2
Pseudoangiosarcoma, 55
Pseudocysts, 169–170, *170*
clinical presentation of, 169
differential diagnosis of, 170
etiology of, 169
histology of, 170
radiologic appearance of, 170
site of, 169–170
treatment of, 170
Psychologic factors, 33–39
attributes of healers, 35
bedside manner, 35
communication, 33–34
"doing everything" vs. "doing nothing," 35
effect of cancer diagnosis on doctor, 33
effect on etiology and course of cancer, 36–39
holistic medicine, 37
inhibited aggression, 38
interactions between etiologic factors, 38
mind-body unity, 36–37
psychoneuroimmunology, 37–38
Simonton approach to disease, 37
empathy, 34
healing relationship, 35
physicians' self-understanding, 36
relaying diagnosis to patient, 34
relaying prognosis to patient, 34–35
reluctance to obtain second opinions, 33
variable responses to healing, 36
Punctate hyperkeratosis, 149, *150*
Pyogenic granuloma, 48, *49*, 151

Radiation, ionizing
bone tumors due to, 25
carcinogenicity of, 13–14
skin cancers due to, 29
Radiotherapy, angiosarcoma after, 54
ras proteins, 2–3
Renal transplant recipients, cytomegalovirus in, 58
Reticulohistiocytoma, 134, 151
cutaneous, 134
differential diagnosis of, 134
etiology of, 134
systemic, 134
Retinoblastoma, 5
Retinoids, 18
Retroviruses, 6–8
acute transforming viruses, 8
genetic structure of, 7
human T cell leukemia viruses, 8
slow transforming viruses, 7–8
Rhabdomyoma, 69–70
classification of, 70
clinical features of, 70
diagnostic procedures for, 70
differential diagnosis of, 70
histology of, 70
recurrence of, 70
treatment of, 70
Rhabdomyosarcoma, 70–75
age and sex distribution of, 70–71
alveolar, 72
botryoid, 71–72
clinical features of, 71

Rhabdomyosarcoma—*continued*
  embryonal, 71
  epidemiology of, 27
  etiology of, 27
  incidence of, 70
  locations of, 71
  pleomorphic, 72–75
    age and sex distribution of, 72
    clinical features of, 72
    diagnostic procedures for, 73–74
    differential diagnosis of, 72–73
    groups I-IV of, 74
    histology of, 72
    incidence of, 72
    locations of, 72
    prognosis of, 75
    treatment of, 74–75
  prognosis of, 71
  subtypes of, 71
RNA tumor viruses, 6–8
  acute transforming viruses, 8
  genetic structure of, 6–7
  hepatitis B virus, 12–13
  human T cell leukemia viruses, 8
  slow transforming viruses, 7–8
Rous sarcoma virus, 2, 6

S-100 protein, 111–112
Scar carcinoma, 152–153, *153*
Scar keratoses, 152
Schwann cells, 100–101
Schwannoma
  age distribution of, 98
  ancient, 106
  benign
    clinical manifestations of, 102
    histopathology of, 107, *107*
    incidence of, 97
    prognosis of, 116
    treatment of, 114, *115*
  cellular
    age distribution of, 98
    clinical manifestations of, 103
    histopathology of, 106–107
    incidence of, 97
    sites of, 99
  diagnosis of, 111–112
  differential diagnosis of, 110, 110t
  glandular, 107
  malignant
    age distribution of, 98
    clinical manifestations of, *102*, 102–103
    histopathology of, 108
    incidence of, 97
    metastatic sites of, 99, 117
    pathologic conditions associated with, 117t
    in patients with neurofibromatosis, 97
    prognosis of, 117
    sex distribution of, 98
    sites of, 99
    treatment of, 114–115
  site of, 99
Scoliosis, in neurofibromatosis, 105
Second opinion, 33
Sever's disease, 87
Sinding-Larsen-Johansson syndrome, 87
Sinus histiocytosis, *15*, 15–16
  definition of, 15

  as prognostic factor, 14, 15
Skin cancer. See Cutaneous tumors
"Soap bubble" lesions, 55
Soft-tissue tumors, 45–77. See also specific types
  of adipose tissue, 143–148
    adiposis dolorosa, 147
    angiomyolipoma, 147
    lipofibromatous hamartoma, 147–148
    lipoma, 143–145
    lipoma arborescens, 147
    liposarcoma, 145–147
    nevus lipomatosus superficialis, 145
    piezogenic papules, 147
  cutaneous, 149–159
    melanocytic, 156–159
    nonmelanocytic, 149–156
  epidemiology of, 26–27
  fibrous, 120–137
    benign, 125–126
    classification of, 120–123
    diagnostic procedures for, 123–124
    fibrohistiocytic, 132–137
    fibromatosis, 128–130
    incidence of, 120
    of infancy and childhood, 126–128
    malignant, 130–132
  muscular, 63–77
    angioleiomyoma, 65–67
    leiomyoma, 64–65
    leiomyosarcoma, 67–69
    myoblastoma, 75–76
    myositis ossificans, 76–77
    rhabdomyoma, 69–70
    rhabdomyosarcoma, 70–75
  neural, 97–118
    age distribution of, 97–98
    classification of, 99–101
    clinical manifestations of, 102–105
    diagnostic procedures for, 110–113
    differential diagnosis of, 109–110
    histopathology of, 105–108
    incidence of, 97
    pathogenesis of, 101–102
    prognosis of, 115–118
    sex distribution of, 98
    sites of, 98–99
    treatment of, 113–115
  tenosynovial, 79–92
    diagnostic procedures for, 80–86
    differential diagnosis of, 86
    giant cell tumor of tendon sheath, 88–90, 90t
    malignant giant cell tumors, 90
    peritendinous fibromas and lipomas, 88
    pigmented villonodular synovitis, 88, 89
    synovial hemangioma, 88
    synovial sarcomas, 90–91, *91–96*
    treatment and prognosis of, 91
  vascular, 45–58
    angiosarcoma, 53–55
    diagnosis of, 45
    diagnostic procedures for, 45–47
    glomangiosarcoma, 52
    glomus tumors, 51
    hemangiomas, 47–51
    hemangiopericytoma, 52
    Kaposi's sarcoma, 55–59
    proliferating angioendotheliomatosis, 53
    pseudo-Kaposi's sarcoma, 59

pseudoangiosarcoma, 55
Spitz nevus, 157
Squamous cell carcinoma, 152–153, *153*
  epidemiology of, 29
  etiology of, 29
Stewart-Treves syndrome, 155
Strawberry nevus, 48
Stucco keratoses, 149, *149*
Subungual exostosis, 191–192, *193–194*
  age distribution of, 191
  clinical features of, 191
  differential diagnosis of, 191
  histology of, 191, *194*
  sites of, 191
  treatment of, 192
Suppressor genes, 5
SV40 virus, 9
Synovial chondromatosis, 87–88
  differential diagnosis of, 87
  etiology of, 87
  radiographic signs of, 87
  symptoms of, 87
Synovial hemangioma, 51, 88
Synovial lining cells, 79–80
Synovial sarcoma, 90–91, *91–95*
  age and sex distribution of, 91
  epidemiology of, 27
  radiographic signs of, 87, 91
  variations of, 90–91
Synovitis, 88
  granulomatous, 88
  pigmented villonodular, 88, *89–90*

Tenalgia, definition of, 80
Tendinitis, 86–87
  definition of, 80
  due to overuse, 86
  on ultrasound, 80, *82*
Tendon cells, 79
Tenosynovial cyst, 86
  definition of, 86
  epidemiology of, 86
  etiology of, 86
  radiographic signs of, 86
Tenosynovial neoplasia, 79–92
  benign, 88–90
    giant cell tumor of tendon sheath, 88–90, 90t
    peritendinous fibromas and lipomas, 88
    pigmented villonodular synovitis, 88, *89–90*
    synovial hemangioma, 88
  diagnostic procedures for, 80–86
    arteriography, 81–83
    computerized tomography, 83
    contrast arthrography, 83
    fine-needle aspiration cytology, 84–86, *85*
    magnetic resonance imaging, 83–84, 84t
    ultrasonography, 80–81, *81–83*
    xeroradiography, 80
  differential diagnosis of, 86
  malignant, 90–91
    giant cell tumor, 90
    sarcomas, 90–91, *91–95*
  vs. nonneoplastic lesions, 86–88
    cyst, 86
    granulomatous synovitis, 88
    osteochondritis dissecans, 87
    synovial chondromatosis, 87
    tendinitis, 86–87

xanthoma, 87–88
  prognosis of, 91
  treatment of, 91
Tibial bowing, in neurofibromatosis, 105
TNM staging system, 44
Transcutaneous electrical nerve stimulation, 114
Transforming growth factors, 3
Trevor's disease, 191, *193*
Tuberous sclerosis, periungual fibromas in, *122*
Tumor suppressor genes, 5
Tumorigenesis, 1–19
  effect on cell cycle, 6
  immunologic theories of, 14–16
    delayed hypersensitivity, *14*, 14–15
    germinal center hyperplasia, 14
    sinus histiocytosis, *15*, 15–16
  nutritional effects on, 17–19
    dietary fiber, 19
    vitamin A, 18–19
    vitamin C, 18
    vitamin E, 18
  role of interferon in, 16–17
  role of ionizing radiation in, 13–14
  role of oncogenes in, 1–6. See also Oncogenes
  role of viruses in, 6–13. See also Viral oncogenesis
Tumors
  definition of, 40
  primary vs. secondary, 44
  TNM staging system for, 44

Ulex europaeus I lectin, 46
Ultrasonography
  of fibrous tumors, 124
  of tenosynovial neoplasia, 80–81, *81–83*
Ultraviolet exposure
  malignant melanoma due to, 29
  nonmelanotic skin cancers due to, 29
Unicameral bone cyst, 165–168, *168*
  active vs. latent, 165
  clinical presentation of, 165
  differential diagnosis of, 165
  etiology of, 165
  histology of, 165
  radiologic appearance of, 165
  site of, 165
  treatment of, 165–168

Vascular neoplasms, 45–59
  biopsy of, 46
  clinical features of, 45
  color of, 45
  diagnostic tests for, 45–47
    angiography, 46–47
    computerized tomography, 47
    immunohistochemistry, 45–46
    magnetic resonance imaging, 47
    plain films, 46
  history taking for, 45
  pain of, 45
  skin temperature over, 45
Verocay bodies, 107
Verrucous carcinoma, 153, *153*
Verrucous hamangioma, 49
Vimentin, 112
Vinculin, 3
Viral oncogenesis, 6–13
  DNA tumor viruses, 8–13
    Epstein-Barr virus, 11–12, *12*

Viral oncogenesis—*continued*
    human papilloma virus, 9–11, *10*
    in humans vs. animals, 8–9
    mechanism of neoplastic transformation by, 9
  historical recognition of, 6
  RNA tumor viruses, 7–8
    acute transforming viruses, 8
    genetic structure of, 6–7
    hepatitis B virus, 12–13
    human T cell leukemia viruses, 8
    slow transforming viruses, 7–8
  viruses involved in, 6, 7t
    classification of, 6
Vitamin A, 18–19
Vitamin C, 18
Vitamin E, 18
von Recklinghausen's disease. See Neurofibromatosis

Xanthelasma, 134–135

Xanthogranuloma, juvenile, 133–134
  differential diagnosis of, 134
  epidemiology of, 133
  histology of, 133–134
  prognosis of, 134
  sites of, 133
Xanthoma, 87–88, 134–135
  classification of, 134
  definition of, 87, 134
  diagnosis of, 135
  eruptive, 134
  normocholesterolemic, 87–88
  plane, 135
  prognosis of, 135
  tendinous, 134
  tuberous, 134
Xeroradiography
  of fibrous tumors, 123
  of tenosynovial neoplasms, 80